NEONATAL NURSING CARE HANDBOOK

Carole Kenner, PhD, NNP, RN, FAAN, is internationally known for her work in neonatal nursing, nursing education, and health policy establishing the rights of the neonate, standards for neonatal nursing care and neonatal nursing education, and the reduction of infant mortality worldwide. Dr. Kenner is the Carol Kuser Loser dean/professor in the School of Nursing, Health, and Exercise Science at the College of New Jersey, Ewing, New Jersey, and the chief executive officer for the Council of International Neonatal Nurses, Inc., Yardley, Pennsylvania. She has published more than 100 peer-reviewed journal articles, 30 books, and nearly 100 book chapters. Dr. Kenner has participated as principle investigator, co-investigator, or consultant on approximately 65 research/education/policy grants. She is a member of four honorary societies, including the American Academy of Nursing (AAN) (elected in 1994), and is a member of numerous review panels, editorial boards, and consultant groups. In 2010, Dr. Kenner received the prestigious Audrey Hepburn Award for Contributions to the Health and Welfare of Children from Sigma Theta Tau International. In 2014, she received a Lifetime Achievement Award for her work in neonatal nursing from the National Association of Neonatal Nurses (NANN).

Judy Wright Lott, PhD, NNP-BC, RN, FAAN, served as the founding dean of the nursing program at Wesleyan College in Macon, Georgia, until 2014. She served as dean, Baylor University Louise Harrington School of Nursing in Dallas, Texas, from 2002 to 2012. Dr. Lott has served as a neonatal nurse practitioner (NNP) from 2004 to 2005, associate professor of nursing and director of the NNP Specialty at the University of Cincinnati College of Nursing from 1996 to 2002, and assistant professor, Neonatal Graduate Specialty University of Florida College of Nursing from 1986 to 1990. She has worked in the clinical setting in various capacities since 1976. Dr. Lott was inducted into the American Academy of Nursing (AAN) in 2003, joined the American Association of Colleges of Nursing (AACN) Fuld Leadership for Academic Nursing Program in 2003, and was named visiting professor for the Perinatal Society of Australia and New Zealand (2001). Dr. Lott has co-authored four editions of *Comprehensive Neonatal Nursing Care* with Dr. Kenner. Dr. Lott has been invited to deliver more than 60 presentations at national and international professional meetings and 17 research presentations. She has published more than 20 peer-reviewed journal articles and 35 book chapters, and has been awarded six funded research grants, including a grant from the National Institute of Nursing Research (NINR).

NEONATAL NURSING CARE HANDBOOK
An Evidence-Based Approach to Conditions and Procedures

Second Edition

Carole Kenner, PhD, NNP, RN, FAAN

Judy Wright Lott, PhD, NNP-BC, RN, FAAN

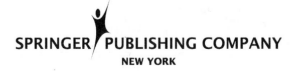

SPRINGER PUBLISHING COMPANY
NEW YORK

Springer Publishing Company, LLC
11 West 42nd Street
New York, NY 10036
www.springerpub.com

Acquisitions Editor: Elizabeth Nieginski
Composition: diacriTech

ISBN: 978-0-8261-7164-1
e-book ISBN: 978-0-8261-7165-8

16 17 18 / 5 4 3 2 1

The author and the publisher of this Work have made every effort to use sources believed to be reliable to provide information that is accurate and compatible with the standards generally accepted at the time of publication. Because medical science is continually advancing, our knowledge base continues to expand. Therefore, as new information becomes available, changes in procedures become necessary. We recommend that the reader always consult current research and specific institutional policies before performing any clinical procedure. The author and publisher shall not be liable for any special, consequential, or exemplary damages resulting, in whole or in part, from the readers' use of, or reliance on, the information contained in this book. The publisher has no responsibility for the persistence or accuracy of URLs for external or third-party Internet websites referred to in this publication and does not guarantee that any content on such websites is, or will remain, accurate or appropriate.

Library of Congress Cataloging-in-Publication Data

Names: Kenner, Carole, editor. | Lott, Judy Wright, 1953-, editor.
Title: Neonatal nursing care handbook : an evidence-based approach to
   conditions and procedures / [edited by] Carole Kenner, Judy Wright Lott.
Other titles: Neonatal nursing handbook.
Description: Second edition. | New York, NY : Springer Publishing Company,
   LLC, [2016] | Preceded by Neonatal nursing handbook / [edited by] Carole
   Kenner, Judy Wright Lott. c2004. | Includes bibliographical references and
   index.
Identifiers: LCCN 2016013689| ISBN 9780826171641 | ISBN 9780826171658 (e-book)
Subjects: | MESH: Neonatal Nursing—methods | Evidence-Based Nursing—methods
   | Handbooks
Classification: LCC RJ253 | NLM WY 49 | DDC 618.92/01—dc23 LC record available at
http://lccn.loc.gov/2016013689

Printed in the United States of America by R.R. Donnelley.

Contents

Contributors

Leslie B. Altimier, DNP, RNc, NE-BC   Director of Clinical Marketing, Mother & Child Care Patient Care & Clinical Informatics, Phillips Healthcare, North Andover, Massachusetts

Donna Armstrong, MSM, CAGS, RN, CCRN   Staff Nurse III, Boston Children's Hospital Neonatal Intensive Care Unit (NICU), Boston, Massachusetts

Susan T. Blackburn, PhD, RN, FAAN   Professor, Department of Family & Child Nursing, University of Washington, Seattle, Washington

Marina Boykova, PhD, RN   Research Coordinator, Council of International Neonatal Nurses, Inc., Yardley, Pennsylvania

Caitlin Bradley, MS, RN, NNP-BC   Neonatal Nurse Practitioner, Boston Children's Hospital NICU, Boston, Massachusetts

Carrie-Ellen Briere, BSN, RN, CLC   Staff Nurse II, Boston Children's Hospital NICU, Boston, Massachusetts

Julie Briere, BSN, RN, CCRN   Neonatal Nurse, Boston Children's Hospital, NICU, Boston, Massachusetts

Beth Brown, RNC, MSN   Adjunct Nursing Instructor, Kettering College, Division of Nursing, Kettering Medical Center, Dayton, Ohio

Monica A. Carleton, BSN, RN   Staff Nurse II, Boston Children's Hospital NICU, Boston, Massachusetts

Denise Casey, MS, RN, CCRN, CPNP   Clinical Nurse Specialist, Boston Children's Hospital NICU, Boston, Massachusetts

Anita Catlin, DNSc, FNAP, FAAN   Ethics and Research Consultant, Pope Valley, California

Xiaomei Cong, PhD, RN   Associate Professor, University of Connecticut School of Nursing, Storrs, Connecticut

Mary Coughlin, RN, MS, NNP   President & Global Learning Officer, Caring Essentials Collaborative, LLC, Boston, Massachusetts

Michele DeGrazia, PhD, RN, NNP-BC, FAAN   Director of Nursing Research, NICU, Boston Children's Hospital NICU, Boston, Massachusetts

Eileen C. DeWitt, RNC, MS, NNP-BC   Neonatal Nurse Practitioner, Boston Children's Hospital NICU, Boston, Massachusetts

Georgia R. Ditzenberger, PhD, NNP-BC, APNP   Assistant Professor, CNHS, Department of Pediatrics, Neonatology Division, University of Wisconsin, School of Medicine and Public Health, Madison, Wisconsin

Noel Dwyer, MBA, RN, CCRN   Staff Nurse II, Boston Children's Hospital NICU, Boston, Massachusetts

Wakako Eklund, DNP, NNP-BC, RN   Neonatal Nurse Practitioner, Pediatrix Medical Group of Tennessee, Nashville, Tennessee

Patricia Fleck, PhD, RN, NNP-BC   Neonatal Nurse Practitioner, Boston Children's Hospital, Boston, Massachusetts, South Shore Hospital, Weymouth, Massachusetts

Tricia Grandinetti, BSN, RN   Staff Nurse II, Boston Children's Hospital NICU, Boston, Massachusetts

Maura Heckmann, DNP, MSN, CPNP, RN   Pediactric Nurse Practitioner, Boston Children's Hospital Medical Surgical ICU, Boston, Massachusetts

Patricia Johnson, DNP, MPH, RN, NNP   Neonatal Nurse Practitioner Coordinator, Maricopa Integrated Health System, Phoenix, Arizona

Carole Kenner, PhD, NNP, RN, FAAN   Carol Kuser Loser Dean/Professor, School of Nursing, Health, and Exercise Science, The College of New Jersey, Ewing, New Jersey

Michelle LaBrecque, MSN, RN, CCRN   Clinical Nurse Specialist, Boston Children's Hospital, Boston, Massachusetts

Judy Wright Lott, PhD, NNP-BC, RN, FAAN   Neonatal Nurse Practitioner, Surrey, British Columbia, Canada

Ruth Lucas, PhD, RNC-IPO, CLS   Assistant Professor, School of Nursing, University of Connecticut, Storrs, Connecticut, Nurse Scientist, Institute for Nursing Research & Evidence-Based Practice, Connecticut Children's Medical Center, Hartford, Connecticut

Carolyn Lund, MS, RN, FAAN   Neonatal Clinical Nurse Specialist, Benioff Children's Hospital Oakland, Oakland, California, Associate Clinical Professor, University of California, San Francisco, School of Nursing, San Francisco, California

Mary-Jeanne Manning, MSN, RN, PNP-BC, CCRN   Clinical Nurse Specialist, Boston Children's Hospital Medical Surgical ICU, Boston, Massachusetts

Samual L. Mooneyham, MSN, NNP, RN   Interim Director of Obstetrics/Nursing Supervisor, Heywood Hospital, Gardner, Massachusetts

Katherine M. Newnam, PhD, RN, NNP-BC, CPNP   Assistant Professor, University of Tennessee Knoxville, College of Nursing, Knoxville, Tennessee, Neonatal Nurse Practitioner, Children's Hospital of the King's Daughters, Norfolk, Virginia

Stephanie Packard, BSN, RN, CCRN   Project Manager, Patient Safety and Quality Cardiovascular and Critical Care Programs, Boston Children's Hospital NICU, Boston, Massachusetts

Leslie A. Parker, PhD, RN, NNP-BC   Clinical Associate Professor, College of Nursing University of Florida, Gainesville, Florida

Ann Gibbons Phalen, PhD, CRNP, NNP-BC   Associate Professor, Associate Dean, Undergraduate Programs, Jefferson College of Nursing, Thomas Jefferson University, Philadelphia, Pennsylvania

Jana L. Pressler, PhD, RN   Assistant Dean & Professor, University of Nebraska Medical Center, College of Nursing Lincoln Division, Lincoln, Nebraska

Melissa Roberts, MSN, RN, CPNP   Pediatric Nurse Practitioner, Shriners Hospital, Boston, Massachusetts

Ann Schwoebel, RNC-NIC, CRNP   Clinical Nurse Educator, Pennsylvania Hospital, Philadelphia, Pennsylvania

Elizabeth (Liz) Sharpe, DNP, ARNP, NNP-BC, VA-BC   Assistant Professor, The University of Alabama at Birmingham School of Nursing, Birmingham, Alabama

Beth Shields, PharmD   Associate Director, Operations, Clinical Specialist, Pediatrics, Rush University Medical Center, Department of Pharmacy, Chicago, Illinois

Tamara Wallace, DNP, RN, NNP-BC   Neonatal Nurse Practitioner, Nationwide Children's Hospital, Columbus, Ohio

Charlotte Wool, PhD, RN   Assistant Professor of Nursing, York College of Pennsylvania, York, Pennsylvania

Ksenia Zukowsky, PhD, CRNP, NNP-BC   Associate Professor, Thomas Jefferson University, Jefferson College of Nursing, Associate Dean Graduate Programs, Coordinator of Neonatal Nurse Practitioner Program, Philadelphia, Pennsylvania

Foreword

The health of newborns in all countries must be at the forefront of all activities (teaching, research, and service) if neonatal nursing is to embrace the post-2015 global development framework. It is within this ethos that the *Neonatal Nursing Care Handbook: An Evidence-Based Approach to Conditions and Procedures* has been written to serve a global cadre of neonatal nurses!

The neonatal handbook provides an explanation of common conditions and focuses on a few procedures that are widely implemented in practice. The editors, Drs. Carole Kenner and Judy Wright Lott, have been mindful that resources may vary significantly in some countries where the handbook will be utilized. The neonatal handbook is therefore available, keeping at the forefront the principles of evidence-based nursing practice while appreciating that clinical decisions will be guided by the best evidence shared in the neonatal handbook, the resources available in the practice setting, the clinical practice skills of the neonatal nurse, and the parents' preference with respect to care provided to their newborn.

There is an appreciation that learners and clinicians in some countries are not able to readily access knowledge or evidence to inform practice. This neonatal handbook has therefore been written with the intent of making evidence easily accessible to learners in the classroom or clinical setting, as well as to practitioners in clinical care who want to improve the quality of care. The authors have anticipated that the need for this knowledge will increase, given the call to end preventable deaths through the Every Newborn Action Plan, which is being coordinated by the World Health Organization and the United Nations Children's Fund. The neonatal handbook will therefore be an important resource for neonatal nurses worldwide.

The neonatal handbook employs a systems approach detailing management of disorders related to each system. Many of the special care considerations can be applied universally; for instance developmental care and breastfeeding. A separate section covers procedures and diagnostic tests.

Evidence-informed practice improves patient outcomes and sharing knowledge about best practices (i.e., current state of evidence) is an important step in this regard. The gift of knowledge will ensure the health and well-being of newborns in all countries.

Shahirose Sadrudin Premji, PhD, MScN, BSc, BScN, RN
Associate Professor, University of Calgary, Faculty of Nursing
Adjunct Associate Professor, University of Calgary
Faculty of Medicine, Department of Community Health Sciences
Calgary, Alberta, Canada

Preface

Neonatal nursing care is taking on an increasing prominence as part of the Every Newborn Action Plan (ENAP) and the United Nations Millennium Development Goals (MDGs). Yet, there is no quick reference for neonatal nurses in many countries, thus making this handbook extremely valuable for nurses working in international communities.

Neonatal nursing professionals need a quick reference for the most common conditions and procedures, which they can use to find the necessary information in a timely manner. The second edition of this handbook is divided into three sections. The first section takes a systems approach, providing a brief description of each of the most common conditions, signs and symptoms, assessment, and brief treatment. The second section focuses on special care considerations. The third section includes procedures, diagnostic tests, lab values, and common drugs that are most frequently needed in the care of neonates. The appendices consist of charts and graphs, such as weight and temperature charts, a list of common abbreviations, and pertinent web resources.

For more complete information please see the fifth edition of Kenner and Lott's (2014) *Comprehensive Neonatal Nursing* published by Springer Publishing Company. **Included in this book are the MedCalc Acid–Base Calculator (http://www.medcalc.com/acidbase .html) and the Neonatal Intensive Care Unit (NICU) Quick Drip Calculator (http://www.medcalc.com/drip.html), pages 55 and 637, respectively.**

Carole Kenner
Judy Wright Lott

Acknowledgments

I wish to first express my appreciation, love, and support for my dad who turned 104 in 2015. He still gets excited when a new edition is published. Thank you, dad, from both of us as Judy also has grown close to you over the years.

I also wish to acknowledge the support from Dr. Marina Boykova, who reminds me what the international neonatal nursing community needs!

Carole

I would like to thank my daughter, husband, and sisters for their love, support, and patience through not only this book, but my other publishing adventures!

Judy

Together we would like to express our appreciation for the assistance of Margaret Zuccarini from Springer Publishing Company, who is a longtime trusted colleague and guided this project to a successful completion. Thank you for believing in this project. A special thank you goes to Elizabeth Nieginski from Springer Publishing Company, for all her assistance and guidance through the development and publication of this project. We really enjoyed working with both of you. Also, we would like to thank Jan Zasada for her tireless efforts to try to keep us organized and on track. And of course, thank you to all the authors who provided their expertise. Finally, we want to thank the professionals across the globe who take care of babies and their families.

Systems Assessment and
Management of Disorders

Respiratory System

Katherine M. Newnam

OVERVIEW

The mechanisms and structures that bring about normal pulmonary function in the fetus and neonate are complex. Pulmonary structures form early in gestation with continued growth well into childhood. The development of the pulmonary system is orderly, along a predetermined sequence throughout gestation (Greenough & Milner, 2005) beginning at the fourth week. Neonatal respiratory compromise can be pulmonary in nature or related to other neonatal comorbidities including congenital heart defects, congenital malformations, metabolic abnormalities, and disorders of the central nervous system (CNS). Regardless of origin, these infants often present in a similar fashion with respiratory distress that includes increased rate and effort of breathing, cyanosis, and oxygen requirement.

Reductions in both neonatal mortality and morbidity have been realized though advances in prenatal care, delivery room resuscitation, and subsequent neonatal care (Goldsmith & Karotkin, 2014). Despite significant therapeutic advances over the past 30 years, the most common and severe diseases of the newborn remain pulmonary in origin. Respiratory distress syndrome (RDS) is the most common diagnosis in nurseries worldwide, representing 7% of term infants, 29% of late preterm infants, and nearly 100% of the extremely low-birth-weight (ELBW) infants (Stoll et al., 2010). Respiratory complications, regardless of cause, can lead to respiratory failure and cardiopulmonary arrest if they are not recognized and management strategies are not instituted (Reuter, Moser, & Baack, 2014).

ANATOMY AND PHYSIOLOGY

Fetal lung development follows an organized and predetermined sequence beginning with out-pouching of the embryonic foregut and continuing with rapid structural changes including the expansion of the gas exchange surface area until around term gestation (Soltau & Carlo, 2014). Pulmonary growth or alveolarization continues well into childhood with ongoing development of both alveolar surfaces and the capillary networks and blood supply to support gas exchange. At term, the neonate possesses an adequate complement of conductive airways and millions of peripheral airspaces, mostly the "saccular" type with thickened walls and capillary structures sandwiched between connective tissue. The term neonate has approximately 50 million alveoli with continued growth over the next several years to lung maturation of about 300 million or more alveoli (Burri, 2006).

The alveolar cell known as type II pneumocytes produces a mixture of proteins and phospholipids called pulmonary surfactant. *Surfactant* is a surface active compound that modifies surface tension, which is a critical component of lung function and compliance at delivery. This is accomplished by coating the alveolus, thereby decreasing surface tension in the small alveoli and increasing the surface tension in the larger airways. This mechanism provides the neonatal lung stability and allows the alveoli to remain open (Soltau & Carlo, 2014). The importance of surfactant is not limited to reducing surface tension in the alveoli; rather, it decreases opening pressure of the alveoli, enhances alveolar fluid clearance, and provides a level of protection for the fragile epithelial cell surface (Gardner, Enzman-Hines, & Dickey, 2011).

Phosphatidylglycerol (PG), which is the second most common phospholipid in surfactant, usually appears at about 36 weeks gestation and continues to increase until term gestation. Surfactant is stored, recycled, and secreted in the neonatal lung; however, under certain conditions, the metabolism and/or effectiveness of surfactant will be altered. These include maternal conditions such as diabetes, infection, hypertension, drug use, and placental insufficiency, as well as infant conditions such as acidemia, hypoxia, mechanical ventilation, hypercapnia, twin gestation, sepsis, and prematurity (Gardner et al., 2011).

Physiologic changes at birth

At birth, a drastic change in the lung environment occurs with pulmonary fluid being rapidly replaced by air. This transition to extrauterine life begins as the infant takes the first breath of air, usually in response to tactile stimulation. This first breath of the term infant requires an opening pressure of 60 to 80 cm of water with subsequent breaths requiring less as the surface tension of the liquid-filled airways and alveoli are stabilized.

Oxygen passively diffuses across the alveolar-capillary membrane, due to the difference in oxygen pressure, which is higher in the alveoli than in the capillary blood supply. Oxygen dissolves in the plasma and then binds to the hemoglobin and circulates systemically. Oxygen is deposited into the tissues in much the same passive manner. The oxygen pressure is higher in the arterial blood supply than in the tissues; therefore, the oxygen moves from the hemoglobin to the tissues.

Importance of maternal and perinatal history

Specifically, certain maternal conditions can greatly influence the development and function of the respiratory system. A thorough and systematic review of the prenatal and birth history will provide the clinician with information regarding specific risk factors that will impact neonatal care and resuscitation requirements. Maternal history is typically separated into three separate time frames: antepartum (during pregnancy), intrapartum (labor and delivery), and postpartum (following delivery). Maternal conditions, both chronic and acute illness that affect the fetal well-being, should also be reviewed. Maternal serologies including blood type, ultrasound findings including estimated fetal weight, and gestation should be identified prior to delivery if possible.

GENERAL FOCUSED ASSESSMENT OF THE RESPIRATORY SYSTEM

Vital signs (temperature, pulse, respiratory rate, heart rate, and blood pressure) will provide needed information to the clinician. Hypothermia or hyperthermia may alter the metabolic load of the neonate. The hypoxic or hypotensive infant may require rapid intervention and is often associated with respiratory compromise.

General observation of the neonate is an important first step in your assessment.

■ Tachypnea or increased respiratory rate (> 60 bpm) is the earliest sign of respiratory compromise. This is a compensatory mechanism in the neonate to maintain alveolar ventilation and gas exchange. However, this increased rate will often expend additional energy, requiring increased oxygen to support the infant. Prolonged tachypnea will often result in fatigue and decreased effort to meet systemic demands, leading to respiratory compromise and eventually respiratory failure.

■ Grunting or the forcing of air through a partially closed glottis on expiration. This is a compensatory method to maintain functional residual capacity (FRC) in order to maintain alveolar distention and promote gas exchange. This may be heard audibly without stethoscope.

■ Use of accessory muscles of respiration is an indication of respiratory distress. This includes nasal flaring, retractions, or the inward pull of the chest wall on inspiration.

■ Symmetry of the chest wall may provide information regarding ongoing or progressive pathology.

■ Seesaw respirations in a compensatory mechanism are used to support the effectiveness of gas exchange. With continued respiratory distress, the infant will appear more barrel- or pigeon-chested.

■ A scaphoid abdomen is a classic sign of a diaphragmatic hernia.

■ Pallor, mottling, or poor color of the infant may indicate hypotension or acidosis. Cyanosis or blue discoloration of the skin and mucous membranes is a classic sign of hypoxemia. This is a late and serious sign of compromise; the infant will require rapid supportive intervention. This is often associated with respiratory distress, leading to respiratory failure.

- Tachycardia, bradycardia, blood pressure, and perfusion are important signs of cardiac compromise from congenital heart disease (CHD) or ongoing respiratory compromise and failure.

- Diminished muscle tone and poor activity are critical signs of profound hypoxia and acidosis.

Auscultation of the chest includes

- Comparing and contrasting bilateral lung sounds
- Quality and volume of air exchange
- Adventitious breath sounds (crackles, rales, and decreased air entry)
- Absence or asymmetric volume of air exchange

Percussion and palpation of the neonatal chest has little diagnosis value.

Brief overview of blood gas analysis

The goal of blood gas analysis in the neonate is to determine the type and degree of disorder and compensation. Indications include all RDSs, metabolic conditions, sepsis, and neurologic concerns. Cord gases may provide the clinician with a specific quantity in which to determine the degree of asphyxia experienced prior to birth (see Figure 1.1). Oxygen moves from the oxygen-rich alveolar-capillary membrane through passive measures to the blood, where the oxygen level is lower. This passive mechanism is the partial pressure of oxygen. The oxygen dissolves into the plasma and binds to the hemoglobin. This measure is reflected in the PaO_2 value.

Carbon dioxide moves rapidly across the cell membrane in response to ventilation. The movement from tissues is more efficient than oxygenation. The PaO_2 is a reflection of ventilation status.

The acid–base balance depends on the interaction between bicarbonate ions and carbon dioxide. Acidosis or low pH is not well tolerated by the neonate and can increase vasoconstriction in sensitive pulmonary vasculature, increasing the state of hypoxemia (see Figure 1.1; also see the MedCalc Acid–Base Calculator at the end of this chapter).

Common conditions of the neonatal respiratory system are listed and described in the following text. Common diagnoses with a decision-making algorithm for the infant who presents with respiratory disease is included (see Figure 1.2). Specific care and treatment of these conditions are described under each topical heading.

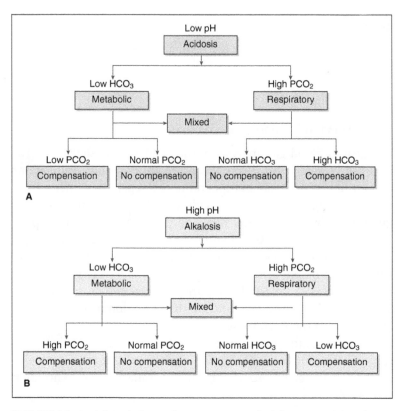

FIGURE 1.1. Acid–base balance: diagnostic approach. (A) Low pH. (B) High pH.
Source: Soltau and Carlo (2014).

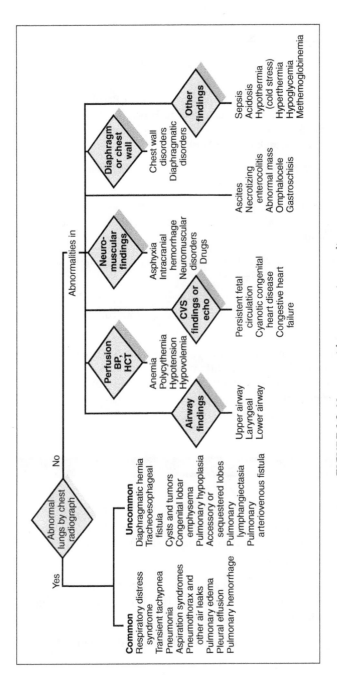

FIGURE 1.2. Neonate with acute respiratory distress.

CVS, cardiovascular system.

REFERENCES

Burri, P. H. (2006). Structural aspects of postnatal lung development—Alveolar formation and growth. *Biology of the Neonate, 89*, 313–322.

Gardner, S. L., Enzman-Hines, M., & Dickey, L. A. (2011). Respiratory diseases. In S. L. Gardner, B. S. Carter, M. Enzman-Hines, & J. A. Hernandez (Eds.), *Merenstein & Gardner's handbook of neonatal intensive care* (7th ed., pp. 581–677). St. Louis, MO: Elsevier Mosby.

Goldsmith, J. P., & Karotkin, E. H. (2014). *Assisted ventilation of the neonate* (5th ed.). Philadelphia, PA: Elsevier Saunders.

Greenough, A., & Milner, A. D. (2005). Pulmonary disease of the newborn. In J. Rennie (Ed.), *Robertson's textbook of neonatology* (4th ed.). London, UK: Churchill Livingstone.

Reuter, S., Moser, C., & Baack, M. (2014). Respiratory distress in the newborn. *Pediatrics in Review, 35*(10), 417–428.

Soltau, T. D., & Carlo, W. A. (2014). Respiratory system. In C. Kenner & J. W. Lott (Eds.), *Comprehensive neonatal nursing care* (5th ed.). New York, NY: Springer Publishing Company.

Stoll, B. J., Hansen, N. I., Bell, E. F., Shankaran, S., Laptook, A. R., Walsh, M. C., & Eunice Kennedy Shriver National Institute of Child Health and Human Development Neonatal Research Network. (2010). Neonatal outcomes of extremely preterm infants from the NICHD Neonatal Research Network. *Pediatrics, 26*, 443–456.

RESPIRATORY DISTRESS SYNDROME

INCIDENCE

- Inverse relationship to gestational age; 98% at 23 weeks gestation, 86% at 28 weeks gestation, 29% at 35 weeks gestation, and 7% of term infants
- Higher occurrence with maternal history of gestational or chronic diabetes (infant of a diabetic mother [IDM] or gestational diabetes mellitus [GDM]), chorioamnionitis, or perinatal asphyxia
- Affects approximately 40,000 infants annually in the United States
- Male to female ratio is 2:1

TABLE 1.1 Stages of Normal Lung Growth		
Phase	**Timing**	**Major Event**
Embryonic	Weeks 4–6	Formation of proximal airway
Pseudoglandular	Weeks 7–16	Formation of conducting airways
Canalicular	Weeks 17–28	Formation of acini
Saccular	Weeks 29–35	Development of gas-exchange sites
Alveolar	Weeks 36 through postnatal life	Expansion of surface area

PHYSIOLOGY

DS is a global term that refers to disorders of the respiratory system that begin at or shortly following birth. Although most common in those infants born prior to term, respiratory distress can result from any neonatal condition that leads to progressive atelectasis, hypoventilation, and/or hypoxia. Diseases that affect the respiratory system in the early neonatal period may extend well into infancy or childhood (see Table 1.1 on the stages of normal lung growth).

If lung compliance is decreased, there is also a decrease in tidal volume. In order for the neonate to achieve sufficient minute ventilation, the respiratory rate will increase (tachypnea). Hypoxemia also will trigger an increased respiratory rate to compensate. Increased work of breathing is the result of mismatched pulmonary mechanics, including increased airway resistance, diminished lung compliance, or both (Reuter, Moser, & Baack, 2014).

PATHOPHYSIOLOGY

The causes of RDS are varied and may reflect disorders of alterations of normal lung development (or lack of development in the preterm infant) or failure to transition to extrauterine life.

Availability of surfactant is usually inadequate (lack of production or inactivated), which leads to diffuse alveolar atelectasis, cell injury, and pulmonary edema (Jackson, 2012).

The injuries to the pulmonary epithelial cells are visible histologically and include: increased eosinophilic material following injury to the cellular structures, alveolar spaces that have areas of collapse, evidence of pulmonary edema, and pulmonary hemorrhage.

The inflammatory cascade is often initiated secondary to the pulmonary cellular injury or globally in the case of perinatal/neonatal asphyxia. Inflammation causes increased metabolic workload on the neonate, including increased oxygen requirement, and can contribute to cell damage and death of the affected and surrounding tissues (Newnam, Gephart, & Wright, 2013).

ASSESSMENT

The assessment of the neonate with RDS should always begin with a detailed maternal and prenatal history (see Overview section). This history may contain critical information that supports your physical findings but leads to a timely diagnosis. Differential diagnoses include both common and uncommon conditions including those with origins in other neonatal systems (see Figure 1.2).

CLINICAL MANIFESTATIONS/DIAGNOSIS

The diagnosis of RDS is based on history, physical findings, blood gas analysis, and x-rays.

Distress is usually present at birth or shortly thereafter. Progressive respiratory difficulty typically coincides with increasing atelectasis of the alveoli and may take place over the first few minutes of life or several hours following birth. Infants with poor or deficient respiratory effort can progress to respiratory failure without rapid and effective intervention.

Physical exam findings

■ Tachypnea (> 60 breaths per minute)

■ Intermittent or continuous expiratory grunting which is caused by the forced air past the glottis to maintain positive end-expiratory pressure (PEEP) at the alveolar level

- Retractions (subcostal, substernal, intercostal, and/or supracla-vicular)
- Nasal flaring
- Hypoxemia with or without cyanosis
- Increasing oxygen requirement to maintain systemic oxygenation at PaO_2 at 50 to 70 mmHg
- Increased adventitious breath sounds (crackles, rales, and decreased air entry)
- Paradoxical seesaw respirations
- If the condition progresses, the infant will have changes in cardiac function including decreased perfusion, pallor, and tachycardia (early) and bradycardia (late)
- If the condition progresses, the infant will demonstrate CNS changes including lethargy, decreased or obtunded response to stimuli, and loss of muscle tone.

Typical findings of diagnostic procedures/tests for RDS are illustrated here.

Laboratory data

- Complete blood count (CBC) including hematocrit to evaluate for anemia or polycythemia
- Blood type and screen (evaluate for ABO incompatibility based on maternal blood type or transfusion in acute blood loss)

Blood gas analysis

- Respiratory acidosis; increased CO_2 levels as the atelectasis progresses.
- Increased acidosis (respiratory and metabolic) ensues as the hypoxemia progresses. The pH decreases, the CO_2 level increases, PaO_2 level decreases, and bicarbonate decreases.
- As cardiac function is altered, the lactic acid increases systemically, precluding the infant to a state of progressive systemic acidosis and lowering the pH and bicarbonate.

Radiographic findings

■ The anteroposterior (AP) view is usually sufficient for initial examination.

TREATMENT

■ Respiratory support includes:
  ■ Surfactant administration
  ■ Nasal continuous positive airway pressure (CPAP), "sigh" synchronized intermittent airway pressure (SiPAP), or noninvasive positive pressure ventilation (NIPPV)
  ■ Mechanical ventilation
  ■ Supplemental oxygen delivery (nasal cannula, high-flow nasal cannula, vapotherm, nasal cannula)
■ Surveillance and management of comorbidities
  ■ Patent ductus arteriosus (PDA)
  ■ Sepsis
  ■ Apnea of prematurity (AOP)
■ Pharmacologic management includes:
  ■ Caffeine administration
  ■ Broad spectrum antibiotics as clinically indicated

PROGNOSIS

Survival rates for the preterm infant with RDS are based on gestational age, birth weight, and degree of RDS. Prolonged use of mechanical ventilation, although lifesaving, has negative consequences for the pulmonary structures. The airway and alveolar pressure created with positive pressure can cause overdistention and scarring of the lung parenchyma, leading to chronic lung disease (CLD). Infants with CLD typically have poorer neurodevelopmental outcomes when compared with infants who did not require mechanical ventilation. Supplemental oxygen for prolonged time frames will contribute to CLD; in addition, systemic oxygen toxicity can lead to or complicate retinopathy of prematurity (ROP).

REFERENCES

Jackson, J. C. (2012). Respiratory distress in the preterm infant. In C. A. Gleason & S. U. Devaskar (Eds.), *Avery's diseases of the newborn* (9th ed., pp. 633–646). Philadelphia, PA: Elsevier Saunders.

Newnam, K. M., Gephart, S. M., & Wright, L. (2013). Common complications of dysregulated inflammation in the neonate. *Newborn & Infant Nursing Reviews*, 13, 154–160.

Reuter, S., Moser, C., & Baack, M. (2014). Respiratory distress in the newborn. *Pediatrics in Review, 35*(10), 417–428.

ADDITIONAL WEB RESOURCES

www.NICUniversity.org

www.pediatrix.com/PediatrixUniversity

TRANSIENT TACHYPNEA OF THE NEWBORN

INCIDENCE

■ Transient tachypnea of the newborn (TTN) occurs in 5.7 per 1,000 live births

■ It occurs in males more often than females (1.3–1 ratio)

PHYSIOLOGY

TTN is a parenchymal lung disease caused by pulmonary edema secondary to retained lung fluid. The fetal lung fluid has a high-chloride concentration, higher than plasma, interstitial fluid, or the amniotic fluid. During labor, chemical release of catecholamines occurs that results in the reduction of active chloride and fluid transport into the fetal lung and the reabsorption of fetal lung fluid via a protein gradient and sodium channels. The fluid is transported to the lymphatic system, with an estimated two thirds of the fetal lung volume removed prior to birth. Increased oxygen tension following infant birth increases the epithelium's capacity to transport sodium further reducing the fetal lung fluid. Infants born without labor or precipitously will not have the feedback mechanism to signal the fluid reabsorption or adequate time for the process to be effective (Abu-Shaweesh, 2011).

PATHOPHYSIOLOGY

Retained fetal lung fluid typically occurs because of a delay in the removal of lung fluid or excessive volume of lung fluid. As noted earlier, infants born without labor, typically via C-section, are at highest risk for TTN. Other conditions that preclude the newborn to TTN include breech delivery, second twin, macrosomia, and delayed cord clamping, which can elevate the central venous pressure secondary to increased systemic blood volume.

The delayed reabsorption of lung fluid at delivery will often fill the interstitial spaces with fluid. This leads to alveolar air trapping and decreased lung compliance (Whitsett, Rice, Warner, Wert, & Pryhuber, 2005). As described in the RDS section, as lung compliance decreases, the tidal volume will decrease. In order for the neonate to achieve sufficient minute ventilation, the respiratory rate will increase (tachypnea). Hypoxemia also will trigger an increased respiratory rate to compensate.

The delayed clearance of the lung fluid by the lymphatics will cause an accumulation of fluid in the peribronchiolar lymphatics and cause bronchiolar collapse. Air trapping is the consequence of this bronchiolar collapse, which causes hyperinflation of the alveoli. Hypoxemia and hypercarbia result from inadequate perfusion at the gas exchange interface. This increased work of breathing is the result of mismatched pulmonary mechanics, including increased airway resistance, diminished lung compliance, or both (Reuter, Moser, & Baack, 2014).

ASSESSMENT

The assessment of the neonate with RDS should always begin with a detailed maternal and prenatal history including the mother's prenatal health and illnesses; prenatal care history; any issues or problems with the mother or baby during pregnancy; labor history, including any problems with mother or baby; and the baby's status immediately after birth, including Apgars and initial care needed. This information may contain critical information that supports your physical findings but leads to a timely diagnosis. Assessment should include general observation, vital signs, and the auscultation of bilateral breath sounds (see general focused assessment section). The differential diagnoses include both common and uncommon conditions including those with origins in other neonatal systems (see Figure 1.2).

CLINICAL MANIFESTATIONS/DIAGNOSIS

The diagnosis of TTN is based on history, physical findings, blood gas analysis, and x-ray findings.

Physical exam findings

- Profound tachypnea (> 60 breaths per minute)
- May have retractions (subcostal, substernal, intercostal, and/or supraclavicular)
- May present with nasal flaring
- May have oxygen requirement to maintain systemic oxygenation at PaO_2 at 50 to 70 mmHg
- Paradoxical or seesaw respirations

Diagnostic procedures/tests

- Blood gas results will typically show mild respiratory acidosis (see previously mentioned blood gas analysis).
- Radiology findings will include diffuse haziness and streakiness in both peripheral lung fields. Fluid-filled interlobar fissures with mild hyperinflation may be visible.

TREATMENT

- As noted previously, this diagnosis is one of exclusion so other disorders should be ruled out.
- Blood gases should be serially monitored (see section Brief Overview of Blood Gas Analysis).

- If history indicates risk factors for infection, broad-spectrum antibiotic therapy should be considered until blood culture results are negative.
- Supportive care includes:
  - Oxygen delivery by nasal cannula or nasal CPAP
  - Continuous oxygen saturation monitoring
  - Thermoregulation to avoid increased metabolic load
  - Adequate fluid intake (mild fluid losses through increased respiratory rate)
  - Adequate nutrition (usually by gavage tube if RR > 60 bpm to prevent aspiration)
  - Serial monitoring and management of blood glucose levels within acceptable range

Fluid restriction and/or the use of diuretics *has not* been supported in the treatment of TTN (Kassab, Khriesat, Bawadi, & Anabrees, 2013; Stroustrup, Trasande, & Holzman, 2012)

PROGNOSIS

TTN is usually self-limiting with excellent prognosis. The need for respiratory support is usually transient and improves steadily over several hours to days. A few infants will demonstrate high pulmonary artery (PA) pressures and symptoms of persistent pulmonary hypertension of the newborn (PPHN), which can complicate or prolong the infant's clinical course and outcome (see section "Persistent Pulmonary Hypertension of the Newborn").

REFERENCES

Abu-Shaweesh, J. M. (2011). Respiratory disorders in the preterm and term infants. In R. Martin, A. A. Fanaroff, & M. C. Walsh (Eds.), *Fanaroff and Martin's neonatal–perinatal medicine: Diseases of the fetus and infant* (9th ed.). Philadelphia, PA: Elsevier Saunders.

Kassab, M., Khriesat, W. M., Bawadi, H., & Anabrees, J. (2013). Furosemide for transient tachypnoea of the newborn. *Cochrane Database of Systematic Reviews, 6*, CD003064.

Reuter, S., Moser, C., & Baack, M. (2014). Respiratory distress in the newborn. *Pediatrics in Review, 35*(10), 417–428.

Stroustrup, A., Trasande, L., & Holzman, I. R. (2012). Randomized controlled trial of restrictive fluid management in transient tachypnea of the newborn. *Journal of Pediatrics, 160*(1), 38–42.

Whitsett, J. A., Rice, W. R., Warner, B. B., Wert, S. E., & Pryhuber, G. S. (2005). Acute respiratory disorders. In M. G. MacDonald, M. D. Mullett, & M. M. K. Seshia (Eds.), *Avery's diseases of the newborn* (5th ed., pp. 553–577). Philadelphia, PA: Elsevier Saunders.

APNEA AND AOP

INCIDENCE

- Apnea in full-term neonates occurs in less than 2% of infants and is typically related to other organic causes (sepsis, obstruction, or neurologic or metabolic influences).

- Apnea occurs in 30% to 90% of preterm infants.

- It is inversely correlated with gestational age (80% in infants < 28-week gestation).

- It is not accompanied by cyanosis or changes in heart rate initially. Bradycardia and hypoxia will ensue if apnea is not corrected rapidly.

- Normal neurologic development reduces the episodes of periodic breathing and apnea around term gestation (Miller, Fanaroff, & Martin, 2011).

PHYSIOLOGY

Apnea represents one of the most common respiratory complications in the preterm infant. It is typically defined as cessation of respiratory effort for longer than 20 seconds in length. Most apnea occurs in the preterm infant, classified as AOP, and occurs independent of other organic causes. This is not to be confused with periodic breathing, which is recurrent sequences of pauses in respiratory effort for 10 to 15 seconds followed by a brief "catch up" phase of tachypnea.

AOP is typically classified into one of four types: central apnea, obstructive apnea, mixed apnea, or idiopathic apnea.

1. Central apnea is the absence of respiratory effort and airflow into the respiratory system and accounts for approximately 15% of apnea. While the causes of central apnea in the preterm infant are not fully understood, contributing factors are chest wall afferent neuromuscular immaturity, chest wall instability, diaphragmatic fatigue, and the immature response to hypoxia and hypercapnia.

2. Obstructive apnea is the absence of airflow with continued respiratory effort; it is thought to contribute to up to 30% of apneic events. This is usually caused by the blockage of the airway at the pharynx or larynx, which can be obstructed due to poor head and neck position of the neonate (Kattwinkel, 2011). Other causes of obstruction may be congenital anomalies of the airway and are described in a later section.

3. Mixed apnea is a combination of obstructive and central apnea.

4. Idiopathic apnea is diagnosed when the baby has apnea that does not result from the other three types of apnea. The cause is unknown.

Both events, periodic breathing and apnea of the preterm infant, subside with neurologic development around the corrected age of 39 to 41 weeks.

PATHOPHYSIOLOGY

Apnea in the premature infant is due to the immature central respiratory center secondary to poor CNS myelinization, decreased number of synapses, and dendritic arborization.

In the term infant, the chemoreceptors that are located centrally within the medulla and peripherally in the carotid and aortic bodies transmit important information regarding the pH and oxygen levels to the respiratory center in the brain via pathways along the vagus and glossopharyngeal nerves. Increased respiratory rate is triggered when these levels are low. In the preterm infant, these pathways are not well established and/or not responsive to systemic hypoxemia (MacFarlane, Ribeiro, & Martin, 2013). This explanation supports the cessation of AOP secondary to the normal maturation of the preterm brain and plasticity/development of neuropathways.

However, apneic events may also be a classic first sign of systemic stress in the preterm infant. Other organic causes should be considered prior to the assumption that events are caused by AOP.

Apnea in the term newborn is always an abnormal finding and should be systemically investigated for other causes.

ASSESSMENT

Vital signs (temperature, pulse, respiratory rate, heart rate, and blood pressure) will provide needed information to the clinician.

General observation of the neonate is an important first step in your assessment.

- Tachypnea or increased respiratory rate (> 60 bpm) is the earliest sign of respiratory compromise.
- Periodic breathing with pauses in the respiratory pattern for less than 15 seconds combined with rapid respiratory rate following pauses may be present.
- Prolonged pauses in respiratory pattern longer than 20 seconds in length may be observed. Bradycardia or pallor will ensue if a spontaneous or assisted respiratory pattern does not occur.
- Use of accessory muscles of respiration is an indication of respiratory distress. This includes nasal flaring, retractions, or the inward pull of the chest wall on inspiration.
- Symmetry of the chest wall may provide information regarding ongoing or progressive pathology.
- Seesaw respirations in a compensatory mechanism are used to support the effectiveness of gas exchange. With continued respiratory distress, the infant will appear more barrel- or pigeon-chested.

■ Pallor, mottling, or poor color of the infant may indicate hypotension or acidosis. Cyanosis or blue discoloration of the skin and mucous membranes is a classic sign of hypoxemia. This is a late and serious sign of compromise, after which the infant will require rapid supportive intervention. This is often associated with respiratory distress, leading to respiratory failure.

Auscultation of the chest includes:

■ Comparing and contrasting bilateral lung sounds

■ Quality and volume of air exchange

■ Adventitious breath sounds (crackles, rales, and decreased air entry)

■ Absence or asymmetric volume of air exchange

■ Grunting or the forcing of air through a partially closed glottis on expiration. This is a compensatory method to maintain FRC in order to maintain alveolar distention and promote gas exchange. This may be heard audibly without a stethoscope.

Percussion and palpation of the neonatal chest has little diagnosis value.

CLINICAL MANIFESTATIONS/DIAGNOSIS

The diagnosis of apnea for the preterm or term infant is based on history, physical findings, x-rays, and blood gas results.

Physical exam findings

■ Periodic breathing with pauses in the respiratory pattern for less than 15 seconds combined with rapid respiratory rate following pauses.

■ Prolonged pauses in respiratory pattern longer than 20 seconds in length.

■ Bradycardia or pallor that will ensue if a spontaneous or assisted respiratory pattern does not occur.

TREATMENT

■ Prompt and gentle tactile stimulation is often sufficient to have the infant respond with spontaneous respiratory effort and avert further therapy.

Pharmacologic interventions

■ Methylxanthine, such as caffeine

   ▨ Signs of toxicity include tachycardia, increased diuresis, gastrointestinal symptoms (increased emesis or clinical gastroesphogeal reflux symptoms).

■ Aminophylline, a methylxanthine that has been used in this population to exert a stimulatory effect on the CNS

   ▨ Caution should be used for signs of toxicities with xanthines, including tachycardia, increased diuresis, and gastrointestinal symptoms (increased emesis).

   ▨ More common and severe side-effect profiles have been reported with aminophylline as compared with caffeine and caffeine citrate (e.g., Cafcit).

■ Apneic event with profound associated bradycardia with or without cyanosis requires more aggressive diagnostic and therapeutic intervention.

   ▨ Close clinical observation and physiologic monitoring including pulse oximeter.

   ▨ Blood gas analysis (see Brief Overview of Blood Gas Analysis section).

   ▨ AP chest x-ray for evaluation of lung structures including atelectasis, ventilation, and presence of air leaks.

   ▨ Sepsis evaluation to include CBC and vital signs with support of hypothermia and hypotension. Blood, urine, and cerebral spinal fluid culture tested as indicated. Antibiotic therapy is performed as suggested by the clinical condition of the infant, lab, and blood gas findings (refer to section on neonatal sepsis).

▨ Increased respiratory support including nasal cannula for stimulation with or without supplemental oxygen has been shown to be beneficial.

▨ Nasal CPAP to provide support of FRC and reduce atelectasis in the preterm neonate may be required.

▨ Intubation and provision of mechanical ventilation to support the infant's respiratory status will be required when other methods prove ineffective.

PROGNOSIS

The overall prognosis for preterm neonates with AOP is excellent and infants will typically cease symptoms by 39 to 41 weeks corrected age. The prognosis for term infants who demonstrate symptoms of apnea is based on the organic cause of the episodes. See the section that follows on pulmonary air leaks.

REFERENCES

Kattwinkel, J. (2011). *Textbook of neonatal resuscitation* (6th ed.). Elk Grove Village, IL: American Academy of Pediatrics and American Heart Association.

MacFarlane, P. M., Ribeiro, A. P., & Martin, R. J. (2013). Carotid chemoreceptor development and neonatal apnea. *Respiratory Physiology & Neurobiology, 185,* 170–176.

Miller, M. J., Fanaroff, A. A., & Martin, R. (2011). Respiratory disorders in the preterm and term infants. In R. Martin, A. A. Fanaroff, & M. C. Walsh (Eds.), *Fanaroff and Martin's neonatal–perinatal medicine: Diseases of the fetus and infant* (9th ed.). Philadelphia, PA: Elsevier Saunders.

AIR LEAK SYNDROME

Air leak syndrome includes pneumothorax, pneumomediastinum, pneumopericardium, pneumoperitoneum, and subcutaneous emphysema.

INCIDENCE

■ Air leaks occur in 1% to 2% of term newborns.

■ Incidence increases to 16% to 36% in those infants requiring delivery room resuscitation, nasal CPAP, bag-mask ventilation, or mechanical ventilation (Fraser, 2015).

PHYSIOLOGY

Air leak syndrome is an overdistention of the alveolar sac that causes rupture. This rupture can occur spontaneously or by mechanical means during assisted ventilation. When the air dissects from the alveolus, it can accumulate in five primary locations: the mediastinum, the pleural space, the space surrounding the heart, the peritoneal cavity, or subcutaneously.

PATHOPHYSIOLOGY

In the healthy term infant, the required opening airway pressure during the first spontaneous breath is 60 to 80 cm of water, with subsequent breaths requiring less as the surface tension of the liquid-filled airways and alveoli are stabilized. If secretions or other mechanical obstructions prevent even air distribution, some areas of the newborn's lung will remain collapsed. The infant will generate additional pressure to open these collapsed areas and spontaneous rupture of the open airways can occur.

Air leaks typically occur when a neonate has underlying RDS and the parenchyma of the lung is noncompliant. This "stiff" and nonresponsive lung status is at risk for air leak syndrome.

In the infant with meconium aspiration syndrome (MAS), the obstructive nature of the meconium may cause a ball-valve trapping of air, allowing air to flow into small airways and alveoli, but not escape. This will cause hyperventilation and rupture in some cases.

Positive pressure or respiratory care that is required to support ventilation and oxygen exceeds the capacity of the alveoli and rupture may result.

CLINICAL MANIFESTATIONS/DIAGNOSIS

Pneumothorax

Based on history, physical findings, x-rays, and blood gas results, physical exam findings include:

- A sudden deterioration that will occur if the air leak is large
- Decreased breath sounds on the affected side or bilaterally
- Hypotension, which often accompanies pneumothorax
- Perfusion changes (mottled or pale coloring with prolonged capillary refill time)

Pneumomediastinum

Based on history, physical findings, x-rays, and blood gas results, physical exam findings include:

- Hypotension
- Muffled heart sounds
- Bradycardia (if cardiac tamponade)

Typical findings of diagnostic procedures/tests for *air leak syndrome* are:

- AP chest x-ray
  - A partial or complete pneumothorax will be a collapse of the lung field bilaterally or unilaterally (affected side). Without air inflation, the lung field is darkened without pulmonary markings. Other structures may be shifted to the right or left (heart, trachea).
  - In pneumomediastinum, the air will be visible encircling the heart (called a *halo appearance*) or develop a "sail sign" indicating the elevation of the thymus with air.
  - In pulmonary interstitial emphysema (PIE), the affected alveoli may be bilateral or unilateral with microcystic areas throughout.

This pattern has been described as a "shot gun" pattern. The lung fields are often hyperinflated with flattened diaphragm.

TREATMENT

■ For pneumothorax:

  ▨ Supportive care is needed.

  ▨ If asymptotic, the treatment is removal of air with thoracentesis (needle aspiration) and chest tube placement until resolution.

  ▨ Thoracostomy (chest) tube is placed in the anterior chest on the affected side(s) and connected to a negative pressure system.

  ▨ If asymptomatic, monitor closely for spontaneous resolution.

  • Administration of oxygen may be beneficial in the absorption of the air leak for term infants (oxygen toxicity caution).

■ For pneumomediastinum:

  ▨ Supportive care is needed.

  ▨ Monitor for worsening clinical condition or pneumothorax.

■ For pneumopericardium:

  ▨ Emergency treatment to include pericardial window performed by a skilled cardiologist or general or cardiac surgeon (may be completed with ultrasound guidance).

■ For PIE:

  ▨ Supportive care is needed.

  ▨ If unilateral, the infant may be placed affected side down to aid in decompression of the hyperventilated areas.

  ▨ One can minimize pressures through mechanical or noninvasive respiratory management.

  ▨ High-frequency ventilation is an option as well.

PROGNOSIS

The overall prognosis will depend on the overall pathology of the lung as well as systematic influences. The newborn with spontaneous pneumothorax may resolve fully without intervention. The mortality rate with pneumopericardium, significant PIE, and/or pneumothorax in the ELBW or newborn with pulmonary hypoplasia is greater than 70%.

REFERENCE

Fraser, D. (2015). Respiratory distress. In M. T. Verklan & M. Walden (Eds.), *Core curriculum for neonatal intensive care nursing* (5th ed.). Philadelphia, PA: Elsevier Saunders.

MECONIUM ASPIRATION SYNDROME

INCIDENCE

- Meconium-stained amniotic fluid (MSAF) occurs in 11% to 14% of all term and near-term deliveries.
- Overall incidence of MAS is 1% to 3%.
- Equal incidence occurs in males and females.
- Cesarean delivery is associated with a higher incidence of MAS.
- Associated mortality is 5% to 37%.

PHYSIOLOGY

MAS has been described as the most common type of neonatal aspiration and is typically characterized by early and significant respiratory distress in the meconium-stained infant. During stress or perinatal asphyxia, intestinal peristalsis is stimulated and rectal tone is decreased. Meconium, containing a mixture of epithelial cells and bile salts, is then passed into the amniotic fluid. Fetal stress will often lead to primary or secondary apnea, where the infant makes gasping respiratory efforts while aspirating the meconium-containing amniotic fluid prior to delivery. Controversy surrounds whether the contact between vulnerable pulmonary structures and irritating bile salts or the stressed state of the fetus ultimately leads to significant respiratory distress. Meconium passage in utero has been correlated with a stressed state or asphyxia event prior to or during labor.

PATHOPHYSIOLOGY

Following aspiration of the meconium-containing amniotic fluid, a partial airway obstruction can occur. As pulmonary structures are obstructed (atelectasis), others are hyperinflated through a ball-valve effect, resulting in ventilation–perfusion mismatch and hypoxemia. Air leak or pneumothorax, a known complication of MAS, occurs in 9.6% of reported cases (Dargaville & Copnell, 2006).

The neonatal inflammatory cascade will be triggered by the chemical pneumonitis. The lung compliance is altered, causing increased pulmonary vascular resistance (PVR) and increased hypoxemia. Meconium decreases the levels or inactivates the surfactant proteins, SP-A and SP-B, and phospholipids, increasing respiratory distress, hypoxemia, acidosis, and/or increased risk for PPHN.

ASSESSMENT

The clinical presentation of this infant is a term or near-term infant born with MASF. These infants may require vigorous resuscitation following delivery for respiratory depression or respiratory failure. Typical signs of mild to severe respiratory distress will include tachypnea, nasal flaring, and subcostal and/or intercostal retractions with or without hypoxemia. A prolonged expiratory phase of respirations may be apparent with a hyperinflated or barrel-shaped chest.

CLINICAL MANIFESTATIONS/DIAGNOSIS

The diagnosis of MAS is based on history, physical findings, and radiographic findings.

Physical exam findings

■ Yellow-green stained skin and nailbeds

■ Symptoms of RDS

■ Rales and rhonchi on auscultation

■ No specific laboratory data for diagnosis

Diagnostic procedures/tests

■ Chest x-ray may be specific for hyperexpanded areas mixed with patchy atelectasis

■ Blood gas results specific for acidosis (both metabolic and respiratory) with low PaO_2

TREATMENT

■ In the delivery room: Prior to stimulation, if the infant shows symptoms of perinatal depression, intubate with suctioning of the trachea with a meconium aspiration device and slowly remove the endotracheal tube (ETT), monitoring for signs of meconium below the vocal cords. Repeat as necessary to clear the airway (American Academy of Pediatrics and the American Heart Association, 2011)

■ Clear the mouth and nares with large gauge suction catheter

■ Proceed with resuscitation efforts; provide warmth, tactile stimulation, and support

■ Measure blood gases serially to monitor respiratory levels and acidosis

■ Provide assisted ventilation and/or supplemental oxygen; consider high-frequency ventilation

■ Consider inhaled nitric oxygen (iNO) if infant demonstrates symptoms of PPHN

- Use surfactant replacement as indicated
- Monitor for signs/symptoms of pneumothorax
- Perform CBC and blood culture and consider broad spectrum antibiotic coverage while blood culture is monitored

PROGNOSIS

The overall prognosis for term neonates with mild MAS is excellent with supportive care. If the clinical picture is complicated with PPHN or severe asphyxia, mortality rates approach 40%.

REFERENCES

American Academy of Pediatrics & the American Heart Association. (2011). *NRP: Neonatal Resuscitation Textbook* (6th ed.). Retrieved from http://ebooks .aappublications.org/content/nrp-neonatal-resuscitation-textbook-6th-edition-english-version

Dargaville, P. A., & Copnell, B. (2006). The epidemiology of meconium aspiration syndrome: Incidence, risk factors, therapies and outcome. *Pediatrics, 117,* 1712–1721.

PNEUMONIA

INCIDENCE

- In developed nations, neonatal pneumonia occurs in the term infant about 1% of the time and about 10% in the preterm infant (Abu-Shaweesh, 2011).
- Rates for ventilated preterm neonates are estimated at 28% (Abu-Shaweesh, 2011).
- The World Health Organization (WHO) estimates 800,000 neonatal deaths annually from pneumonia.
- Neonatal pneumonia can have early (congenital) or late (acquired) onset.
- Numbers of reported cases and causative agents vary by institution.
- Ventilator-associated pneumonia (VAP) rates are 0.7 to 2.2 per 1,000 ventilator days (Edwards et al., 2009).

■ Congenital pneumonia is typically caused by maternal enteric organisms and frequently accompanies chorioamnionitis and/or funisitis (Barnett & Klein, 2006).

PHYSIOLOGY

Pneumonia is an infection of the fetal or newborn lung and may be classified as congenital or acquired. Congenital pneumonia occurs from an intrauterine infection, passing the infecting agent to the fetus through transplacental transmission or ascending through the amniotic fluid. Postnatally acquired infections are opportunistic in an immune-deficient host.

PATHOPHYSIOLOGY

Infants born following maternal conditions such as chorioamnionitis or prolonged rupture of membranes (> 18 hours) are at a higher risk for congenital or prenatally acquired pneumonia. Systemic fetal infection can be caused by organisms that cross the placenta and enter the fetal circulation prior to delivery. Infants will often show symptoms of illness at birth or shortly thereafter.

Infection can occur several days to weeks following birth. Typical causative organisms are acquired from other infected patients, personnel, or family visitors. Inflammation will cause the alveoli to become edematous and fluid filled, complicating air exchange. Macrophages, in response to the invading organisms, will invade the pulmonary parenchyma in order to remove debris. Some organisms, specifically *Staphylococcus aureus* and *Klebsiella*, may lead to increased lung cell death with or without abscess formation.

The causative organisms responsible for neonatal pneumonia are primarily group B streptococci and gram-negative organisms (*Escherichia coli, Klebsiella, Pseudomonas,* and *Serratia marcescens*). Other possible organisms include *S. aureus, Staphylococcus epidermidisa, Streptococcus pneumonia,* and *Candida.* Viral causative agents have also been reported (herpes, respiratory syncytial virus [RSV], enterovirus, adenovirus, and parainfluenza virus).

CLINICAL MANIFESTATIONS/DIAGNOSIS

The diagnosis of pneumonia is based on history, physical findings, x-rays, and lab values.

Maternal history should be reviewed for significant findings to include:

- Maternal serologies
- History of maternal illness or fever
- Evidence of chorioamnionitis
- Antenatal antibiotic therapy
- Gestational age

General history

- Postnatal history (intubation, prematurity, recent exposures to illness)

Physical exam findings

- Symptoms of respiratory distress (cyanosis, hypoxemia, hypercapnia, grunting, retractions, and tachypnea)
- Diminished breath sounds with or without rales

Diagnostic procedures/tests

- Lab testing
  - A CBC may be specific for neutropenia, leukopenia, or left shift (abnormal ratio of immature to total neutrophils).
  - Samples of blood for viral and bacterial culture should be obtained and monitored during treatment. Results are often negative unless systemic bacterial/viral sepsis is present.
- Radiographic findings are variable:
  - Unilateral or bilateral infiltrates
  - Diffuse interstitial pattern

- Pleural effusions
- Similar in appearance to neonates with RDS

TREATMENT

- Thermoregulation
- Monitor glucose levels and correct hypoglycemia or hyperglycemia as appropriate
- Monitor blood pressure and perfusion
  - Treat anemia
  - Treat hypotension
  - Close monitoring of intake/output
- Supportive respiratory management
  - Supplemental oxygen
  - Assisted ventilation (nasal cannula [NC], nasal CPAP, SiPAP, vapotherm, NIPPV)
  - Intubation and mechanical ventilation as indicated
  - Monitor blood gases and adjust therapy as indicated
  - Consider surfactant replacement as warranted
- Pharmacologic management includes:
  - Broad spectrum antibiotics
  - Vasopressors as indicated

PROGNOSIS

The overall mortality rate for prenatally acquired pneumonia is estimated at 10% with postnatally acquired rates as high as 50% (Hoffman et al., 2003).

REFERENCES

Abu-Shaweesh, J. M. (2011). Respiratory disorders in the preterm and term infants. In R. Martin, A. A. Fanaroff, & M. C. Walsh (Eds.), *Fanaroff and Martin's neonatal–perinatal medicine: Diseases of the fetus and infant* (9th ed.). Philadelphia, PA: Elsevier Saunders.

Barnett, E. D., & Klein, J. O. (2006). Bacterial infections of the respiratory tract. In J. S. Remington & J. O. Klein (Eds.), *Infectious diseases of the fetus and newborn infant* (6th ed., pp. 297–317). Philadelphia, PA: Elsevier Saunders.

Edwards, J. R., Peterson, K. D., Mu, Y., Banerjee, S., Allen-Bridson, K., Morrell, G., … Horan, T. C. (2009). National Healthcare Safety Network (NHSN) report: Data summary for 2006 through 2008, issued 2009. *American Journal of Infection Control, 37*(10), 783–805.

Hoffman, J., Mason, E., Schultz, G., Tan, T. Q., Barson, W. J., Givner, L. B., … Kaplan, S. L. (2003). Streptococcus pneumonia infections in the neonate. *Pediatrics, 112,* 1095.

PERSISTENT PULMONARY HYPERTENSION OF THE NEWBORN

INCIDENCE

- The condition occurs in 1.9% per 1,000 live births (Roofthooft, Elema, Bergman, & Berger, 2011).

- 77% are diagnosed within the first 24 hours, 97% by 72 hours of life (Gardner, Enzman-Hines, & Dickey, 2011).

- Typically occurs in term or near-term infants.

PHYSIOLOGY

PPHN or persistent fetal circulation is a condition where high right-sided pressure at the PA is combined with right-to-left shunting through fetal pathways (foramen ovale and/or ductus arteriosus). The increased pressure at the PA is caused by an elevated PVR, which is a process of maladaptation between fetal and adult circulation. The pulmonary vascular bed and heart is structurally normal. This vasoconstriction may be transient or persistent and reactive or resistant to therapy.

PATHOPHYSIOLOGY

Following delivery, the infant takes that initial breath and the lungs inflate. Oxygenation depends on the lung inflation, closure of fetal shunts, decreasing PVR, and increasing pulmonary blood flow. The PVR usually falls by about 50% in the first 24 hours of life; however, when the PVR remains high, the transition from fetal to adult circulation is delayed. The PAs in the neonate are reactive and respond to hypoxia or acidosis with vasoconstrictive properties. This high PVR further restricts pulmonary blood flow, which increases this acidotic state and makes oxygenation difficult.

Certain fetal and newborn conditions increase the risk for PPHN and include MAS, congenital diaphragmatic hernia (CDH), RDS, asphyxia, sepsis, pneumonia, hypoglycemia, or other neonatal stressors. Conditions that increase the acidotic state in the newborn, like hypothermia, can also contribute to pulmonary vasoconstriction. These infants share several characteristics: elevated PVR, abnormal pulmonary vasoreactivity, diminished response to vasodilators (oxygen, medications), and increased blood levels of endothelin, a potent vasoconstrictor (Delaney & Cornfield, 2012).

CLININCAL MANIFESTATIONS

Vital signs (temperature, pulse, respiratory rate, heart rate, and blood pressure) will provide needed information to the clinician. Hypothermia or hyperthermia may alter the metabolic load of the neonate. The hypoxic or hypotensive infant may require rapid intervention and is often associated with respiratory compromise.

General observation/impression of the neonate:

■ Tachypnea or increased respiratory rate (> 60 bpm) is the earliest sign of respiratory compromise. This is a compensatory mechanism in the neonate to maintain alveolar ventilation and gas exchange.

- Use of accessory muscles of respiration is an indication of respiratory distress. This includes nasal flaring, retractions, or the inward pull of the chest wall on inspiration.
- Symmetry of the chest wall during inspiration may provide information regarding ongoing or progressive pathology.
- Seesaw respirations in a compensatory mechanism are used to support the effectiveness of gas exchange. With continued respiratory distress, the infant will appear more barrel- or pigeon-chested.
- Pallor, mottling, or poor color of the infant may indicate hypotension or acidosis.
- Cyanosis or blue discoloration of the skin and mucous membranes is a classic sign of hypoxemia. This is a late and serious sign of compromise and the infant will require rapid supportive intervention. This is often associated with respiratory distress, leading to respiratory failure.
- Tachycardia, bradycardia, blood pressure, and perfusion are important signs of cardiac compromise from CHD or ongoing respiratory compromise and failure.
- Diminished muscle tone and poor activity are critical signs of profound hypoxia and acidosis.

  Auscultation of the chest includes:

- Comparing and contrasting bilateral lung sounds
- Quality and volume of air exchange
- Adventitious breath sounds (crackles, rales, and decreased air entry)
- Absence or asymmetric volume of air exchange
- Grunting or the forcing of air through a partially closed glottis on expiration is a compensatory method to maintain FRC in order to maintain alveolar distention and promote gas exchange. This may be heard audibly without a stethoscope.

See earlier discussion for assessment of the neonatal respiratory system.

DIAGNOSIS

The diagnosis of PPHN is based on history, physical findings, x-rays, and echocardiogram.

Significant prenatal and delivery findings

■ Meconium-stained fluid, maternal infection, tight nuchal cord, hypovolemia (placental abruption, accrete, or previa cord accident), maternal sedation

■ History of hypoxia or asphyxia at delivery (low Apgar scores, required resuscitation, acidotic cord blood gases)

Physical exam findings

■ Near-term or term infant

■ Symptoms of RDS (see RDS assessment section for findings)

■ Hypoxemia with or without cyanosis

■ Low PaO_2 despite high levels of delivered supplemental oxygen

Diagnostic procedures or tests

■ AP chest x-ray may be abnormal or normal. Usually obtained to rule out other pathology that could contribute to the state of hypoxia.

■ Arterial blood gas is a good serial monitoring method to determine oxygenation and state of acidosis.

■ Prepost ductal oxygen saturation monitoring will be valuable to determine differences between the preductal measurement (right upper extremity) with postductal locations (left upper extremity or lower extremities). If PaO_2 measurements are more than 15 mmHg, this is an indication of ductal shunting (Orlando, 2012).

■ Echocardiogram will rule out CHD and evaluate the structure and function of the heart and myocardium. Also helpful is the PA pressure measurement, report of septal flattening, and/or distention of the right heart and flow direction at the level of PDA and/or patent foramen ovale (PFO).

■ Hyperoxia test is placing the infant in 100% FIO_2 (fraction of inspired oxygen) and monitoring the oxygen saturations (postductal) or arterial PaO_2. If the infant's oxygenation does not significantly change, this is a clear sign of CHD or PPHN.

■ Serum electrolytes are important to monitor glucose and serum CO_2 levels.

■ Lactate will measure the state of systemic acidosis.

■ CBC and blood cultures should be obtained for sepsis evaluation.

TREATMENT

■ Minimal stimulation occurs as infants demonstrate significant alterations in PVR with even gentle handling and touch.

■ Supportive care (based on the cause of PPHN) may include antibiotic therapy, cooling protocol, and thermoregulation.

■ A central arterial line is placed to monitor systemic blood pressure and obtain serial arterial blood gases.

■ A central venous line is placed to administer fluids and vasopressors as indicated.

■ Ventilation and oxygenation are supported with intubation, mechanical ventilation (conventional, high-frequency jet, high-frequency oscillatory ventilator), and supplementation oxygen (a potent vasodilator) as indicated.

■ iNO, a selective pulmonary vasodilator, has been shown to improve oxygenation in approximately 50% of infants with PPHN (Finer & Barrington, 2006).

■ Surfactant replacement should be considered for infants with parenchymal lung disease (Orlando, 2012).

■ Correct acidosis through ventilation or the administration of bases (sodium bicarbonate) or fluids.

- Close evaluation and fluid adjustments are made based on urine output; avoid pulmonary edema.
- Extracorporeal membrane oxygenation (ECMO) should be considered when conventional therapies are not successful.
- Pharmacologic intervention:
  - Sedatives to maintain calm state
  - Vasopressors to increase systemic blood pressure, thereby reducing PVR; this will decrease right-to-left shunting
  - iNO as discussed earlier
  - Sildenafil as an adjunct therapy to iNO to promote pulmonary vasodilation (Gardner et al., 2011)
  - Analgesics as an adjunct to sedatives to maintain calm state and reduce metabolic need during acute phase of illness

PROGNOSIS

The overall prognosis for term neonates with PPHN is based on the underlying cause or disease process. Residual effects from PPHN include CLD from prolonged ventilation requirement, symptoms of withdrawal secondary to long-term narcotic/sedative requirement, sensorineural hearing loss, learning disabilities, and feeding challenges.

REFERENCES

Delaney, C., & Cornfield, D. N. (2012). Risk factors for persistent pulmonary hypertension of the newborn. *Pulmonary Circulation, 2*(1), 15–20.

Finer, N. N., & Barrington, K. J. (2006). Nitric oxide for respiratory failure in infants born at or near term. *Cochrane Database of Systematic Reviews, 4*, CD000399.

Gardner, S. L., Enzman-Hines, M., & Dickey, L. A. (2011). Respiratory diseases. In S. L. Gardner, B. S. Carter, M. Enzman-Hines, & J. A. Hernandez (Eds.), *Merenstein & Gardner's handbook of neonatal intensive care* (7th ed., pp. 581–677). St. Louis, MO: Elsevier Mosby.

Orlando, S. (2012). Pathophysiology of acute respiratory distress. In D. Fraser (Ed.), *Acute respiratory of the neonate* (3rd ed., pp. 29–50). Santa Rosa, CA: NICU INK Books.

Roofthooft, M. T,. Elema, A., Bergman, K. A., & Berger, R. M. (2011). Patient characteristics in persistent pulmonary hypertension of the newborn. *Pulmonary Medicine, 2011*(2011), 858154.

ADDITIONAL WEB RESOURCE

NeonatalGoldenHours.org (free streaming videos on the topic of PPHN)

CONGENITAL AIRWAY DEFECTS

PULMONARY HYPOPLASIA

INCIDENCE

- 9 to 11 in 10,000 live births
- Mortality rates 71% to 95%
- Equal incidence in male/female
- Frequently associated with oligohydramnios

PHYSIOLOGY

Pulmonary hypoplasia is a rare but often lethal condition in which the lungs are underdeveloped, usually secondary to a space occupying mass, renal, or urinary tract anomalies with oligohydramnios. Diaphragmatic hernia and diaphragmatic eventration also present with symptoms of RDS secondary to pulmonary hypoplasia, as the displaced bowel occupies pulmonary space that prevents adequate growth (see the following section).

PATHOPHYSIOLOGY

Hypoplastic lungs have a decrease in lung volume/mass under conditions of restricted space to develop in utero. This decrease occurs in both number of airway generations and smaller peripheral alveoli than normal term or preterm infants. The unaffected area of the lung has a structure that is appropriate for gestational age.

Infants who are affected by oligohydramnios have lung parenchyma that are structurally and biochemically immature for gestational age, although the exact mechanism for this is still undetermined. These infants have poor epithelial maturation, a lack of elastic tissue development, and low concentrations of lung phospholipids (Chen, Wang, Chou, & Lang, 2010). It is uncertain if this condition is secondary to a lack of exposure to fetal lung fluid, which provides lung tissue the mechanical stretching necessary for development, or if it is a lack of growth factor secretion.

ASSESSMENT

Assessment is similar to other conditions of acute respiratory distress noted in the previous sections.

CLINICAL MANIFESTATIONS/DIAGNOSIS

The diagnosis of pulmonary hypoplasia is based on history, physical findings, blood gas results, and x-rays.

Physical exam findings

■ Tachypnea (> 60 bpm)

■ Intermittent or continuous expiratory grunting which is caused by the forced air past the glottis in an effort to maintain PEEP at the alveolar level

■ Retractions (subcostal, substernal, intercostal, and/or supraclavicular)

■ Nasal flaring

■ Hypoxemia with or without cyanosis

- Increasing oxygen requirement to maintain systemic oxygenation at PaO_2 at 50 to 70 mmHg
- Increased adventitious breath sounds (crackles, rales, and asymmetrical decreased air entry)
- Paradoxical seesaw respirations
- If the condition progresses, the infant will have changes in cardiac function including decreased perfusion, pallor, tachycardia (early), and bradycardia (late)
- If the condition progresses, the infant will demonstrate CNS changes including lethargy, decreased or obtunded response to stimuli, and loss of muscle tone.

Diagnostic procedures/tests

- Arterial blood gas (analysis as described earlier)

Radiographic findings

- AP view, which is usually sufficient for initial examination
- Computed tomography (CT) of the chest (if mass is suspected)

TREATMENT

- Respiratory support as indicated (may require intubation)
- High index of suspension for signs/symptoms of pneumothorax
- Symptomatic care
- Palliative support for genetic anomalies

PROGNOSIS

The overall prognosis for term neonates with pulmonary hypoplasia is poor, with mortality rates ~70% to 90%.

REFERENCE

Chen, C. M., Wang, L. F., Chou, H. C., & Lang, Y. D. (2010). Mechanism of oligohydramnious-induced pulmonary hypoplasia. *Journal Experimental Clinical Medicine, 2*(3), 104–110.

PULMONARY HEMORRHAGE

INCIDENCE

- Occurs in 2% to 12% of preterm infants who weigh less than 1,500 g
- Occurs most frequently day 2 to 4 of life
- May be associated with other complications (PDA, sepsis)
- Following surfactant administration increases incidence
- Appears in males more than females

PHYSIOLOGY

Pulmonary hemorrhage is the presence of blood fluid from the trachea or lung fields. The event can be a massive event or slow leak into the alveoli.

PATHOPHYSIOLOGY

This acute event can be life threatening secondary to airway obstruction and/or hypovolemia. This condition will often accompany or be the complication of a comorbid condition such as disseminated intravascular coagulation (DIC), PDA, RDS, or CHD. Pulmonary hemorrhage is a known complication of surfactant administration or tracheal suctioning.

ASSESSMENT

- Presents with sudden deterioration (vital sign changes, oxygen saturations)
- Significant RDS from obstruction
- Bright red blood or pink-tinged secretions noted

CLINICAL MANIFESTATIONS/DIAGNOSIS

The diagnosis of pulmonary hemorrhage is based on history, physical findings, and x-ray.

Physical exam findings

■ Symptoms of severe RDS

■ Hypotension

■ Anemia

■ Shock

TREATMENT

■ Provide blood or blood products based on clotting studies

■ Support respiratory requirements

■ Suction/clear ETT; replacement may be indicated but risk for poor outcome

■ Correct acidosis and anemia

■ Assess for and treat PDA

■ Treat underlying causes (sepsis)

PROGNOSIS

The overall prognosis for term neonates with pulmonary hemorrhage is poor if massive bleeding is not stopped or slowed. If hemorrhage is small, the infant will recover unless the underlying cause is significant.

CONGENITAL ANOMALIES THAT AFFECT THE RESPIRATORY SYSTEM

CONGENITAL DIAPHRAGMATIC HERNIA

INCIDENCE

■ 1 in 2,500 live births

■ Most symptomatic at birth with severe RDS

■ Left-sided defect 90% of the time

PHYSIOLOGY

This defect is caused by the herniation of abdominal contents, primarily intestine, into the chest cavity.

PATHOPHYSIOLOGY

The diaphragmatic herniation usually occurs early in gestation, which promotes pulmonary hypoplasia secondary to compression. Although the etiology is unclear, the contralateral side also will have some degree of pulmonary hypoplasia.

ASSESSMENT

■ The infant with CDH will classically present with scaphoid abdomen.

■ Some degree of RDS may be severe.

■ Bowel sounds may be heard in the chest.

■ Heart sounds may be shifted to the right side.

CLINICAL MANIFESTATIONS/DIAGNOSIS

The diagnosis of diaphragmatic hernia is based on history, physical findings, x-rays, and lab values.

Physical exam findings

■ Symptoms of respiratory distress (cyanosis, hypoxemia, hypercapnia, grunting, retractions, and tachypnea)

■ Diminished breath sounds (asymmetrical)

■ May auscultate bowel sounds in chest

■ Dextrocardia may be present

Typical findings of diagnostic procedures/tests for diaphragmatic hernia are:

■ Radiographic findings are significant for bowel presence above the diaphragm.

- A CBC is performed.
- Samples of blood for viral and bacterial culture should be obtained and monitored during treatment. Results are often negative unless systemic bacterial/viral sepsis is present.

TREATMENT

- DO NOT ADMINISTER PPV (avoid gastric air delivery)
- Intubate infant and provide respiratory support with supplemental oxygen
- Use a decompression tube to suction (prevent bowel from filling with air)
- Offer respiratory support including high-frequency ventilation and supplemental oxygen
- Consider iNO for symptoms of PPHN
- Suggest a surgical consult

PROGNOSIS

The overall prognosis for term neonates with diaphragmatic hernia is poor with a high incidence of PPHN and ECMO sometimes used for management.

CHOANAL ATRESIA

INCIDENCE

- 50% of cases have bilateral blockages.
- Affected infants have associated anomalies such as CHARGE syndrome (coloboma, heart defects, atresia of the choanae, retardation of growth and development, genital/urinary abnormalities, ear abnormalities and/or hearing deficit).
- It affects females more than males.

PHYSIOLOGY

Infants are obligate nasal breathers in order to breathe effectively during oral feedings. When nasal passages are blocked or obstructed by tissue or mucus, the infant will exhibit symptoms of RDS.

PATHOPHYSIOLOGY

Choanal atresia causes upper airway obstruction as the choanae or nasal passages do not connect to the nasopharynx. The bucconasal membrane which normally opens during gestation blocks the passage and therefore obstructs the passage of air.

ASSESSMENT

The degree of respiratory compromise at delivery usually determines the severity of the obstruction. If both nares are obstructed, the infant will require assistance to support oral airway patency and air exchange. If a single naris is obstructed, respiratory compromise may only be detected when the infant is feeding and the oral airway is obstructed with breast or bottle.

CLINICAL MANIFESTATIONS/DIAGNOSIS

The diagnosis of choanal atresia is based on history and physical findings.

History and physical exam

- Benign prenatal history and ultrasound results unless CHARGE association
- Severe respiratory distress (retractions, poor aeration)
- Cyanosis that becomes pink with crying
- Failure to pass a nasogastric tube (NGT) in one or both nares

TREATMENT

- Oral airway
- Tracheal intubation as indicated
- Maintain calm state with comfort measures
- Evaluation for CHARGE association (echocardiogram, renal ultrasound, eye exam, hearing evaluation)
- Eventual surgical correction

PROGNOSIS

The overall prognosis for term neonates with choanal atresia is excellent. The mortality rate for surgical correction is less than 1%, and complications are rare.

ADDITIONAL WEB RESOURCE

Choanalatresia.org/aboutccaf.html

PIERRE ROBIN SEQUENCE

INCIDENCE

- 60% of affected patients have a cleft palate.
- It can be seen in isolation (50%–70%) or in combination with other anomalies (Stickler, 22q deletion and Treacher Collins, primarily).
- It occurs in 1 per 8,500 to 14,000 live births (Lee & Bradley, 2014).
- Increased risk occurs in families with other children affected by Pierre Robin sequence (1%–5% chance).
- 13% to 27.7% of other family members are affected with cleft lip with or without cleft palate.

PHYSIOLOGY

The major feature of Pierre Robin sequence is micrognathia or small mandible, glossoptosis, and upper airway obstruction. The tongue is posteriorly placed close to the oropharynx and will obstruct the airway (Kenner & Lott, 2014). The mandible is formed at about the fourth week of gestation from the first pharyngeal arch and migrating neural crest cells. At about 6 weeks gestation, the trigeminal nerve innervates the area and promotes osteogenesis, forming the major structures of the mandible. Prenatal or genetic factors disrupt the normal growth of the mandible and micrognathia occurs.

Postnatal growth of the mandible occurs secondary to the coordinating and oppositional forces at two major sites (Lee & Bradley, 2014).

PATHOPHYSIOLOGY

Pierre Robin sequence without other genetic syndrome may be the result from intrauterine forces acting on the mandible, which restrict its growth. Due to the poor mandibular growth, the tongue is displaced between the palatal shelves. Cases of Pierre Robin sequence have been associated with oligohydramnios with an unclear etiology. In these cases, the micrognathia results from intrauterine molding and the mandibular growth can continue following delivery. When Pierre Robin sequence is combined with other genetic causes, varied responses to extrauterine growth is possible without surgical intervention. Higher incidence occurs in families with other cleft deformities.

ASSESSMENT

■ Cyanosis and respiratory distress following delivery is common secondary to airway obstruction.

CLINICAL MANIFESTATIONS/DIAGNOSIS

The diagnosis of Pierre Robin sequence is based on history and physical findings.

Physical exam findings

- Small mandible
- RDS that may be relieved when the infant is placed prone
- Tongue that appears large for mouth

TREATMENT

- Prone position to allow tongue to fall forward. Positioning will resolve the airway obstruction in ~70% of cases.
- Surgical tongue-lip adhesion, where the tongue is affixed to the lip with sutures to prevent airway obstruction from the tongue position.
- Oral feedings in a prone or side-lying position may be tolerated. Nasogastric feedings are often required initially.
- Mandibular distraction osteogenesis is an established technique used to treat infants with Pierre Robin sequence associated with severe airway obstruction. Mandibular distraction has shown favorable results with a 50% reduction in tracheostomy placement (Lee & Bradley, 2014).

PROGNOSIS

Excellent survival rates are noted for these infants. Mandibular growth contributes to resolution by 6 to 12 months of age. Prognostic outcomes in infants with comorbidities including syndromes or genetic diseases have various results based on those genetic conditions.

REFERENCES

Kenner, C., & Lott, J. W. (2014). *Comprehensive neonatal nursing care* (4th ed.). New York, NY: Springer Publishing Company.

Lee, J. C., & Bradley, J. P. (2014). Surgical considerations in Pierre Robin sequence. *Clinical Plastic Surgery, 41*, 211–217.

ADDITIONAL WEB RESOURCE

http://www.cleftline.org/parents-individuals/publications/pierre-robin-sequence

CONGENITAL PULMONARY MALFORMATIONS

Congenital pulmonary malformations (CPMs) are a group of rare abnormalities that affect different parts of the neonatal lung or supporting structures, including the main or terminal airways, the parenchyma, and the supportive vasculature. These abnormalities are typically caused by aberrant embryologic lung development at various stages and can be self-limiting or cause significant respiratory distress at birth or shortly thereafter (Nadeem, Elnazir, & Greally, 2012). The following is a brief description of the most common forms of CPMs; these include congenital pulmonary airway malformation (CPAM), bronchial or bronchogenic cyst, and pulmonary sequestration.

CONGENITAL PULMONARY AIRWAY MALFORMATION

This condition was previously known as congenital cystic adenomatoid malformation (CCAM).

INCIDENCE

- It occurs in 1 per 8,300 to 35,000 live births.
- Males and females are affected equally.

PATHOPHYSIOLOGY

The lesion of CPAM is characterized by solid, closely packed structures that resemble terminal bronchioles without alveoli, similar to the histologic fetal lung around 16 weeks gestation. Because of the space occupied by this mass, pulmonary hypoplasia may result in severe cases; however, only three out of 29 cases exhibit symptoms of respiratory distress in the first week of life. Associations between CPAM and malignancy, specifically bronchoalveolar carcinoma, have been reported.

ASSESSMENT

- Classic symptoms of RDS are observed in severe cases (see the RDS section).
- Large cystic formations can present with acute respiratory failure.
- Acute deterioration secondary to pneumothorax has been reported.

CLINICAL MANIFESTATIONS/DIAGNOSIS

The diagnosis of CPAM is based on history, physical findings, and radiologic evaluation.

Physical exam findings

- Ranges from normal respiratory exam when the mass is small to acute distress.

Typical findings of diagnostic procedures/tests for CPAM are:

- AP chest x-ray will be specific for the location and size of the CPAM.
- Chest (thoracic) CT scan is required to identify subtle structures of the CPAM.

TREATMENT

- Surgical intervention with excision is typically recommended.
- Of note: In fetal cases with CPAM and nonimmune hydrops, fetal resection, or thoracoamniotic shunt, have reportedly been effective.

PROGNOSIS

Prognosis depends on the size and location of the CPAM and to what degree lung hypoplasia is present at birth (Akinkuotu et al., 2014).

Access the MedCalc Acid–Base Calculator at
http://www.medcalc.com/acidbase.html

Arterial Blood Gas (ABG) values:			Anion Gap values:		
pH:		7.36 - 7.44	Sodium (Na⁺):		mEq/L
P$_{CO2}$:	mm Hg	36 - 44 mm Hg	Bicarbonate (HCO₃⁻):		mEq/L
HCO₃⁻:	mEq/L	22 - 26 mEq/L	Chloride (Cl⁻):		mEq/L
			Albumin:		g/dL
Acid–Base Interpretation:			Anion Gap:	< 16	mEq/L Normal:

DISCLAIMER: All calculations must be confirmed before use. The authors make no claims of the accuracy of the information contained herein; and these suggested doses are not a substitute for clinical judgement. Neither MedCalc.com nor any other party involved in the preparation or publication of this site shall be liable for any special, consequential, or exemplary damages resulting in whole or part from any user's use of or reliance upon this material.

Copyright © 1999-2016 MedCalc.com
Created by: Charles Hu
Created: Monday, October 4, 1999
Last Modified: Wednesday, January 27, 2010

REFERENCES

Akinkuotu, A., Sheikh, F., Cass, D. L., Zamora, I. J., Lee, T. C., Cassady, C. I., ... Olutoye, O. O. (2014). Are all pulmonary hypoplasias the same? A comparison of pulmonary outcomes in neonates with congenital diaphragmatic hernia, omphalocele and congenital lung malformations. *Journal of Pediatric Surgery*, *50*, 55–59.

Barnett, E. D., & Klein, J. O. (n.d.). Bacterial infections of the respiratory tract. In J. S. Remington (Ed.), *Infectious diseases of the fetus and the newborn* (7th ed.). Philadelphia, PA: Elsevier Saunders.

Nadeem, M., Elnazir, F., & Greally, P. (2012). Congenital pulmonary malformation in children. *Scientifica*, *2012*, 107. doi:10.6064/2012/209896

Cardiovascular System

Samual L. Mooneyham

OVERVIEW

Fetal circulation differs from extrauterine circulation because of the following in utero characteristics:

■ Pulmonary vascular resistance is higher than systemic vascular resistance.

■ Gas exchange for the fetus occurs in the placenta and bypasses the lungs.

■ Lungs are filled with fluid.

■ Fetal structures such as the foramen ovale, ductus arteriosus (DA), and ductus venosus are present.

Fetal circulation is shown in Figure 2.1.

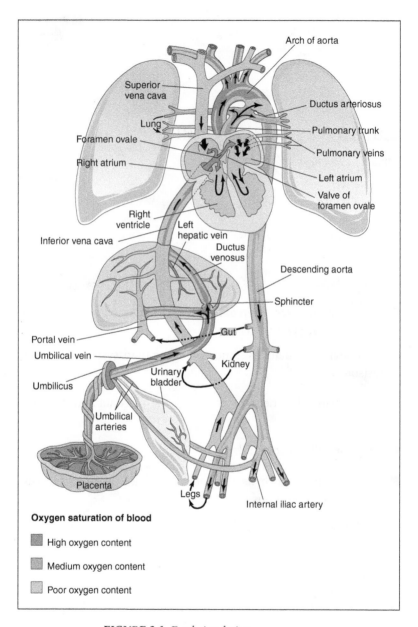

FIGURE 2.1. Fetal circulation.

Adapted and modified from Ross Laboratories (1985).

TRANSITION OF EXTRAUTERINE CIRCULATION

- Pulmonary vascular resistance decreases and systemic vascular resistance increases
- DA and ductus venosus closure
- Left-to-right shunting through the foramen ovale
- Foramen ovale closure

Anatomy of the normal heart is shown in Figure 2.2.

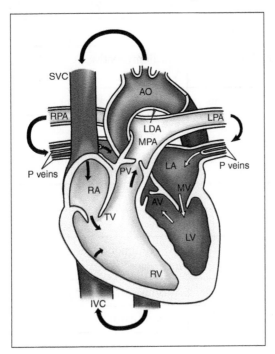

FIGURE 2.2. Normal cardiac anatomy and circulation. AO, aorta; AV, aortic valve; IVC, inferior vena cava; LA, left atrium; LDA, ligamentum ductus arteriosus; LPA, left pulmonary artery; LV, left ventricle; MPA, main pulmonary artery; MV, mitral valve; PV, pulmonary valve; P veins, pulmonary veins; RA, right atrium; RPA, right pulmonary artery; RV, right ventricle; SVC, superior vena cava; TV, tricuspid valve.

Adapted and modified from Ross Laboratories (1985).

IMPORTANCE OF MATERNAL AND PERINATAL HISTORY

There are several maternal conditions that can affect a newborn's cardiovascular system. See Table 2.1 for heart defects associated with maternal history.

TABLE 2.1 Maternal Condition and Associated Congenital Heart Defects	
Condition	Defect
Maternal Disease	
Diabetes mellitus	Cardiomyopathy, TGA, VSD, PDA
Lupus erythematosus	Congenital heart block
Collagen disease	Congenital heart block
Congenital heart defect	Increased risk for congenital heart defect (3%–4%)
Viral Disease	
Rubella	
First trimester	PDA, pulmonary artery branch stenosis
Later	Various cardiac and other defects
Cytomegalovirus	Various cardiac and other defects
Herpesvirus	Various cardiac and other defects
Coxsackie B virus	Various cardiac and other defects
Drugs	
Amphetamines	VSD, PDA, ASD, TGA
Phenytoin	PS, AS, COA, PDA

(continued)

TABLE 2.1 Maternal Condition and Associated Congenital Heart Defects (*continued*)	
Condition	Defect
Trimethadione	TGA, TOF, HLHS
Progesterone/ estrogen	VSD, TOF, TGA
Alcohol	VSD, PDA, ASD, TOF

AS, aortic stenosis; ASD, atrial septal defect; COA, coarctation of the aorta; HLHS, hypoplastic left heart syndrome; PDA, patent ductus arteriosus; PS, pulmonary stenosis; TOF, tetralogy of Fallot; TGA, transposition of the great arteries; VSD, ventricular septal defect.

Source: Lott (2014, p. 155).

GENERAL FOCUSED ASSESSMENT OF THE CARDIOVASCULAR SYSTEM

Complete the history by reviewing maternal, family, and other birth histories to see what risk factors could contribute to cardiovascular diseases. The initial cardiovascular assessment should include general appearance and behavior. Inspect the skin and mucous membranes of the newborn for color and temperature; these can be early signs of cardiac defects. Cyanosis is bluish color of the skin, lips, earlobes, nailbeds, and scrotum in males with significant arterial oxygen desaturation. The two types of cyanosis are central and peripheral (bluish color in hand, feet, and around mouth). Peripheral cyanosis is a normal finding in newborns until around day two of life. Pallor and mottling can also be signs of cardiac defects. Pallor is caused by vasoconstriction and shunting blood from the skin to vital organs. Mottling can be associated with cardiogenic shock; this may be caused by a decrease in cardiac output or hypovolemia. Be aware that you might see mottling with normal newborns that are stressed or cold. Perfusion is also important; looking at capillary filling time, greater than 3 to 4 seconds is abnormal. Peripheral pulse should be assessed and measured (Tappero & Honeyfield, 2009). See Table 2.2 for grading of pulses.

TABLE 2.2 Grading of Pulses	
Grade	Description
0	Not palpable
+1	Difficult to palpate, thready, weak, easily obliterated with pressure
+2	Difficult to palpate, may be obliterated with pressure
+3	Easy to palpate, not easily obliterated with pressure (NORMAL)
+4	Strong, bounding, not obliterated with pressure

Source: Hockenberry and Wilson (2011).

REFERENCES

Hockenberry, M., & Wilson, D. (2011). *Wong's nursing care of infants and children* (9th ed., p. 149). St. Louis, MO: Mosby/Elsevier.

Lott, J. W. (2014). Cardiovascular system. In C. Kenner & J. W. Lott (Eds.), *Comprehensive neonatal nursing care* (5th ed., pp. 152–188). New York, NY: Springer Publishing Company.

Vargo, L. (2009). Cardiovascular Assessment. In E. P. Tappero & M. E. Honeyfield (Eds.), *Physical assessment of the newborn: A comprehensive approach to the art of physical examination* (4th ed.). Santa Rosa, CA: NICU Ink Book.

ATRIAL SEPTAL DEFECT

Samual L. Mooneyham

INCIDENCE

▪ Accounts for 5% to 10% of all congenital heart defects (CHDs)

PHYSIOLOGY

Atrial septal defect (ASD) is an opening in the atrial septum that develops as a result of improper septal formation early in fetal cardiac development.

There are three types of ASDs (Park, 2007; Webb, Smallhorn, Therrien, & Reddington, 2011):

■ Ostium, commonly associated with mitral valve

■ Ostium primum, an endocardial cushion defect (ECD) associated with anomalies of one or both atrioventricular (AV) valves

■ Sinus venosus, often associated with partial anomalous pulmonary venous connection

ASD is shown in Figure 2.3.

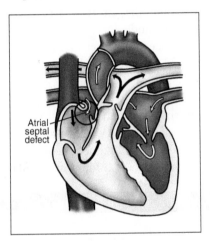

FIGURE 2.3. Atrial septal defect is a communication between the right and left atria.

Adapted and modified from Ross Laboratories (1985).

HEMODYNAMICS

ASD usually does not produce symptoms until pulmonary vascular resistance begins to decrease and right ventricular end-diastolic and right atrial pressure decline. ASDs produce some blood flow alterations. Blood shunts from left to right through the defect because the right ventricle offers less resistance to fill it. The left-to-right shunt increases right ventricular volume and decreases pulmonary vascular resistance, so the pulmonary artery pressure is almost normal. The large pulmonary blood flow gradually leads to increased pulmonary artery pressure.

CLINICAL MANIFESTATIONS/DIAGNOSIS

Newborns with ASDs are usually asymptomatic, although there may be grade 2/6 to 3/6 systolic ejection murmurs (SEMs); see Table 2.3 for a grading scale of murmurs, which can best be heard at the upper left sternal border (ULSB). In a large ASD, there can be middiastolic rumble caused by the relative tricuspid stenosis audible at the lower left sternal border (LLSB) (Park, 2007; Webb et al., 2011). On a chest radiograph, the heart is enlarged, with a prominent main pulmonary artery segment and increased pulmonary vascularity. Echocardiogram enhances detection of the ASD; it shows a right axis deviation and mild right ventricular hypertrophy. There may be an incomplete right bundle branch block (Danford, Gumbiner, Martin, & Fletcher, 2000; Park, 2007).

Echocardiogram shows increased tight ventricular dimension and paradoxical movement of the ventricular septum. Diagnosis can be made by two-dimensional echocardiogram, which shows the location and size of the defect. Children with ASDs are usually thin

TABLE 2.3 Grading Scale of Murmurs	
Grade 1	Barely heard
Grade 2	Soft but easily audible
Grade 3	Moderately loud, no thrill
Grade 4	Loud, thrill present
Grade 5	Loud, audible with stethoscope barely on chest
Grade 6	Loud, audible with stethoscope near chest

Source: Kenner and Lott (2014).

and may be easily fatigued. By late infancy, there may be a precordial bulge caused by an enlarged right side of the heart.

MANAGEMENT

Untreated ASD can lead to congestive heart failure (CHF), pulmonary hypertension, and atrial dysrhythmias in adulthood. Spontaneous closure of ASDs occurs in the first 5 years of age in up to 40% of children (Park, 2007). Medical management of ASD consists of prevention or treatment of CHF. There is no need to limit activity. Closure of the ASD may be accomplished through insertion of a device that covers the ASD and is attached to the atrial septum during cardiac catheterization. This approach does not require cardiopulmonary bypass.

Surgical correction is reserved for infants for whom the transcatheter approach is contraindicated or unsuccessful. The surgical process is done during open-heart surgery by placing a patch or with direct closure. This process requires cardiopulmonary bypass. Surgery usually occurs between 2 and 5 years, but depends on the severity of the defect and the significance of left-to-right shunting. Mortality rate of surgery is less than 1%, with the highest risk for infants with CHF or increased pulmonary vascular resistance (Park, 2007; Webb et al., 2011).

REFERENCES

Danford, D., Gumbiner, C., Martin, A., & Fletcher, S. (2000). Effects of electrocardiography and chest radiography on the accuracy of preliminary diagnosis of common congenital cardiac defects. *Pediatric Cardiology, 21*(4), 334–340.

Kenner, C., & Lott, J. (2014). *Comprehensive neonatal nursing care* (5th ed.). New York, NY: Springer Publishing Company.

Park, M. (2007). *Pediatric cardiology for practitioner.* Chicago, IL: Mosby.

Webb, G., Smallhorn, J., Therrien, J., & Reddington, A. (2011). Congenital heart disease. In R. Bonow, D. Mann, D. P. Zipes, P. Libby, & E. Braunwald (Eds.), *Braunwald's heart disease: A textbook of cardiovascular medicine* (pp. 1411–1467). Philadelphia, PA: WB Saunders.

VENTRICULAR SEPTAL DEFECT

Samual L. Mooneyham

INCIDENCE

■ Accounts for 20% to 25% of all CHDs. It is the most common defect.

PHYSIOLOGY

Ventricular septal defect (VSD) is a defect or opening of the ventricular septum. VSD results from imperfect ventricular division during early fetal development. It can occur anywhere on the muscular or membranous septum. This size and degree of pulmonary vascular resistance may vary. This is more important than where it is located. Small defects have a large resistance to the left-to-right shunting and shunting is not dependent on pulmonary vascular resistance. Large defects have little resistance to the left-to-right shunting and are dependent on the level of pulmonary vascular resistance (Park, 2007; Turner, Hunter, & Wyllie, 1999; Webb, Smallhorn, Therrien, & Reddington, 2011). VSD is shown in Figure 2.4.

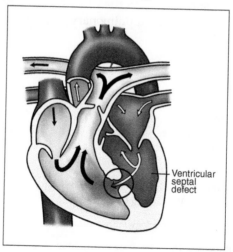

FIGURE 2.4. VSD is a communication between the right and left ventricles.

VSD, ventricular septal defect.

Adapted and modified from Ross Laboratories (1985).

HEMODYNAMICS

The hemodynamic considerations depend on the size of the VSD.

■ Small VSD—these produce minimal shunting and may not show any signs or symptoms. A chest radiograph and echocardiogram may appear normal. During auscultation, a loud, harsh pansystolic murmur may be heard at the third and fourth left intercostal space at the sternal border (Park, 2007; Turner et al., 1999; Webb et al., 2011).

■ Moderate VSD—there is shunting from the left to right ventricle because of the high pressure of the left ventricle and higher systemic vascular resistance. The shunting occurs during systole, when the right ventricle contracts, moving blood to the pulmonary artery versus staying in the right ventricle. This prevents right ventricular hypertrophy.

■ Large VSD—there is shunting from the left to right ventricle; the amount depends on the size of the VSD. The larger the size, the greater the amount of shunting; this creates higher pressure in the right ventricle and pulmonary artery. When there is significantly increased pressure in the pulmonary artery, the walls of the pulmonary arterioles thicken and increased resistance may decrease the left-to-right shunting. Pulmonary vascular disease can lead to right-to-left shunting and cyanosis.

CLINICAL MANIFESTATIONS/DIAGNOSIS

Manifestations depend on the size/shunting. Smaller VSDs may be asymptomatic with no change in hemodynamics. Larger VSDs are associated with decreased exertional tolerance, recurrent pulmonary infections, poor growth, and symptoms of CHF. Pulmonary hypertension and cyanosis are seen in severe VSDs.

A systolic thrill may be palpated at the LLSB. A precordial bulge may appear with larger VSDs. Grade 2/6 to 5/6 regurgitant systolic murmurs can be heard at LLSB. During auscultation, you may hear an apical diastolic rumble and perhaps loud pulmonary heart sounds.

X-ray testing can detect moderate to large VSDs (Danford, Gumbiner, Martin, & Fletcher, 2000). Radiographs show cardiomegaly that involves the left atrium, left ventricle, maybe the right ventricle, and increased pulmonary vascularity. Echocardiogram may show left ventricular hypertrophy and, in severe cases, right hypertrophy. Two-dimensional echocardiogram shows the size and location of the defect as well as other defects (Park, 2007; Webb et al., 2011). MRI shows the volume of blood flow to the lungs.

With large VSDs not detected in the neonatal period, physical examination in the infant may show inadequate weight gain, cyanosis, and clubbing of the digits.

MANAGEMENT

Treatment depends on the severity and symptoms of the VSD. Small VSDs usually spontaneously close by the age of 6, as long as it causes no compromise and can be observed. The highest spontaneous closure rate with VSDs is muscular versus perimembranous (29% vs. 69%) (Turner et al., 1999).

Medical management for significant VSDs is monitored for CHF and prompt initiation of therapy. CHF is treated with diuretics and digitalis in older infants, unless there is pulmonary hypertension. Activities are not restricted; if indicated, prophylaxis is used against bacterial endocarditis.

Surgical management involves closure of the defect, but the time of this surgery depends on the severity of the circulatory and pulmonary compromise. Significant left-to-right shunting and evidence of severe compromise indicate surgery. If the infant does not improve sufficiently to medical management, surgical intervention is required. Surgery for VSD requires cardiopulmonary bypass. Moderate VSDs that require surgical intervention usually occur between 2 and 4 years.

The mortality rate for VSD corrections is about 5%, with the higher rate in small infants and those with multiple VSDs.

REFERENCES

Danford, D., Gumbiner, C., Martin, A., & Fletcher, S. (2000). Effects of electrocardiography and chest radiography on the accuracy of preliminary diagnosis of common congenital cardiac defects. *Pediatric Cardiology, 21*(4), 334–340.

Park, M. (2007). *Pediatric cardiology for practitioner.* Chicago, IL: Mosby.

Turner, S., Hunter, S., & Wyllie, J. (1999). The natural history of ventricular septal defects. *Archives of Disease in Childhood, 81*(1), 49–52.

Webb, G., Smallhorn, J., Therrien, J., & Reddington, A. (2011). Congenital heart disease. In R. Bonow, D. Mann, D. P. Zipes, P. Libby, & E. Braunwald (Eds.), *Braunwald's heart disease: A textbook of cardiovascular medicine* (pp. 1411–1467). Philadelphia, PA: WB Saunders.

PATENT DUCTUS ARTERIOSUS

Judy Wright Lott

INCIDENCE

- 5% to 10% of all CHDs in term newborns
- Higher occurrence in females (3:1)
- More common in infants with trisomy 21 or Down syndrome
- Infants of mothers with rubella during pregnancy (Lott, 2014)

PHYSIOLOGY

The ductus arteriosus (DA) is a wide muscular connection between the pulmonary artery and the aorta that originates from the left pulmonary artery and enters the aorta below the subclavian artery. The purpose of the DA is to allow oxygenated blood from the placenta to bypass the nonfunctional lungs and enter the fetal circulation. The DA should close functionally by about 15 hours postbirth. Intermittent shunting of blood is quite common during the first 24 hours in response to changes in the systemic or pulmonary vascular resistance, such as infusion of fluids or handling the neonate. Increased arterial oxygen concentration after the neonate begins to breathe causes ductal closure. Decreased prostaglandin E (PGE) and increased acetylcholine and bradykinin contribute to the closure (Lott, 2014).

PATHOPHYSIOLOGY

Failure of the DA to close, allowing shunting of blood in the term neonate after 24 hours postdelivery, is considered a patent ductus arteriosus (PDA) in the term neonate. PDA in the preterm neonate presents a different clinical problem that is discussed separately.

After birth, blood flow through the DA is reversed. Blood flows from left to right through the PDA, reentering the pulmonary system (Figure 2.5). The amount of blood that flows through the PDA and the effects of the increased flow depend on the difference between systemic and pulmonary vascular resistance and the diameter and length of the ductus. Prolonged increased pulmonary blood flow

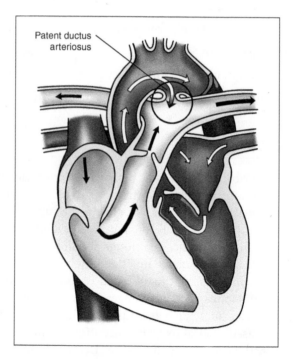

FIGURE 2.5. PDA is a communication between the pulmonary artery and the aorta.

PDA, patent ductus arteriosus.

Adapted and modified from Ross Laboratories (1985).

can cause increased pulmonary vascular resistance, pulmonary hypertension, and right ventricular hypertrophy (Lott, 2014).

ASSESSMENT

The severity of the PDA is determined by the diameter and length of the DA and the amount of blood shunted into the pulmonary system. A small PDA may be asymptomatic. A large PDA with significant shunting causes signs of congestive heart failure, such as tachypnea, dyspnea, and hoarse cry. Infants with uncorrected PDA may have frequent lower respiratory tract infections, coughing, and poor weight gain (Lott, 2014).

CLINICAL MANIFESTATIONS/DIAGNOSIS

The diagnosis of PDA is based upon history, physical findings, x-rays, and echocardiogram.

Physical exam findings

- Bounding peripheral pulses
- Widened pulse pressure of more than 25 mmHG
- Hyperactive precordium
- Systolic thrill at ULSB
- Murmur (grade 1/6–4/6) at ULSB or infraclavicular area
- Murmur heard throughout the cardiac cycle
- Definitive diagnosis made by echocardiogram

Typical findings of diagnostic procedures/tests for PDA are illustrated in Table 2.5.

TREATMENT

Pharmacologic closure occurs through administration of medications that cause constriction of the ductus.

- Indomethacin
- Ibuprofen

- Cardiac catheterization and insertion of coil or device is placed into ductus to obstruct flow.
- Definitive treatment of a large PDA with significant shunting is surgical ligation (Lott, 2014).

PROGNOSIS

The overall prognosis for term neonates with PDA is excellent. The mortality rate for surgical ligation is less than 1%, and complications are rare (Lott, 2014). Medical closure is not effective in older infants.

REFERENCE

Lott, J. W. (2014). Cardiovascular system. In C. Kenner & J. W. Lott (Eds.), *Comprehensive neonatal nursing care* (5th ed., pp. 152–188). New York, NY: Springer Publishing Company.

TETRALOGY OF FALLOT

Samual L. Mooneyham

INCIDENCE

- This accounts for 10% of all CHD.
- It is the most common cyanotic heart defect beyond infancy because repair is usually carried out after the patient becomes a 1 year old.

PHYSIOLOGY

Tetralogy of Fallot (TOF) is developed as a lack of subpulmonary conus during fetal life. It consists of a large VSD, pulmonary stenosis (PS) or other right ventricular outflow tract obstruction, overriding aorta, and right ventricle hypertrophy, although initially the right ventricle may not be hypertrophied. TOF is shown in Figure 2.6.

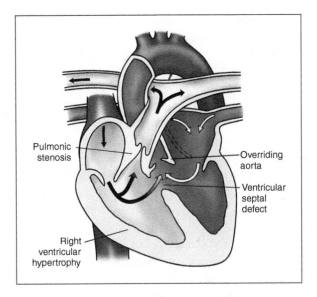

FIGURE 2.6. Tetralogy of Fallot consists of PS, ventricular septal defect, overriding aorta, and hypertrophy of the right ventricle.

PS, pulmonary stenosis.

Adapted and modified from Ross Laboratories (1985).

HEMODYNAMICS

The VSD in TOF causes pressures in the ventricles to be equal. The obstruction of the pulmonary artery causes oxygenated blood to flow into the aorta through the VSD.

CLINICAL MANIFESTATIONS/DIAGNOSIS

The cardinal signs of TOF are cyanosis, hypoxia, and dyspnea. Newborns may present with a loud murmur or may be cyanotic. Severe decompensation or "tet" spells are common in infants and children; they can occur in the neonatal period, too. Instinctively children will squat; this decreases systemic venous return by trapping venous blood in the legs. Chronic arterial desaturation stimulates erythropoiesis, leading to polycythemia. Increased red blood cells and microcytic anemia increase the viscosity of blood and can lead to cerebrovascular accident (stroke). Chronic hypoxemia and polycythemia cause an increased risk of hemorrhagic diathesis because reduced platelet aggregation and decreased platelet survival time cause thrombocytopenia and impaired synthesis of vitamin K–dependent clotting factors.

TOF exhibit varying degrees of cyanosis, depending on the obstruction of blood flow to the right ventricular outflow. A very loud grade 3/6 to 5/6 SEM is heard at the middle and upper left sternal border. In severe TOF, a PDA may be heard (Park, 2007).

A chest radiograph may show decreased or normal heart size with decreased pulmonary vascularity. The heart may be boot-shaped because of a concaved main pulmonary artery segment with upturned apex. It may also show an enlarged right atrial and a right aortic arch.

An echocardiogram will show a large VSD and overriding aorta. A two-dimensional echocardiogram identifies the right ventricular outflow tract and pulmonary valve.

TOF may show clubbing of fingers.

MANAGEMENT

The definitive treatment for TOF is surgical correction. This procedure requires cardiopulmonary bypass. Surgical correction may be delayed with medical management. Decreasing pulmonary vascular resistance may improve mild cyanosis. Medical management is used to prevent or treat hypoxemia, polycythemia, infection, and microcytic hypochromic anemia. Continuous follow-up is needed, as well as parent education and support for home management (Dipchand, Giuffre, & Freedom, 1999; Park, 2007). Parents need education in recognizing early signs and symptoms of decompensation. They also need to recognize and treat hypercyanotic or "tet" spells. See Table 2.4 for recognition and treatment of "tet" spells. Lowering the systemic vascular resistance and a large right-to-left ventricular shunt leads to a "tet" spell. Increased activity, crying, nursing, or defecation can trigger hypoxemic episodes. A right-to-left shunt results in a decrease in PaO_2, increase in PCO_2, and decrease in pH. This stimulates the respiratory system and causes an increase in rate and depth of respiration, known as hyperpnea. This causes an increase in systemic venous return. The right ventricular outflow tract obstruction prevents the increased blood flow from entering the pulmonary artery, so it is shunted to the aorta. This further decrease in PaO_2 with severe uninterrupted hypercyanotic spells can lead to seizures, hypoxemia, loss of consciousness, and even death.

TABLE 2.4 Recognition and Treatment of Tet Spells		
Manifestations	Treatment	Rationale
Irritability, crying, hyperpnea	Knee to chest or squatting position	Traps blood in the lower extremities to decrease systemic venous return; increases pulmonary blood flow
Cyanosis	Oxygen administration	Improves arterial oxygen saturation
Diaphoresis, loss of consciousness	Morphine sulfate (0.1–0.2 mg/kg/ dose)	Suppresses respiratory center to decrease hyperpnea
Seizures	Bicarbonate	Corrects acidosis and eliminates stimulation of respiratory center
Decreased murmur	Propranolol (Inderal; 0.15–0.25 mg/kg/dose)	May decrease spasm of right ventricular outflow tract or may act peripherally to stabilize

Source: Lott (2014).

An indication for immediate surgical treatment is the presence of "tet" spells; this increases hypoxemia, increases metabolic acidosis, leads to inadequate systemic perfusion, increases cyanosis, and increases polycythemia. Systemic perfusion evaluation occurs by observing peripheral pulse intensity, urine output, capillary refill time, blood pressure, or peripheral vasoconstriction.

Surgical management is divided into palliative or corrective procedures. Palliative procedure is used to create a pathway between the systemic and pulmonary system. This also allows for the right and left pulmonary arteries to grow. This procedure is indicated when newborns have TOF, PA, severe cyanosis while younger than 6 months, unmanageable "tet" spells, or hypoplastic pulmonary artery where corrective surgery is difficult (Park, 2007). The corrective procedure is performed after 6 months of age. It can be delayed until ages 2 to 4 years in asymptomatic children or those who have received the palliative procedure. This procedure requires cardiopulmonary bypass and consists of closure of the VSD, excision of the PS, and widening of the right ventricular outflow tract. The postoperative mortality rate is 5% to 10%, with the first 2 years in uncomplicated TOF and higher in more severe cases.

REFERENCES

Dipchand, A., Giuffre, M., & Freedom, R. (1999). Tetralogy of Fallot with non-confluent pulmonary arteries and aortopulmonary septal defect. *Cardiology in the Young, 9*(1), 75–77.

Lott, J. W. (2014). Cardiovascular system. In C. Kenner & J. W. Lott (Eds.), *Comprehensive neonatal nursing care* (5th ed., pp. 152–188). New York, NY: Springer Publishing Company.

Park, M. (2007). *Pediatric cardiology for practitioner.* Chicago, IL: Mosby.

COARCTATION OF THE AORTA

Samual L. Mooneyham

INCIDENCE

■ It accounts for 8% of all CHDs.

■ It is found in 30% of newborns with Turner syndrome (Park, 2007).

■ Male to female ratio is 2:1.

PHYSIOLOGY

Coarctation of the aorta (COA) is the narrowing or constriction of the aortic arch. It is more commonly seen below the left subclavian artery. COA can occur as a single lesion related to improper development of the aorta or because of the constriction of the DA. The severity depends on the degree of constriction and location. Preductal COA (proximal to the DA) accounts for 40% of cases. Other defects associated with preductal COA are VSD, transposition of the great arteries (TGA), and PDA. Collateral circulation is more effective with postductal COA versus preductal COA. There are normally no other defects with postductal COA and they are usually asymptomatic. In newborns with COA, there is a greater than 50% chance that they will have a bicuspid valve (Park, 2007). COA is shown in Figure 2.7.

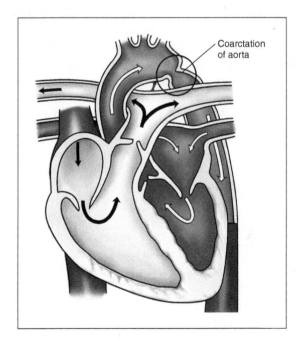

FIGURE 2.7. COA is a narrowing or constriction of the aorta near the DA.

COA, coarctation of the aorta; DA, ductus arteriosus. Adapted and modified from Ross Laboratories (1985).

HEMODYNAMICS

COA causes an obstruction to blood flow, which causes varying pressure across the aortic arch. An obstruction proximal to the constriction of the aorta results in elevated pressure and causes increased left ventricular pressure. This increased pressure results in left ventricular hypertrophy and dilation. The compensatory mechanism is collateral circulation (develops proximal to distal arteries to bypass the constriction). This increases blood flow to the lower extremities and abdomen, which produces a lower pulse (Park, 2007).

CLINICAL MANIFESTATIONS/DIAGNOSIS

The severity depends on the degree of constriction and location as well as the time of appearance of symptoms and the presence of associated cardiac defects. Some symptoms of COA include signs of CHF, as well as weak, absent, or delayed lower extremity pulses. If CHF is present, then all pulses may be weak. With severe COA, auscultation will reveal a loud and single S2, an ejection click may be audible at the apex if a bicuspid aortic valve or systemic hypertension is present, and a grade 2/6 to 3/6 SEM is heard at the upper right and middle or lower left sternal border and left interscapular area in newborns. In newborns, greater than 50% will have no murmurs in COA (Park, 2007).

Diagnosis is based on history, physical findings, radiograph, ECG, and echocardiograph.

Radiograph

■ Asymptomatic newborns—may show a normal or slightly enlarged heart and may see dilation of the ascending aorta. On a barium swallow study an "E" sign may appear. The "E" sign is due to the large proximal aortic segment or prominent subclavian artery above the poststenotic dilation of the descending aorta below the constricted segment (Park, 2007).

■ Symptomatic newborns—reveals cardiomegaly and increased pulmonary venous congestion.

Echocardiogram

■ Asymptomatic newborns—may show left axis deviation of the QRS and left ventricular hypertrophy.

■ Symptomatic newborns—reveals normal or right axis deviation of the QRS, right ventricular hypertrophy, or right bundle branch block in newborns. In older children, a left ventricular hypertrophy is present.

A two-dimensional echocardiogram reveals the location and degree of constriction and other associated cardiac defects.

MANAGEMENT

The definitive treatment is surgical correction. Surgery may be delayed until the patient is 3 to 5 years of age if medically controlled; however, severe symptomatic newborns require immediate surgery. Medical management is used to provide adequate oxygenation, prevent or treat CHF, and prevent subacute infective endocarditis (SAIE). Prostaglandin (PGE1) may be used if the constricted segment is at the DA to maintain ductal patency (Park, 2007).

Surgical intervention involves excision of the constricted segment with end-to-end anastomosis, patch graft, bypass tube graft, or Dacron graft (Park, 2007). Another alternative may be a subclavian flap aortoplasty. If CHF is present, then surgery is indicated even without circulatory shock. The mortality rate for surgical correction is less than 5%. Almost 20% of postoperative complications include renal failure and recoarctation.

TABLE 2.5 Diagnosis of Congenital Heart Defects

Defect	Chest Radiograph	EKG	Echocardiogram	Catheterization	Lab Tests
PDA	Increased pulmonary vascularity; cardiac enlargement; left aortic arch	Left atrial and ventricular enlargement; abnormal QRS axis for age	LA:AO ratio > 1.3 (term); 1 (preterm); increased left atrium and ventricle (2D)	Increased O_2 saturation in pulmonary artery; increased right ventricular and pulmonary artery pressure (with pulmonary hypertension)	NA
ASD	Mild heart enlargement; prominent main pulmonary artery; increased pulmonary vascularity	Right axis deviation; incomplete right bundle branch block; right ventricular hypertrophy	Dilated right ventricle; paradoxical movement of ventricular septum	Increased O_2 in right atrium; normal right side atrium; normal right side pressure; 10%; PAPVR	NA

VSD	Enlarged heart; increased pulmonary markings	Left and right ventricular hypertrophy	Large left atrium (M-mode); presence or absence of other defects (2D)	Increased O_2 in right ventricle; increased systolic pressure in right ventricle and pulmonary artery	NA
TOF	Normal heart size; boot-shaped contour; decreased pulmonary markings; prominent aorta; right aortic arch in 13 cases	Right axis deviation; right ventricular hypertrophy	Large VDS, aortic dextroposition, and PS; size of main, right, and left pulmonary arteries (2D)	Demonstrates anatomy of right ventricular outflow region; microcytic anemia	Increased Hgb and HCT clotting time

(continued)

TABLE 2.5 Diagnosis of Congenital Heart Defects (*continued*)

Defect	Chest Radiograph	EKG	Echocardiogram	Catheterization	Lab Tests
PS	Normal heart size; normal pulmonary vascularity; enlarged pulmonary artery; right ventricle filling (lateral)	Right axis deviation; right atrial enlargement; right ventricular hypertrophy	Decreased valve leaflet motion; small changes in right ventricular wall thickness	Elevated right ventricular pressure; normal or slightly lowered pulmonary artery pressure	NA
TGA	Enlarged heart with narrow base; enlarged ventricles; increased pulmonary vascularity	Right axis deviation; right ventricular hypertrophy	Abnormal origin of great vessels	Increased right ventricular pressure; catheter can enter aorta from right ventricle; pulmonary artery can be entered only through PDA or ASD	Increased Hgb and HCT; polycythemia

| COA | Cardiomegaly; postcoarctation dilation (by age 5 years); notching of ribs from collateral vessels | Left ventricular hypertrophy; inverted T waves in left precordial leads; right ventricular hypertrophy (severe) | Visualization of narrowed aorta and location of associated defects; allows evaluation of aortic valve movement, structure, and function and left ventricular size and function | Performed to determine exact location and evaluation | NA |

ASD, atrial septal defect; COA, coarctation of the aorta; HCT, hematocrit test; PAPVR, partial anomalous pulmonary venous return; PDA, patent ductus arteriosus; PS, pulmonary stenosis; TOF, tetralogy of Fallot; TGA, transposition of the great arteries; VSD, ventricular septal defect.

Source: Adapted from Lott (2014).

REFERENCES

Lott, J. W. (2014). Cardiovascular system. In C. Kenner & J. W. Lott (Eds.), *Comprehensive neonatal nursing care* (5th ed., pp. 152–188). New York, NY: Springer Publishing Company.

Park, M. (2007). *Pediatric cardiology for practitioners*. Chicago, IL: Mosby.

Neurologic System

Georgia R. Ditzenberger, Susan T. Blackburn, Beth Brown, and Leslie B. Altimier

OVERVIEW

Neurologic development begins in the third week of gestation with the formation of the neural plate, neural folds, and neural tube. Once the tube is formed and becomes a closed system, different regions of the brain begin to develop. At 4 weeks gestation the brain differentiates into the forebrain, midbrain, and hindbrain. The forebrain translates input from the senses and is responsible for memory formation, thinking, reasoning, and problem solving. The midbrain functions as a relay station, coordinating messages to their final destination. Regulating the heart, breathing, and muscle movements is the function of the hindbrain. At 7 weeks gestation, the brain has the first detectable brain waves. By weeks 9 to 11, the basic brain structure is complete. As these different regions of the brain begin to form, the development of the central nervous system (CNS) is characterized by the following distinct overlapping processes: neurulation, prosencephalic development, neuronal proliferation, neuronal and glial cell migration, organization, and myelination. These processes, especially organization and myelinization, continue past birth.

Congenital anomalies that arise during the period of neurulation result in neural tube defects (NTDs), a common and devastating birth defect. Failure of the neural tube to close occurs at either the cranial or caudal end 80% of the time (Blackburn, 2013; Volpe, 2008). Failure to close the neural tube in the cranial region (exencephaly, also called anencephaly after degradation of the exposed neural tissue) leads to death before or at birth. Infants born with caudal NTDs (e.g., myelomeningocele or spina bifida) have increased risk of mortality, and those that survive often face lifelong disabilities and neurologic, cognitive, urologic, and gastrointestinal complications. NTDs occur in approximately one in 1,000 live births in the United States and resulted in 71,000 deaths globally in 2010 (CDC, 2011; Lozano et al., 2012).

The majority of NTDs in humans are thought to have a multifactorial and complex etiology in which disturbances in more than one gene affect closure. Moreover, environmental factors can also alter the risk of NTDs (Wilde, Petersen, & Niswander, 2014).

- Genetic syndromes (trisomy for chromosome 3, 18, and X) (Goetzinger et al., 2008)
- Maternal diabetes (Rasmussen, Chu, Kim, Schmid, & Lau, 2008; Stothard, Tennant, Bell, & Rankin, 2009)
- Maternal obesity
- Maternal hyperthermia (Wilde, Petersen, & Niswander, 2014)
- Maternal alcohol consumption (De Marco et al., 2011)
- Maternal smoking and maternal exposure to environmental tobacco smoke (ETS) (Wang, Amin, Jallo, & Ahn, 2014)

A few genetic syndromes are associated with NTDs in humans, including trisomy for chromosome 3, 18, and the X chromosome (Goetzinger et al., 2008). In the general population, the genetic risk for having a second child with an NTD is only 2% to 5% (Deak et al., 2008; Joó et al., 2007). Growing evidence suggests that environmental factors have the ability to alter the epigenetic landscape and, therefore, transcriptional activity.

Maternal diabetes and maternal obesity have been linked to an increased risk for NTDs (Rasmussen et al., 2008; Stothard et al., 2009). Another identified risk factor is maternal fever in early pregnancy (Wilde et al., 2014). A National Birth Defects Prevention Study from 1997 to 2005 showed the risk for anencephaly increased by 1.7-fold for women who reported using hot tubs during early pregnancy. However, only hot tub sessions lasting more than 30 minutes had a significant effect (Duong et al., 2011).

Maternal alcohol consumption has also been linked to NTDs (De Marco et al., 2011). Maternal smoking and maternal exposure to ETS have also been studied epidemiologically with respect to risk for an NTD-affected pregnancy, with conflicting conclusions. Maternal smoking confers a small increased risk for spina bifida, and a moderately increased NTD risk in cases of maternal ETS exposure (Wang et al., 2014).

NTDs are a complex disease impacted by genetic susceptibility, epigenetic influences, and environmental insults. Therefore, understanding neural tube development and the causes of NTDs are of critical importance. The CNS forms early in gestation but is not completely mature at birth even in a full-term infant.

REFERENCES

Blackburn, S. (2013). Maternal, fetal, & neonatal physiology (4th ed.). St. Louis, MO: Saunders.

Centers for Disease Control and Prevention. (2011). CDC Birth Defects Data/ Statistics Registry. Atlanta, GA.

De Marco, P., Merello, E., Calevo, M. G., Mascelli, S., Pastorino, D., Crocetti, L., ... Capra, V. (2011). Maternal periconceptional factors affect the risk of spina bifida-affected pregnancies: An Italian case-control study. *Child's Nervous System, 27*(7), 1073–1081.

Deak, K. L., Siegel, D. G., George, T. M., Gregory, S., Ashley-Koch, A., Speer, M. C., & NTD Collaborative Group. (2008). Further evidence for a maternal genetic effect and a sex-influenced effect contributing to risk for human neural tube defects. *Birth Defects Research Part A: Clinical and Molecular Teratology, 82*(10), 662–669.

Duong, H. T., Shahrukh Hashmi, S., Ramadhani, T., Canfield, M. A., Scheuerle, A., Kim Waller, D., & National Birth Defects Prevention Study. (2011). Maternal use of hot tub and major structural birth defects. *Birth Defects Research Part A: Clinical and Molecular Teratology, 91*(9), 836–841.

Goetzinger, K. R., Stamilio, D. M., Dicke, J. M., Macones, G. A., & Odibo, A. O. (2008). Evaluating the incidence and likelihood ratios for chromosomal abnormalities in fetuses with common central nervous system malformations. *American Journal of Obstetrics and Gynecology, 199*(3), 235.e1–235.e6.

Joó, J. G., Beke, A., Papp, C., Tóth-Pál, E., Csaba, A., Szigeti, Z., & Papp, Z. (2007). Neural tube defects in the sample of genetic counseling. *Prenatal Diagnosis, 27*(10), 912–921.

Lozano, R., Naghavi, M., Foreman, K., Lim, S., Shibuya, K., Aboyans, V., ... Memish Z. A. (2012). Global and regional mortality from 235 causes of death for 20 age groups in 1990 and 2010: A systematic analysis for the Global Burden of Disease Study 2010. *Lancet, 380*(9859), 2095–2128.

Rasmussen, S. A., Chu, S. Y., Kim, S. Y., Schmid, C. H., & Lau, J. (2008). Maternal obesity and risk of neural tube defects: A meta-analysis. *American Journal of Obstetrics and Gynecology, 198*(6), 611–619.

Stothard, K. J., Tennant, P. W. G., Bell, R., & Rankin, J. (2009). Maternal over-weight and obesity and the risk of congenital anomalies: A systematic review and meta-analysis. *Journal of the American Medical Association, 301*(6), 636–650.

Volpe, J. J. (2008). *Neurology of the newborn* (5th ed.). Philadephia, PA: Saunders/ Elsevier.

Wang, J., Amin, A., Jallo, G., & Ahn, E. (2014). Ventricular reservoir versus ventriculosubgaleal shunt for posthemorrhagic hydrocephalus in preterm infants: Infection risks and ventriculoperitoneal shunt rate. *Journal of Neurosurgery: Pediatrics* [serial online], *14*(5), 447–454 (8p.).

Wilde, J. J., Petersen, J. R., & Niswander, L. (2014). Genetic, epigenetic, and environmental contributions to neural tube closure. *Annual Review of Genetics, 48*, 583–611. doi:10.1146/anmirev-genet-120213-092208

CNS DEVELOPMENT

Development of the CNS is divided into six overlapping stages. Development progresses at different rates in various sections of the CNS. Many disorders of the neurologic system are related to defects in the development of the CNS. The stages of CNS development are as follows.

- Neurulation is the process by which the brain and spinal cord are formed via inductive events within the dorsal area of the embryo. The inductive events are separated into two stages:

    - Primary neurulation (formation of the brain and spinal cord excluding the caudal segments of the lumbar region) during the first 3 to 4 weeks of gestation

▨ Secondary neurulation (caudal neural tube formation) from 4 to 7 weeks. The brain and spinal cord develop from the neural plate and neural folds, which fuse to eventually form the forebrain, midbrain, hindbrain, and spinal cord. Closure of the neural tube takes place between 22 and 28 days gestation. Failure of part of the neural tube to close leads to NTDs (Ditzenberger & Blackburn, 2014; Moore, Persaud, & Torchia, 2013; Volpe, 2008).

■ Prosencephalic development, or ventral induction, involves early development of the brain and ventricular system during the second to third month of gestation. The brain develops from the cranial end of the neural tube beginning at the end of the fourth week. Since development of the face is associated with prosencephalic development, alterations in brain development often result in facial malformations (Back & Plawner, 2012; Ditzenberger & Blackburn, 2014; Kanekar, Kaneda, & Shively, 2011; Volpe, 2008; Volpe, Campobasso, De Robertis, & Rembouskos, 2009).

■ Neuronal proliferation involves development and proliferation of neurons and glial cells in the subependymal germinal matrix. The peak period of neuronal proliferation is from 2 to 4 months gestation. Proliferation of other glia and derivatives (including astrocytes and oligodendrocytes) occurs intensively at 5 to 8 months gestation. During the most intense period of proliferation, before 32 to 34 weeks gestation, the periventricular area receives a large proportion of the cerebral blood flow. This area is vulnerable to germinal matrix (periventricular)-intraventricular hemorrhage (GM-IVH or, commonly, IVH) in preterm infants (Blackburn, 2013; Ditzenberger & Blackburn, 2014; Volpe, 2008).

■ Neuronal migration is characterized by the movement of millions of cells from their origin in the germinal matrix of the periventricular region to their eventual loci in the cerebral cortex. Neuronal migration is critical to the formation of the cortex, gyri, and deep nuclear structures. Errors or exogenous insults before or after birth can alter migration. The preterm infant may be especially vulnerable to gyral alterations. Rapid development of the gyri begins at 26 to 28 weeks gestation and continues through the third trimester into the postbirth period. Gyra development markedly increases cerebral surface area (Back & Plawner, 2012; Ditzenberger & Blackburn, 2014; Guerrini & Parrini, 2010; Valiente & Marín, 2010; Volpe, 2008).

▪ Organization allows the nervous system to act as an integrated whole. Organizational processes include:

  ▨ Attainment of the proper alignment, orientation, and layering of cortical neurons

  ▨ Arborization or differentiation and branching of axons and dendrites

  ▨ Differentiation of the glial cells

  ▨ Development of synaptic connections ("wiring" of the brain)

  ▨ Balancing of excitatory and inhibitory synapses

  ▨ Cell death and selective elimination of excess neuronal processes

The peak period for organization is about the fifth month of gestation to a few years after birth. However, organizational processes continue throughout childhood. Some processes, such as synaptogenesis, continue throughout life. A marked increase in cerebral cortical volume and gyri occurs during this stage, especially from around 28 to 40 weeks gestation. Organization of the brain is susceptible to insults from errors of metabolism, abnormal chromosomes, and perinatal insults and is particularly vulnerable in the preterm infant being cared for in an intensive care unit during this period (Blackburn, 2013; Ditzenberger & Blackburn, 2014; Volpe, 2008; Volpe, Kinney, Jensen, & Rosenberg, 2011).

▪ Myelinization involves development of myelin sheaths around nerve fibers in the nervous system. Myelinization of fiber tracts tends to occur before maturation of functional ability. Myelinization begins during gestation and continues to adulthood, with the peak period thought to be occurring within the first 8 postnatal months of life. Myelinization is susceptible to damage from diverse exogenous influences, particularly malnutrition, which can lead to a range of neurologic deficits in which hypoplasia of the cerebral white matter occurs (Ditzenberger & Blackburn, 2014; Moore et al., 2013; Volpe, 2008).

REFERENCES

Back, S., & Plawner, L. L. (2012). Congenital malformations of the central nervous system. In H. W. Taeusch, R. A. Ballard, & C. A. Gleason (Eds.), *Avery's diseases of the newborn* (9th ed., pp. 844–867). Philadelphia, PA: Elsevier/Saunders.

Blackburn, S. T. (2013). *Maternal, fetal and neonatal physiology: A clinical perspective* (4th ed.). St. Louis, MO: Saunders/Elsevier Science.

Ditzenberger, G. R., & Blackburn, S. T. (2014). Neurologic system. In C. Kenner & J. W. Lott (Eds.), *Comprehensive neonatal nursing care* (5th ed., pp. 393–437). New York, NY: Springer Publishing Company.

Guerrini, R., & Parrini, E. (2010). Neuronal migration disorders. *Neurobiology of Disease, 38*(2), 154–166.

Kanekar, S., Kaneda, H., & Shively, A. (2011). Malformations of dorsal induction. *Seminars in Ultrasound, CT, and MRI, 32*(3), 189–199.

Moore, K. L., Persaud, T. V. N., & Torchia, M. G. (2013). *The developing human: Clinically oriented embryology* (9th ed.). Philadelphia, PA: Saunders/Elsevier.

Valiente, M., & Marín, O. (2010). Neuronal migration mechanisms in development and disease. *Current Opinion in Neurobiology, 20*(1), 68–78.

Volpe, J. J. (2008). *Neurology of the newborn* (5th ed.). Philadephia, PA: Saunders/Elsevier.

Volpe, J. J., Kinney, H. C., Jensen, F. E., & Rosenberg, P. A. (2011). The developing oligodendrocyte: Key cellular target in brain injury in the premature infant. *International Journal of Developmental Neuroscience, 29*(4), 423–440.

Volpe, P., Campobasso, G., De Robertis, V., & Rembouskos, G. (2009). Disorders of prosencephalic development. *Prenatal Diagnosis, 29*(4), 340–354.

NEUROLOGIC ASSESSMENT

Assessment of neurologic function is an initial step in evaluating an infant's response to the transition to extrauterine life and the impact of perinatal events and pathophysiologic problems on the central and peripheral nervous systems. Assessment of neurologic function and identification of dysfunction encompass several components: history, physical examination, neurologic examination, laboratory tests, and other diagnostic techniques.

History

■ Family history: NTDs, chromosomal or genetic abnormalities, or other malformations

■ Maternal history: substance abuse, chronic health problems, age, nutritional status, exposure to teratogens

■ Obstetrical history: prematurity, postmaturity, placental problems (e.g., abruptio placentae and placenta previa), use of analgesia or anesthesia, maternal problems (e.g., infection, hypertension, and substance abuse), large-for-gestational-age infant, prolonged labor, precipitate labor, forceps delivery, abnormal presentation, intrauterine growth restriction, polyhydramnios, fetal distress, hypoxia, ischemia, low Apgar scores

■ Postnatal history: status at birth, required resuscitation, hypoxic episodes, shock, hypoperfusion ± subsequent reperfusion, hemorrhage, infection, metabolic or electrolyte aberrations

Physical examination

■ Vital signs: temperature, heart rate, respiratory pattern, blood pressure, color

■ Signs of infection, birth trauma: ecchymosis, edema, lacerations, fractures

■ Signs of vascular alterations

■ Seizures; alterations in activity, tone, and state

■ Infant's cry: robustness, presence in response to aversive stimuli, and pitch

■ Head size, shape, growth

  ■ Occipital–frontal (head) circumference (OFC; HC): at birth, daily, or weekly per underlying condition

- Term infants: average 32.6 to 37.2 cm
- Infants 24 to 40 weeks gestation, average growth: 0.1 to 0.6 cm/week

▨ Sutures: proximity, widened, overlapping

- Normal: 4- to 5-mm separation of all sutures except squamosal (temporoparietal)
- Squamosal suture: no more than 2 to 3 mm
- Overriding bone-plates, molding; resolve after first few days postbirth
- Abnormal: persistent suture separation, increased separation
- Increased/increasing separation: increased intracranial pressure (ICP)
- Craniosynostosis: premature closure of one or more sutures

▨ Fontanelles

- Anterior: diamond shaped, 3 to 4 cm long by 1 to 3 cm wide in term infants
  - Closes at 8 to 16 months of age
  - May bulge slightly when the infant cries
  - May be slightly depressed in upright position
- Posterior: if open, triangular shaped, 1 to 3 cm wide
  - Closes 8 months gestation to 2 months after birth
- "Third fontanelle": parietal bone defect; rare
  - Can be palpated in normal infants
  - Often present with Down syndrome or hypothyroidism
- Sunken, depressed: dehydration
- Bulging: increased ICP

▨ Presence/absence of major and/or minor anomalies

- Low-set or abnormally shaped ears, micrognathia, hypertelorism
- Hydrocephalus

- ■ Vertebral column: NTDs; hair tufts, dimples, fistulae
- ■ Cranial bones: fractures, extradural hemorrhage, edema, and areas of uneven ossification

Neurologic examination

- ■ Goal: evaluate for presence, determining the extent of neurologic dysfunction; monitor recovery; prognostic indicator
- ■ Consider when interpreting findings: gestational age, health status, infant state, medications, and feeding timing
- ■ Optimum infant state during exam: quiet and alert
- ■ Level of consciousness: hyper-alert, lethargy, and stupor or coma
  - ■ Hyper-alert: increased sensitivity to sensory stimulation, wide-open eyes, diminished blink response, diminished ability to fixate and follow
  - ■ Lethargy: delayed response to tactile or noxious stimuli
  - ■ Stupor (obtunded): limited response to tactile or noxious stimuli
  - ■ Coma: no response to tactile or noxious stimuli
- ■ Posture, tone, and activity
  - ■ Normal posture, tone, and activity requires integrated functioning of the entire nervous system
  - ■ Disturbances in either the central or peripheral nervous system manifest in alterations in neonatal position, tone, and activity
  - ■ Assess resting position
  - ■ Quality symmetry of activity with spontaneous and elicited movement
  - ■ Alterations in symmetry of trunk, face, and extremities at rest or with spontaneous movement: congenital anomalies, birth injury, or neurologic insult
  - ■ Abnormal findings: tight fisting, persistent cortical thumb; opisthotonos; decerebrate or decorticate posturing
  - ■ Abnormal movements: jitteriness, tremors

- May be normal if infrequent in newborns
- Must be differentiated from seizures
- Tremors: vary with the underlying disorder
  - Metabolic abnormalities, asphyxia, or drug withdrawal: low-amplitude, high-frequency movements
  - CNS complications: high-amplitude, low-frequency movements
- Jitteriness: common finding due to lack of myelinization of pyramidal tracts
  - Stimulus sensitive; not marked by gaze or eye deviations
  - Predominant movement in jitteriness is tremulousness
  - Stops with passive flexion
  - Can be initiated with spontaneous or elicited movement
▨ Tone: resting, passive, active; hypotonia, hypertonia
  - Resting: observe supine infant at rest
  - Passive: evaluate extensibility through righting reactions of legs and trunk and examination of neck flexors and extensors
  - Active: alter infant's posture to obtain directed motor responses
  - Hypotonia with muscle weakness: peripheral nerve injuries, neuromuscular disorders, alterations at the neuromuscular junction, and spinal cord injuries
  - Hypotonia without muscle weakness: CNS disturbances secondary to asphyxia, intracranial hemorrhage, chromosomal disorders or other genetic defects, or metabolic disturbances
  - Marked extensor hypertonia, opisthotonus: severe hypoxic–ischemic injury, bacterial meningitis, or massive IVH
■ Reflexes
  ▨ Primary reflexes: affected by gestational age, present to some degree by 28 to 32 weeks gestation

- Sucking, grasping, crossed extension, automatic walking (stepping), Moro reflex
  - Present, symmetric, and reproducible
  - Gradually disappear during infancy
- Tendon reflexes: biceps, knee, and ankle jerk
  - Present after about 33 weeks gestation
  - Not very helpful beyond confirming symmetry

■ Selected cranial nerves

   ▪ Fixation and following, pupillary responses, doll's eye response, hearing, vestibular response, suck/swallow

Laboratory tests, other diagnostic techniques

■ Laboratory tests:

   ▪ Cerebrospinal fluid (CSF): hemorrhage (increased red blood cells, increased protein, decreased glucose, xanthochromia); rule out infection (culture, turbidity of the fluid, increased or decreased white cells, protein, and/or glucose)

   ▪ Blood: complete blood count with differential, serum glucose, calcium levels, electrolyte levels, blood gases, acid–base status

   ▪ Sepsis workup; screening for toxoplasmosis, rubella, cytomegalovirus, herpes simplex, and syphilis (suspect infection)

   ▪ Genetic workup and other metabolic studies (suspect inborn errors of metabolism, inherited conditions)

■ Other diagnostic techniques:

   ▪ Electroencephalogram (EEG); ≥ 24 hour with video

   ▪ Bedside amplitude-integrated EEG (aEEG)

   ▪ Head ultrasonography (HUS), computed tomography (CT), and magnetic resonance imaging (MRI)

   ▪ Doppler sonography (part of complete HUS)

   ▪ Brainstem auditory evoked responses, visual evoked responses, somatosensory evoked responses

GENERALIZED NURSING CARE

■ Monitor: infant's state, activity level, responsiveness, eye movements, head circumference, and vital signs; seizure activity; signs of increased ICP

■ Monitor fluid and electrolyte status

■ Maintain adequate ventilation and perfusion

■ Position in alignment and change position regularly

■ Promote skin integrity

■ Maintain head in midline, slightly elevated to reduce ICP

■ Massage skin gently to stimulate circulation

■ Maintain an appropriate thermal environment

■ Reduce environmental stressors: minimal handling, decreased noise, light

■ Use sterile technique for dressing changes, wound care

■ Monitor for signs of localized infection or neonatal sepsis

■ Provide parent/family support including condition-specific information and teaching; discharge preparation

(Amiel-Tison & Gosselin, 2009; Ditzenberger, 2010; Ditzenberger & Blackburn, 2014; DuPlessis, 2008; Fenichel, 2007; Heaberlin, 2009; Lehmann, 2009; Simbruner, Mittal, Rohlmann, Muche, & neo. nEURO.network Trial Participants, 2010; Smith, 2012; Trollmann, Nüsken, & Wenzel, 2010; Volpe, 2008)

NEURAL TUBE DEFECTS

INCIDENCE

■ Occur in 0.5 to 5 per 1,000 live births (Back & Plawner, 2012; Kanekar, Shively, & Kaneda, 2011b).

■ Varies with ethnicity, diet, geographical area, socioeconomic status

◼ Folic acid supplementation at conception reduces the rate of NTDs (American Academy of Pediatrics Committee on Genetics, 1999; reaffirmed 2012)

PHYSIOLOGY/PATHOPHYSIOLOGY

NTDs include anencephaly, encephalocele, spina bifida occulta, and spina bifida cystica (meningocele, myelomeningocele, and myeloschisis). NTDs are usually accompanied by alterations in vertebral, meningeal, vascular, and dermal structures. NTDs arise from genetic, nutritional, and/or environmental influences. NTDs can be diagnosed prior to birth using maternal serum alphafetoprotein (AFP, a fetal glycoprotein) screening at 15 to 20 weeks, ultrasound examination, and/or measurement of the AFP level of the amniotic fluid (Blackburn, 2013; Ditzenberger & Blackburn, 2014; Stoll, Dott, Alembik, & Roth, 2011; Volpe, 2008).

REFERENCES

American Academy of Pediatrics Committee on Genetics. (1999, reaffirmed 2012). Folic acid for the prevention of neural tube defects. *Pediatrics, 100*(2), 143–152.

Amiel-Tison, C., & Gosselin, J. (2009). Clinical assessment of the infant nervous system. In M. I. Levene & F. A. Chervenak (Eds.), *Fetal and neonatal neurology and neurosurgery* (4th ed., pp. 128–154). Edinburgh, Scotland: Churchill Livingstone/Elsevier.

Back, S., & Plawner, L. L. (2012). Congenital malformations of the central nervous system. In H. W. Taeusch, R. A. Ballard, & C. A. Gleason (Eds.), *Avery's diseases of the newborn* (9th ed., pp. 844–867). Philadelphia, PA: Elsevier/Saunders.

Blackburn, S. T. (2013). *Maternal, fetal and neonatal physiology: A clinical perspective* (4th ed.). St. Louis, MO: Saunders/Elsevier Science.

Ditzenberger, G. R. (2010). Nutritional management. In M. T. Verklan & M. Walden (Eds.), *Core curriculum for neonatal intensive care nursing* (4th ed., pp. 182–207). St. Louis, MO: Saunders/Elsevier.

Ditzenberger, G. R., & Blackburn, S. T. (2014). Neurologic system. In C. Kenner & J. W. Lott (Eds.), *Comprehensive neonatal nursing care* (5th ed., pp. 393–437). New York, NY: Springer Publishing Company.

DuPlessis, A. J. (2008). Neonatal seizures. In J. P. Cloherty, E. C. Eichenwald, & A. R. Stark (Eds.), *Manual of neonatal care* (6th ed., pp. 483–498). Philadelphia, PA: Wolters Kluwer/Lippincott Williams & Wilkins.

Fenichel, G. M. (2007). *Neonatal neurology* (4th ed.). Philadelphia, PA: Churchill/Livingstone/Elsevier.

Heaberlin, P. D. (2009). Neurologic assessment. In E. P. Tappero & M. E. Honeyfield (Eds.), *Physical assessment of the newborn: A comprehensive approach to the art of physical examination* (4th ed., pp. 159–184). Santa Rosa, CA: NICU Ink.

Kanekar, S., Shively, A., & Kaneda, H. (2011). Malformations of ventral induction. *Seminars in Ultrasound, CT, and MRI, 32*(3), 200–210.

Lehmann, C. U. (2009). Studies for neurologic evaluation. In T. L. Gomella (Ed.), *Neonatology: Management, procedures, on-call problems, diseases, and drugs* (6th ed., pp. 155–162). New York, NY: McGraw-Hill Companies/Lange.

Simbruner, G., Mittal, R. A., Rohlmann, F., Muche, R., & neo.nEURO.network Trial Participants. (2010). Systemic hypothermia after neonatal encephalopathy: Outcomes of neo.nEURO.network RCT. *Pediatrics, 126*(4), e771–e778.

Smith, J. B. (2012). Initial evaluation: History and physical examination of the newborn. In C. A. Gleason & S. Devaskar (Eds.), *Avery's diseases of the newborn* (9th ed., pp. 277–299). Philadelphia, PA: Saunders/Elsevier.

Stoll, C., Dott, B., Alembik, Y., & Roth, M.-P. (2011). Associated malformations among infants with neural tube defects. *American Journal of Medical Genetics Part A, 155A*(3), 565–568.

Trollmann, R., Nüsken, E., & Wenzel, D. (2010). Neonatal somatosensory evoked potentials: Maturational aspects and prognostic value. *Pediatric Neurology, 42*(6), 427–433.

Volpe, J. J. (2008). *Neurology of the newborn* (5th ed.). Philadephia, PA: Saunders/Elsevier.

DISORDERS OF PRIMARY NEURULATION

ANENCEPHALY

RISK FACTORS

■ Genetic predisposition accounts for most of the risk of NTDs, and genes that regulate folate one-carbon metabolism and planar cell polarity have been strongly implicated (Copp, Stanier, & Greene, 2013).

■ Environmental factors also appear to be involved in the development of anencephaly; many of these infants have other anomalies (Gole et al., 2014; Volpe, 2008)

■ Increase risk with low socioeconomic status and history of affected siblings

■ More common in Whites

■ More common in females

INCIDENCE

■ Occurs in 0.2 out of 1,000 live births in the United States (Volpe, 2008)

■ Occurs one out of 1,000 live births worldwide (Cook, Erdman, Hevia, & Dickens, 2008)

■ 75% are stillborn

PATHOPHYSIOLOGY

■ Anencephaly occurs when the neural tube fails to close anteriorly. Malfunction is of primary neurulation. It most commonly involves the forebrain and variable amounts of the upper brainstem. Because the anterior neural tube forms the forebrain, failure of fusion causes minimal development of brain tissue (cerebrum, cerebellum, brainstem, and spinal cord). The brain tissue that does develop is poorly differentiated and becomes necrotic with exposure to amniotic fluid. In this defect, much of the posterior skull is missing.

■ Anencephaly begins within the first 24 to 26 days of gestation. Since the advent of folic acid therapy, the incidence has declined (Williams et al., 2015).

CLINICAL MANIFESTATIONS

■ Exposed neural tissue

DIAGNOSTIC EVALUATION

■ Amniotic fluid reveals high levels of AFP in the first trimester.

■ The primary screening test for the detection of fetal structural abnormalities including open/closed NTDs (anencephaly, encephalocele, spina bifida) is a second trimester anatomical ultrasound with detailed fetal intracranial and spinal imaging and assessment. Prenatal detection of anencephaly by ultrasound is possible in almost 100% of cases (Cameron & Moran, 2009; Johnson et al., 1997).

■ It is apparent upon visual inspection after birth.

TREATMENT/MANAGEMENT

■ Prevention: Folic acid was proven in 1991 to prevent most cases of spina bifida and anencephaly; in 1998, the United States mandated fortification of enriched cereal grain products (Williams et al., 2015). In 2008, less than 10% of folic acid-preventable spina bifida and anencephaly (FAPSBA) was prevented through folic acid fortification programs. The proportion of FAPSBA prevented globally with various types of folic acid fortification as of 2012 is estimated to be 25% (Youngblood et al., 2013).

■ Because anencephaly is a lethal condition, pregnancy with anencephaly may be interrupted at any gestational age on the woman's request.

■ Management of infants with anencephaly is supportive, involving provision of warmth and comfort until the infant dies.

■ Families require emotional support and assistance in coping with their grief over the birth of an infant with a defect and the death of their infant.

PROGNOSIS

■ 75% of anencephalic infants are stillborn.

■ Live-borns die in the first days or month of life, generally by the end of the first week (Volpe, 2008).

ENCEPHALOCELE

RISK FACTORS

■ Environmental and genetic factors

INCIDENCE

■ 0.8 to 5.6 per 10,000 live births
■ Occurs in association with chromosomal abnormalities, such as trisomy 13, 18, and 21, Meckel–Gruber syndrome, or Walker–Warburg syndrome
■ 70% occurs in males

ANATOMY AND PHYSIOLOGY

■ Encephalocele is a congenital anomaly in which intracranial structures (brain tissue, meninges, and CSF) protrude out of the cranium.

PATHOPHYSIOLOGY

■ Encephaloceles form within the first 24 to 26 days of gestation.
■ Encephaloceles arise from the failure of closure of the anterior portion of the neural tube in restricted areas, but are also possibly postclosure defects.
■ 70% to 80% occur in the occipital region.
■ Less commonly, it occurs in the frontal, temporal, or parietal regions.
■ Hydrocephalus is a common complication, occurring at birth or developing after the repair of the encephalocele.

ASSESSMENT/CLINICAL MANIFESTATIONS

■ Protruding midline skin-covered sac is observed from the head or base of the neck.

■ The protruding sac may vary greatly in size; the size of the defect does not always correlate with the presence of neural tissue, and is connected to the CNS by a narrow stalk.

■ Majority of sacs occur in the occipital region.

■ Encephalocele mostly results with spontaneous abortion.

DIAGNOSIS

■ Second trimester intrauterine ultrasonography

■ Cranial ultrasonography

■ CT scan

■ MRI

TREATMENT/MANAGEMENT

■ Maintain normal body temperature

■ If the defect is covered by skin, surgery is delayed pending a full evaluation

■ If the sac is leaking CSF at birth, immediate surgical repair is necessary

■ Insert a ventriculoperitoneal shunt if a hydrocephalus is present

■ Treat seizure activity

■ Prevent infection

■ Position infant to avoid pressure on the defect

■ Support the neonate and family along with the surgical care that may be required

PROGNOSIS

- Mortality rate and later outcome are significantly better for infants with anterior defects than for those with posterior defects.
- Prognosis is poor if significant brain tissue is contained within the sac (Back & Plawner, 2012).

SPINA BIFIDA

RISK FACTORS

- Family history exists of a previous pregnancy resulting in an NTD.
- Women with insulin-dependent diabetes are at increased risk of giving birth to an infant with an NTD.
- Maternal obesity may be a risk factor as a result of hyperinsulinemia.
- Maternal folic acid deficiency before conception and in early pregnancy may significantly increase the risk of NTD.
- Maternal malabsorption may result in nutritional deficiencies that will increase the risk of NTDs.

INCIDENCE

- Spina bifida occulta is estimated to occur in 3% to 20% of the normal population (Moore et al., 2016).
- Spina bifida cystica occurs in approximately one in 1,000 live births (Moore et al., 2016).

ANATOMY AND PHYSIOLOGY

Spina bifida is a defect in caudal neurulation associated with malformations of the spinal cord and vertebrae. The two major forms are spina bifida cystica (failure of closure of the caudal portion of the neural tube during primary neurulation) and spina bifida occulta (alterations in secondary neurulation).

■ Spina bifida occulta is a vertebral defect at L5 or S1 that arises from failure of the vertebral arch to grow and fuse between 5 weeks gestation and the early fetal period. The dermal layer is intact over the vertebral defect; occasionally, the defect is indicated by a dimple, lipoma, or tuft of hair. Many are unrecognized due to minimal/no physical problems arising from the presence of this defect.

■ Spina bifida cystica is an NTD characterized by a cystic sac containing meninges or spinal cord elements, or both, along with vertebral defects. The level of the impairment of the spinal cord determines the severity of the neurologic deficit with impairment of nerve tissues below the sac. If the sac is covered with meninges, there is a risk of rupture and leakage of CSF during delivery with the risk of infection and dehydration.

  ▨ Occurs anywhere along the spinal column; seen most often in lumbar or lumbosacral area

  ▨ Three main forms: meningocele, myelomeningocele (most common), and myeloschisis

    • Meningocele: sac containing meninges and CSF; spinal cord and nerve roots in normal position

      ◦ Not typically associated with neurologic deficits

    • Meningomyelocele: In this type, CNS cord tissue extends into the meningocele sac. This is the most significant and common type, accounting for 94% of cases.

    • Myeloschisis: severe defect; no cystic covering; spinal cord open and exposed

      ◦ Poor prognosis; significant neurologic deficits; many die of sepsis in neonatal period

(Blackburn, 2013; Ditzenberger & Blackburn, 2014; Moore et al., 2013; Sandler, 2010; Volpe, 2008)

ASSESSMENT/CLINICAL MANIFESTATIONS/DIAGNOSIS

■ Prenatal ultrasound

■ Maternal serum alpha fetoprotein

■ Amniocentesis

■ Prenatal magnetic resonance imaging

■ Lesions that are usually apparent at birth

■ Often altered lower extremity tone and activity; may assume a froglike posture

■ If bowel and bladder involved, dribbling of urine and feces

■ Frequently associated with Chiari malformation type II (alterations of lower portion of brain) with noncommunicating hydrocephalus

■ Monitor for associated anomalies including renal dysfunction, as well as cardiac, intestinal, orthopedic, and other neurologic anomalies

■ Ultrasonography, CT, or MRI can be used to determine the size of the ventricular system, to rule out Chiari type II malformation, and to monitor ventricular status and the development of hydrocephalus

(Blackburn, 2013; Ditzenberger & Blackburn, 2014; Gressens & Huppi, 2014; Moore et al., 2013; Sandler, 2010; Volpe, 2008)

TREATMENT

■ Immediate management for spina bifida includes:

  ▪ Stabilize in delivery room: prevent trauma to or infection of sac and contents

  ▪ Provide warmth and hydration and monitor fluid and electrolyte status

■ Immediate closure of meningomyelocele for most infants; reduces infection risk, improves prognosis by reducing further deterioration of the spinal cord and nerve tracts; facilitates caregiving (Piatt, 2010; Volpe, 2008)

■ Multidisciplinary follow-up: neurologic, urologic, orthopedic, psychologic

■ In utero repair of myelomeningocele, performed before 26 weeks gestation, has been reported with mixed results to reduce the need for postnatal shunting, improve motor outcomes, and reduce postnatal complications such as hindbrain herniation, hydrocephalus, and urologic dysfunction (Adzick et al., 2011; Danzer, Johnson, & Adzick, 2012; Ditzenberger & Blackburn, 2014; Hockley & Salanki, 2009)

SPECIFIC NURSING CARE (IN ADDITION TO GENERALIZED NURSING CARE)

■ Monitor: signs of infection, including signs of sepsis or meningitis and localized infection, including redness or discharge from the sac

■ Provide comfort measures including gentle handling, pacifiers, sucrose, and medications as ordered

■ Position prone or on the side to reduce tension on the sac

■ Change position from prone to side-lying or side-to-side

■ Provide range-of-motion exercises; prevents skin breakdown, contractures

■ Keep lumbar/sacral defects free of fecal or urine contamination

  ■ Observe the timing and characteristics of urination and stool excretion: help determine degree of deficit

■ Provide meticulous skin care

■ Provide family teaching regarding skin care, positioning, exercises, handling, and feeding techniques, as well as provision of activities to promote development (Ditzenberger & Blackburn, 2014)

PROGNOSIS

■ Varies with the level and severity of the defect

■ Prognosis of infants with meningomyelocele has improved with the current early and aggressive treatment of infants without major cerebral lesions, hemorrhage, infection, high spinal cord lesions, or advanced hydrocephalus (Ditzenberger & Blackburn, 2014; Thompson, 2009; Volpe, 2008).

REFERENCES

Adzick, N. S., Thom, E. A., Spong, C. Y., Brock, J. W., Burrows, P. K., Johnson, M. P., … Farmer, D. L. (2011). A randomized trial of prenatal versus postnatal repair of myelomeningocele. *New England Journal of Medicine, 364*(11), 993–1004.

Back, S., & Plawner, L. L. (2012). Congenital malformations of the central nervous system. In H. W. Taeusch, R. A. Ballard, & C. A. Gleason (Eds.), *Avery's diseases of the newborn* (9th ed., pp. 844–867). Philadelphia, PA: Elsevier/Saunders.

Blackburn, S. T. (2013). *Maternal, fetal and neonatal physiology: A clinical perspective* (4th ed.). St. Louis, MO: Saunders/Elsevier Science.

Cameron, M., & Moran, P. (2009). Prenatal screening and diagnosis of neural tube defects. *Prenatal Diagnosis, 29*(4), 402–411.

Cook, R. J., Erdman, J. N., Hevia, M., & Dickens, B. M. (2008). Prenatal management of anencephaly. *International Journal of Gynaecology & Obstetrics, 102*(3), 304–308.

Copp, A. J., Stanier, P., & Greene, N. E. (2013). Neural tube defects: Recent advances, unsolved questions, and controversies. *The Lancet Neurology, 12*(8), 799–810. doi:10.1016/S1474-4422(13)70110-8

Danzer, E., Johnson, M. P., & Adzick, N. S. (2012). Fetal surgery for myelomeningocele: Progress and perspectives. *Developmental Medicine & Child Neurology, 54*(1), 8–14.

Ditzenberger, G. R., & Blackburn, S. T. (2014). Neurologic system. In C. Kenner & J. W. Lott (Eds.), *Comprehensive neonatal nursing care* (5th ed., pp. 393–437). New York, NY: Springer Publishing Company.

Gole, R. A., Meshram, P. M., & Hattangdi, S. S. (2014). Anencephaly and its associated malformations. *Journal of Clinical and Diagnostic Research, 8*(9), AC07–AC9. doi:10.7860/JCDR/2014/10402.4885

Gressens, P., & Huppi, P. S. (2014). The central nervous system, part 1: Normal and abnormal brain development. In R. J. Martin, A. A. Fanaroff, & M. C. Walsh (Eds.), *Neonatal and perinatal medicine: Diseases of the fetus and infant* (10th ed). Philadelphia, PA: Mosby/Elsevier.

Hockley, A. D., & Salanki, G. A. (2009). Surgical management of neural tube defects. In M. I. Levene & F. A. Chervenak (Eds.), *Fetal and neonatal neurology and neurosurgery* (4th ed., pp. 847–855). Edinburgh, Scotland: Churchill Livingstone/Elsevier.

Johnson, D. D., Pretorius, D. H., Riccabona, M., Budorick, N. E., & Nelson, T. R. (1997). Three-demensional ultrasound of the fetal spine. *Obstetrics & Gynecology, 89*, 434–438.

Moore, K. L, Persaud, T. V. N., & Torchia, M. G. (2016). *The developing human: Clinically oriented embryology* (10th ed.). Philadelphia, PA: Saunders/Elsevier.

Piatt, J. H. (2010). Treatment of myelomeningocele: A review of outcomes and continuing neurosurgical considerations among adults. *Journal of Neurosurgery: Pediatrics, 6*(6), 515–525.

Sandler, A. D. (2010). Children with spina bifida: Key clinical issues. *Pediatric Clinics of North America, 57*(4), 879–892.

Sullivan, R., Perry, R., Sloan, A., Kleinhaus, K., & Burtchen, N. (2011). Infant bonding and attachment to the caregiver: Insights from basic and clinical science. *Clinics in Perinatology, 38*, 643–656.

Thompson, D. N. P. (2009). Postnatal management and outcome for neural tube defects including spina bifida and encephalocoeles. *Prenatal Diagnosis, 29*(4), 412–419.

Volpe, J. J. (2008). *Neurology of the newborn* (5th ed.). Philadephia, PA: Saunders/Elsevier.

Williams, J., Mai, C. T., Mulinare, J., Isenburg, J., Flood, T. J., Ethen, M., ... Kirby, R. S. (2015). Updated estimates of neural tube defects prevented by mandatory folic acid fortification—United States, 1995–2011. *Morbidity and Mortality Weekly Report, 64*(1), 1–5.

Youngblood, M. E., Williamson, R., Bell, K. N., Johnson, Q., Kancherla, V., & Oakley, G. J. (2013). 2012 Update on global prevention of folic acid-preventable spina bifida and anencephaly. *Birth Defects Research. Part A, Clinical and Molecular Teratology, 97*(10), 658–663. doi:10.1002/bdra.23166

DISORDERS OF PROENCEPHALIC DEVELOPMENT

Holoprosencephaly, holotelencephaly, congenital hydrocephaly, microcephaly, and facial anomalies may all be seen with disorders of proencephalic development (Back & Plawner, 2012; Ditzenberger & Blackburn, 2014; Volpe, 2008; Volpe et al., 2009).

HOLOPROSENCEPHALY

RISK FACTORS

■ Maternal diabetes mellitus

■ Trisomy 13 and 18

INCIDENCE

■ Holoprosencephaly is the most common human brain malformation

■ Prevalence of one in 250 in the developing embryo

■ Occurs one in 10,000 to 20,000 live births

ANATOMY AND PHYSIOLOGY

■ Abnormality in cleavage of the hemispheres that arises from genetic or possibly environmental alterations.

■ Defect involves a variable degree of incomplete cleavage of the proencephalon along one or more of its three major planes (horizontal, transverse, and/or sagittal).

■ The spectrum includes alobar, semilobar, and lobar types, all of which have the unifying diagnostic feature of a single ventricular cerebral mass enclosed by a membrane; aplasia of the optic tract with absence of the olfactory tracts and bulbs; and agenesis of the corpus callosum.

PATHOPHYSIOLOGY

■ Cyclopia (a single central eye) with a nose-like structure (proboscis) above the eye

■ Cebocephaly (a flattened single nostril situated centrally between the eyes)

■ Median cleft lip

■ Mildly affected infants may display a single central incisor or hypotelorism

CLINICAL MANIFESTATIONS

■ Neurologic impairment (degree relates to severity of the cerebral malformation)

■ Apneic episodes in association with intractable seizures

■ Temperature instability and hypothermia

■ Hypernatremia or hyponatremia (diabetes insipidus, inappropriate secretion of antidiuretic hormone, or both)

■ Failure to thrive (impaired suck and swallow)

■ Abnormalities of other systems (cardiac, genitourinary, gastrointestinal)

■ Microcephaly is the norm

■ Persistent primitive reflexes

■ Lack of social smile

DIAGNOSIS

■ CT scan

■ MRI

TREATMENT

■ Supportive and comfort measures

PROGNOSIS

■ Survival correlates with the severity of the brain malformations.

■ Severely affected infants often are stillborn or rarely survive beyond the first year of life.

HOLOTELENCEPHALY

Parts of the brain that develop from the telencephalon form a single spheroid structure; the diencephalon and its derivatives are less affected.

CONGENITAL HYDROCEPHALUS

At about 6 weeks gestation, three critical events occur that are related to the formation and circulation of the CSF: (a) development of secretory epithelium in the choroid plexus, (b) perforation of the roof of the fourth ventricle, and (c) formation of the subarachnoid space. Alterations in the second and third events give rise to a communicating form of hydrocephalus (Ditzenberger & Blackburn, 2014; Volpe, 2008).

RISK FACTORS

■ Congenital hydrocephalus—increased risk in:
  ■ First borns
  ■ Mothers utilizing antidepressants during the first trimester
  ■ Male gender, multiples, and maternal diabetes

INCIDENCE

■ Incidence depends on etiology of the hydrocephalus.

ANATOMY AND PHYSIOLOGY

■ Hydrocephalus, which is usually associated with NTDs, develops as a result of outflow tract obstruction of the CSF from the ventricular system because of downward displacement of the brain.
■ Excess CSF in the ventricles of the brain occurs due to a decrease in reabsorption or overproduction.

PATHOPHYSIOLOGY

■ Excessive CSF production
■ Inadequate CSF absorption secondary to abnormal circulation
■ Excess ventricular CSF secondary

CLINICAL MANIFESTATIONS

■ Large head
■ Widened sutures

- Full (bulging) and tense fontanelles
- Increased or increasing frontal-occipital circumference (FOC)
- Setting-sun eyes
- Vomiting, lethargy, irritability
- Visible scalp veins

DIAGNOSIS

- Increase in FOC measurements
- CT scan
- Cranial ultrasonography
- MRI

TREATMENT

- Maintain lumbar or ventricular pressure at approximately 5 cm H_2O while evaluating for shunt placement
- Ventriculoperitoneal (VP) shunt

PROGNOSIS

- Poor outcomes are likely when cerebral decompression does not occur after VP shunt placement.
- Motor and cognitive deficits are likely.

REFERENCES

Back, S., & Plawner, L. L. (2012). Congenital malformations of the central nervous system. In H. W. Taeusch, R. A. Ballard, & C. A. Gleason (Eds.), *Avery's diseases of the newborn* (9th ed., pp. 844–867). Philadelphia, PA: Elsevier/Saunders.

Ditzenberger, G. R., & Blackburn, S. T. (2014). Neurologic system. In C. Kenner & J. W. Lott (Eds.), *Comprehensive neonatal nursing care* (5th ed., pp. 393–437). New York, NY: Springer Publishing Company.

Volpe, J. J. (2008). *Neurology of the newborn* (5th ed.). Philadephia, PA: Saunders/Elsevier.

Volpe, P., Campobasso, G., De Robertis, V., & Rembouskos, G. (2009). Disorders of prosencephalic development. *Prenatal Diagnosis, 29*(4), 340–354.

DISORDERS OF NEURONAL PROLIFERATION

Alterations in neuronal proliferation can lead to increases or decreases in the number and size of cells in the brain and associated structures. The actual number of neurons is determined early in gestation, because mature neurons cannot divide. Insults may alter the neuronal-glial stem cells, which reduces the number of neuronal or glial cells, or may alter cell growth, which results in smaller cells (Ditzenberger & Blackburn, 2014). The resulting disorders include micrencephaly, macrencephaly, and neurofibromatosis (Abuelo, 2007; Olney, 2007; Volpe, 2008).

MICRENCEPHALY

RISK FACTORS

- Maternal:
  - Viral infections (TORCH spectrum)
  - Exposure to radiation
  - Metabolic conditions
    - Diabetes mellitus
    - Hyperphenylalaninemia in nonphenylketonuric infants
  - Use of prescription and/or street drugs (alcohol, cocaine, etc.), especially in first trimester
  - Genetic (autosomal recessive, autosomal dominant, X-linked, or translocation)
  - Malnutrition is the most common etiology worldwide

- Fetal:
  - Prenatal/perinatal insult: inflammation; hypoxia; birth trauma
- Neonatal:
  - Very-low-birth-weight infant
  - Hypoxic–ischemic encephalopathy (HIE)
  - Nutrition: most common worldwide cause

ANATOMY AND PHYSIOLOGY

Micrencephaly is a disorder in which the primary defect is a marked reduction in the size of the brain or of the cerebral hemispheres. Microcephaly denotes a small cranial vault (defined as a frontal–occipital circumference ≥ 2 standard deviations below the normative curves for age) that is associated with either micrencephaly or acquired brain atrophy. Micrencephaly arises from a decrease in size or number of neuronal-glial stem cell units (Abuelo, 2007; Back & Plawner, 2012; Blackburn, 2013; Ditzenberger & Blackburn, 2014; Volpe, 2008). Small brain implies neurologic impairment (Verklan & Walden, 2010).

PATHOPHYSIOLOGY

- Neuronal proliferation defect
- Occurs between 3 and 4 months gestation
- Destructive micrencephaly occurs when the normal brain suffers prenatal/perinatal insult

CLINICAL MANIFESTATIONS

- Small head, backward sloping of the forehead, small cranial volume

■ Do not have marked neurologic deficits or seizures during neonatal period

■ Mental delays manifest later in infants

DIAGNOSIS

■ Complete physical assessment with thorough neurologic assessment

■ Maternal history

■ CT scan or MRI

TREATMENT/PATIENT CARE MANAGEMENT

■ Record accurate measurement of FOC, length, and weight weekly (note percentiles)

■ Genetic counseling

■ Infectious disease consult

■ Supportive and comfort measures

PROGNOSIS

■ Dependent on severity

■ Frequently associated with developmental delays

MACRENCEPHALY

Excessive proliferation (macrencephaly) may have a familial base, occur with growth disturbances and chromosomal disorders, or have unknown causes. Macrencephaly results in a large brain size because of excessive proliferation of neuronal elements, nonneuronal elements, or a combination of both (Ditzenberger & Blackburn, 2014).

RISK FACTORS

- Maternal:
  - Genetic disorders
    - Beckwith–Wiedemann syndrome
    - Sturge–Weber syndrome
    - Weaver syndrome
    - Achondroplasia
  - Chromosomal disorders
    - Klinefelter and fragile X syndromes
    - Partial trisomy of chromosome 7
  - Multiple hemangiomas
  - Neurocutaneous disorders
    - Neurofibromatosis (autosomal dominant genetic disorder involving excessive proliferation of nonneuronal elements in the CNS and mesodermal structures of the body with cutaneous stigmata (Back & Plawner, 2012; Blackburn, 2013; Ditzenberger & Blackburn, 2014; Isaacs, 2010; Jett & Friedman, 2010; Kanekar et al., 2011; Volpe, 2008).
      - Clinical manifestations include:
        - Altered skin pigmentation (café-au-lait macules)
        - Lisch nodules of the iris
        - Bupthalmos (enlarged eyeball)
        - Skin nodules
        - Multiple benign neurofibromas
        - Associated with learning disabilities
        - Skeletal abnormalities
        - Vascular disease
        - CNS tumors
        - Malignant peripheral nerve sheath tumors

ANATOMY AND PHYSIOLOGY

■ Macrencephaly refers to a diverse group of conditions characterized by a large brain size, believed to arise from excessive proliferation of neuronal elements, nonneuronal elements, or a combination of both. Macrencephaly manifests most commonly as an isolated finding in familial (autosomal dominant or autosomal recessive) and sporadic causes.

PATHOPHYSIOLOGY

■ Neuronal proliferation defect

■ Occurs between 3 and 4 months gestation

CLINICAL MANIFESTATIONS

■ Large brain size—At birth, head circumference in 50% of cases is greater than 90th percentile.

■ Autosomal-dominant macrencephaly (macrocephaly in either parent) is generally associated with favorable outcome.

■ Autosomal-recessive inheritance is commonly associated with mental retardation and epilepsy.

■ Extracerebral fluid collections enlarge the subarachnoid spaces (rarely requires shunt) (Alvarez, Maytal, & Shinnar, 1986).

DIAGNOSIS

■ Complete physical assessment with thorough neurologic assessment

■ Parental history (macrocephaly in either parent)

   ■ CT scan or MRI

TREATMENT/PATIENT CARE MANAGEMENT

■ Record accurate measurement of FOC, length, and weight weekly (note percentiles)

- Genetic counseling
- Supportive and comfort measures

PROGNOSIS

- Dependent on severity
- Frequently associated with developmental delays

REFERENCES

Abuelo, D. (2007). Microcephaly syndromes. *Seminars in Pediatric Neurology, 14,* 118–127.

Alvarez, L. A., Maytal, J., & Shinnar, S. (1986). Idiopathic external hydrocephalus: Natural history and relationship to benign familial macrocephaly. *Pediatrics, 77*(6), 901–907.

Back, S., & Plawner, L. L. (2012). Congenital malformations of the central nervous system. In H. W. Taeusch, R. A. Ballard, & C. A. Gleason (Eds.), *Avery's diseases of the newborn* (9th ed., pp. 844–867). Philadelphia, PA: Elsevier/Saunders.

Blackburn, S. T. (2013). *Maternal, fetal and neonatal physiology: A clinical perspective* (4th ed.). St. Louis, MO: Saunders/Elsevier Science.

Ditzenberger, G. R., & Blackburn, S. T. (2014). Neurologic system. In C. Kenner & J. W. Lott (Eds.), *Comprehensive neonatal nursing care* (5th ed., pp. 393–437). New York, NY: Springer Publishing Company.

Isaacs, H. (2010). Perinatal neurofibromatosis: Two case reports and review of the literature. *American Journal of Perinatology, 27,* 285–292.

Jett, K., & Friedman, J. M. (2010). Clinical and genetic aspects of neurofibromatosis. *Genetics in Medicine, 362,* 2185–2193.

Kanekar, S., Kaneda, H., & Shively, A. (2011). Malformations of dorsal induction. *Seminars in Ultrasound, CT, and MRI, 32*(3), 189–199.

Olney, A. H. (2007). Macrocephaly syndromes. *Seminars in Pediatric Neurology, 14*(3), 128–135.

Verklan, M. T., & Walden, M. (2010). *Core curriculum for neonatal intensive care nursing* (4th ed.). St. Louis, MO: Saunders, Elsevier.

Volpe, J. J. (2008). *Neurology of the newborn* (5th ed.). Philadephia, PA: Saunders/Elsevier.

DISORDERS OF NEURONAL MIGRATION

■ Disorders of migration alter gyral development and lead to hypoplasia or agenesis of the corpus callosum. Gyral development is most dominant during the last 3 months of gestation with the most rapid increase between 26 and 28 weeks and enlarges from 15 to 34 weeks (Blackburn, 2009; McQuillen & Ferriero, 2005).

■ There are three distinctive layers of the brain that develop as the brain matures: the brainstem, limbic system, and cerebral cortex. The brainstem (medulla, cerebellum, pons) is first fashioned around the 33rd day of gestation and is nearly complete around the seventh month of gestation. The brainstem receives sensory messages and relays the information to the cerebral cortex. It processes vestibular sensations necessary for hearing, balance, vision, and focusing attention. It also regulates autonomic functions of internal organs, such as breathing, heartbeat, and digestion.

■ The limbic system (basal ganglia, hippocampus, amygdala, and hypothalamus) is located in the center of the brain.

■ The cognitive brain (cerebrum) is known as the cerebral cortex and performs the most complex organizing of sensory input. The cerebral cortex is highly specialized and contains specific areas for dealing with voluntary functions in the body. Although the neurologic system is one of the earliest systems to develop in the embryo, it is not fully matured until adulthood (Altimier & White, 2014).

NEONATAL SEIZURES

The neonatal period is the most frequent time of life to have epileptic seizures. However, neonates can also exhibit unusual movements that are not epileptic seizures. Differentiating between epileptic and nonepileptic movements can be difficult. Most neonatal epileptic seizures are provoked by an underlying condition, such as hypoxic brain injury, hemorrhage, hypoglycemia, head trauma, electrolyte imbalance, or cerebral infections (Glass, 2014). These are called acute symptomatic seizures and are not epilepsy. Epileptic seizures are a group of conditions in which the seizures are unprovoked. Because neonates exhibit a wide range of paroxysmal movements, which may or may not be epileptic seizures, a thorough neurophysiologic assessment should be performed before treatment is instigated (Hart, Pilling, Alix, & Alix, 2015).

INCIDENCE

- 1.8 to 5 per 1,000 live term births
- 30 to 130 per 1,000 live preterm births

PHYSIOLOGY/PATHOPHYSIOLOGY

- Result of excessive, synchronous electrical discharge, or depolarization in the brain; produces stereotypic, repetitive behaviors
  - Nerve depolarization–repolarization caused by movement of sodium and potassium across the cell membrane
- Specific mechanism causing neonatal seizures unknown, might be the result of one or more:
  - Disturbances in energy production and the Na^+–K^+ pump
  - Altered neuronal membrane permeability to sodium
  - Imbalances in excitatory and inhibitory neurotransmitters
- Biochemical effects
  - Increased energy expenditure
  - Increased blood pressure
  - Increased cerebral blood flow
  - Marked decrease in brain glucose concentrations
- Seizure activity in neonates: arise from temporal lobe, subcortical, limbic area
  - Limbic area involved in sucking, drooling, chewing, swallowing, oculomotor deviations, and apneic episodes; subtle seizures in infant seizures

■ Seizure activity may be acute, recurrent, or chronic.

  ■ Usually acute: one third occur on the first day of life, another one third on the second day of life, then disappear within the first few weeks after birth

■ Perinatal hypoxia–ischemia accounts for 50% to 60% of all neonatal seizures.

■ It is a signal of underlying disease processes resulting in acute disturbance in brain.

  ■ Primary CNS disorders, hypoxic–ischemic events, hypoglycemia, hypocalcemia, intracranial hemorrhage, infection (meningitis, congenital viral infections, viral encephalopathy), congenital anomalies, other metabolic disturbances (alkalosis, hypomagnesemia, hypernatremia, hyponatremia)

  ■ Less common: drug withdrawal (opiates or barbiturates), inborn errors of metabolism, kernicterus, hyperviscosity, local anesthetic intoxication

■ If left untreated, can lead to permanent CNS damage or other issues

■ Types: subtle, tonic, clonic (multifocal or migratory, and focal), and myoclonic

  ■ Subtle: most common

    • Horizontal deviations of the eyes with or without nystagmoid jerking; repetitive blinking or eyelid fluttering; drooling, sucking, or tongue thrusting; swimming or rowing movements of arms; and bicycling movements of legs

    • Apnea, increased blood pressure

  ■ Generalized tonic: more common in preterm infants

    • Extremity extension; sometimes limited to one extremity

    • Eye deviations, apnea, occasional clonic movements, and decerebrate-type postures

  ■ Clonic, multifocal or focal: more frequent in term infants; occasionally observed in older preterm infants

- Rhythmic, jerky clonic movements of one or more limbs; migrate to other parts of the body randomly
- Can be confused with jitteriness
- Associated with focal traumatic CNS injuries: cerebral contusions and infarcts; severe metabolic disturbance or asphyxia

■ Myoclonic: uncommon in term infants, rare in preterm infants

- Single or multiple sudden jerks with flexion of the upper (most common) or lower extremities; occasionally observed on the trunk and neck
- Associated with inborn errors of metabolism and other metabolic problems

ASSESSMENT

■ Determine cause: perinatal and neonatal history, a physical examination, laboratory evaluation, other diagnostic studies

■ Physical examination: general health and neurologic status

CLINICAL MANIFESTATIONS/DIAGNOSIS

■ Difficult to recognize in neonates: often subtle; can be associated with other disorders or masked by seemingly normal newborn behaviors (grimacing, startle, sucking, and twitching); can occur with minimal or no outward sign

■ Abnormal movements or altered tone of trunk or extremities

■ Abnormal, repetitive facial, oral, tongue, or ocular movements: blinking, lip-smacking, or chewing motions

■ Increased blood pressure; apneic events

■ Laboratory studies: electrolyte levels; glucose, calcium, magnesium, and blood urea nitrogen levels; hematocrit value; blood gases; and pH; blood culture and lumbar puncture; screening for congenital viral infections; amino acid screening (for inborn errors of metabolism)

■ Diagnostic studies: CT, ultrasonography, MRI, skull radiography, EEG, and continuous video-EEG

TREATMENT

■ Treatment of the underlying cause of the seizure is a priority for preventing more seizures and neurologic damage

■ Continual monitoring: blood gases, acid–base status, serum glucose, and fluid and electrolyte status

■ Intravenous glucose administration; seizure activity depletes brain glucose and energy supplies

■ Fluid and electrolyte management should be appropriate to the underlying cause of the seizures

■ Anticonvulsant drugs

 ▪ Phenobarbital, phenytoin, and fosphenytoin doses are given incrementally to reach therapeutic blood levels

 • Blood levels monitored carefully to maintain therapeutic effect and prevent toxicity

 ▪ Refractory seizure may require alternative agents: clonazepam, lidocaine, carbamazepine, diazepam, valproate, primidone

SPECIFIC NURSING CARE (IN ADDITION TO GENERALIZED NURSING CARE)

■ Document seizure activity

 ▪ Time the seizure begins and ends

 ▪ Body parts involved (e.g., extremities, eyes, head)

 ▪ Description of movement, eye deviations, pupillary reactions

 ▪ Respiratory status, color, state, level of consciousness, postictal status

 ▪ Protect from injury during the seizure: do not force anything into the infant's mouth or try to restrain the infant's extremities

■ Maintain infant's head to the side during seizure, if possible

■ Parent teaching: help family understand cause, significance of seizures, diagnostic tests; recognition of seizure activity, care during and after a seizure, anticonvulsants (dosage and side effects) if continued after discharge

PROGNOSIS

■ Mortality: less than 15%

■ Morbidity: two thirds of infants with seizures: adverse neurologic sequelae, epilepsy (20%–25%), motor deficits, mental retardation, learning disabilities, or poor social adjustment in teen years

■ Preterm infants tend to recover more rapidly from a seizure than do term infants; however, mortality and later morbidity are higher in preterm infants

■ Prognosis influenced by time of onset, cause, EEG results, treatment response, frequency, duration

　■ Good prognosis: onset after 4 days of life; benign seizures in otherwise healthy infants during first week of life; associated with late hypocalcemia, hyponatremia, uncomplicated subarachnoid hemorrhage (SAH)

　■ Clonic seizures have a better prognosis than other types of seizures

　■ Poor prognosis: onset less than 48 hours after birth

　■ Poorest prognosis: seizures associated with severe hypoxic–ischemic injury, grade III or grade IV IVH, herpes infection, some bacterial meningitis, CNS malformations

　■ Infants with seizures secondary to late hypocalcemia, hyponatremia, and uncomplicated SAH seem to have the best prognosis

　■ EEG results appear to be better prognostic sign in term than in preterm infants

(Bassan et al., 2008; Blackburn, 2009; Bonifacio, Glass, Peloquin, & Ferriero, 2011; Ditzenberger & Blackburn, 2014; Fenichel, 2007; Glass & Wirrell, 2009; Hellstrom-Westas & deVries, 2007; Jensen, 2009; Rennie & Boylan, 2009; Scher, 2012a; Scher, 2012b; Shah, Boylan, & Rennie, 2012; Tao & Mathur, 2010; Toet & deVries, 2012; Toet & Lemmers, 2009; Volpe, 2008)

REFERENCES

Altimier, L., & White, R. (2014). The neonatal intensive care unit (NICU) environment. In C. Kenner & J. W. Lott (Eds.), *Comprehensive neonatal nursing care* (5th ed., pp. 722–738). New York, NY: Springer Publishing Company.

Bassan, H., Bental, Y., Shany, E., Berger, I., Froom, P., Levi, L., & Shiff, Y. (2008). Neonatal seizures: Dilemmas in workup and management. *Pediatric Neurology, 38*(6), 415–421.

Blackburn, S. T. (2009). Central nervous system vulnerabilities in preterm infants, part II. *Journal of Perinatal & Neonatal Nursing, 23* (2), 108–110.

Bonifacio, S. L., Glass, H. C., Peloquin, S., & Ferriero, D. M. (2011). A new neurological focus in neonatal intensive care. *Nature Review Neurology, 7*(9), 485–494.

Ditzenberger, G. R., & Blackburn, S. T. (2014). Neurologic system. In C. Kenner & J. W. Lott (Eds.), *Comprehensive neonatal nursing care* (5th ed., pp. 393–437). New York, NY: Springer Publishing Company.

Fenichel, G. M. (2007). *Neonatal neurology* (4th ed.). Philadelphia, PA: Churchill/Livingstone/Elsevier.

Glass, H. C. (2014). Neonatal seizures: Advances in mechanisms and management. *Clinics in Perinatology, 41*, 177–190.

Glass, H. C., & Wirrell, E. (2009). Controversies in neonatal seizure management. *Journal of Child Neurology, 24*, 591–599.

Hart, A. R., Pilling, E. L., Alix, J. J., & Alix, J. P. (2015). Neonatal seizures-part 1: Not everything that jerks, stiffens and shakes is a fit. *Archives of Disease in Childhood—Education & Practice Edition, 100*(4), 170–175 (6p.). doi:10.1136/archdischild-2014-306385

Hellstrom-Westas, L., & deVries, L. S. (2007). EEG and evoked potentials in the neonatal period. In M. I. Levene & F. A. Chervenak (Eds.), *Fetal and neonatal neurology and neurosurgery* (4th ed., pp. 192–221). Edinburgh, Scotland: Churchill Livingstone/Elsevier.

Jensen, F. E. (2009). Neonatal seizures: An update on mechanisms and management. *Clinics in Perinatology, 36*(4), 1–20.

McQuillen, P. S., & Ferriero, D. M. (2005). Perinatal subplate neuron injury: Implications for cortical development and plasticity. *Brain Pathology, 15*(3), 250–260.

Rennie, J. M., & Boylan, G. B. (2009). Seizure disorders of the neonate. In M. I. Levene & F. A. Chervenak (Eds.), *Fetal and neonatal neurology and neurosurgery* (4th ed., pp. 698–710). Edinburgh, Scotland: Churchill Livingstone/Elsevier.

Scher, M. S. (2012a). Diagnosis and treatment of neonatal seizures. In J. M. Perlman (Ed.), *Neurology* (2nd ed., pp. 109–141). Philadelphia, PA: Saunders/Elsevier.

Scher, M. S. (2012b). Neonatal seizures. In C. A. Gleason & S. Devaskar (Eds.), *Avery's diseases of the newborn* (9th ed., pp. 901–919). Philadelphia, PA: Saunders/Elsevier.

Shah, D. K., Boylan, G. B., & Rennie, J. M. (2012). Monitoring of seizures in the newborn. *Archives of Disease in Childhood—Fetal and Neonatal Edition, 97*(1), F65–F69.

Tao, J. D., & Mathur, A. M. (2010). Using amplitude-integrated EEG in neonatal intensive care. *Journal of Perinatology, 30*(S1), S73–S81.

Toet, M. C., & deVries, L. S. (2012). Amplitude-integrated EEG and its potential role in augmenting management within the NICU. In J. M. Perlman (Ed.), *Neurology* (2nd ed., pp. 263–284). Philadelphia, PA: Saunders/Elsevier.

Toet, M. C., & Lemmers, P. M. A. (2009). Brain monitoring in neonates. *Early Human Development, 85*(2), 77–84.

Volpe, J. J. (2008). *Neurology of the newborn* (5th ed.). Philadephia, PA: Saunders/Elsevier.

BRAIN INJURY IN PRETERM INFANTS

Multiple brain lesions are seen in preterm infants. The most common are the result of IVH, white matter injury (WMI; periventricular leukomalacia [PVL]), and cerebellar injury. These disorders are the leading causes of neurologic disability in preterm infants with motor, cognitive, learning, and behavioral sequelae.

GERMINAL MATRIX-INTRAVENTRICULAR HEMORRHAGE

INCIDENCE

■ Most common type of intracranial hemorrhage seen in the neonatal period

■ Seen almost exclusively in preterm infants, particularly those less than 1,500 g

■ Incidence of IVH in premature infants measuring less than 1,500 g is 15% to 25%; 10% to 15% suffer more severe IVH, particularly those less than 1,000 g.

(Ballabh, 2010; Bassan, 2009; Ditzenberger & Blackburn, 2014; Inder & Volpe, 2011; McCrea & Ment, 2008; Perlman, 2011; Pettorini, Keh, Ellenbogen, Williams, & Zebian, 2014; Takenouchi & Perlman, 2012; Volpe, 2008)

PHYSIOLOGY

In preterm infants, IVH generally arises from the periventricular subependymal germinal matrix (site where neurons and glial cells originate before migrating to the cortex) at the head of the caudate nucleus near the foramen of Monro. IVH is rare after 35 to 36 weeks gestation due to involution of the germinal matrix and changes in cerebral blood flow patterns. If IVH occurs later, bleeding usually arises from the choroid plexus (Bassan, 2009; Ditzenberger & Blackburn, 2014; Volpe, 2008).

PATHOPHYSIOLOGY

The major risk factors for IVH in the neonate are prematurity and hypoxic events interrelated with the anatomic and physiologic processes that make the periventricular (germinal matrix) site particularly vulnerable. Any perinatal or neonatal event that results in hypoxia or alters cerebral blood flow or intravascular pressure increases the risk of IVH. Classification is made by the location and severity of the hemorrhage:

- Grade I: isolated germinal matrix hemorrhage
- Grade II: small IVH (extends into the ventricle) with normal ventricular size
- Grade III: moderate IVH with acute ventricular dilation
- Grade IV: severe hemorrhage involving both intraventricular and brain parenchyma hemorrhage with acute ventricular dilatation

The neuropathophysiology of IVH involves a complex interaction of intravascular, vascular, and extravascular factors. In many preterm infants, the hemorrhage begins as a microvascular event in the germinal matrix and may be confined to the subependymal area. The original hemorrhage may also rupture into the lateral ventricles and then into the third and fourth ventricles. The blood eventually collects in the subarachnoid space of the posterior fossa, often extending into the basal cistern. Progressive ventricular dilation may occur as the result of obstruction of CSF flow by an obliterative arachnoiditis or as the result of blood clots at the aqueduct of Sylvius or the foramen of Monro. With severe hemorrhages, blood may also be found in the periventricular white matter. This usually is due not to extravasation of blood from the ventricles but to an associated insult in the white matter that increases the risk of adverse neuromotor outcome.

Neuropathologic consequences of IVH include (a) destruction of the germinal matrix and its glial precursor cells, (b) infarction and necrosis of periventricular white matter, and (c) posthemorrhagic hydrocephalus. As the IVH moves from the germinal matrix area into the surrounding white matter, periventricular hemorrhagic infarction and intraparenchymal echodensities develop. The appearance of this parenchymal lesion is associated with increased mortality and neurodevelopmental sequelae. Infants with IVH may also have PVL. PVL may be a consequence of hypoxic–ischemic injury and not directly the result of the IVH.

(Ballabh, 2010; Bassan, 2009; Bonifacio, Gonzalez, & Ferriero, 2012; Ditzenberger & Blackburn, 2014; McCrea & Ment, 2008; Perlman, 2011; Volpe, 2008)

ASSESSMENT

Risk factors for IVH

■ Perinatal events associated with fetal and neonatal hypoxia, such as maternal bleeding, fetal distress, perinatal hypoxia–ischemia, prolonged labor, maternal infection, preterm labor, and abnormal presentation.

■ Neonatal hypoxic events, such as respiratory distress, apnea, and hypotension, which further increase the risk of IVH.

■ Events leading to impairment of venous return or increased venous pressure, such as assisted ventilation, high positive inspiratory pressure, prolonged duration of inspiration, continuous positive airway pressure, and air leak.

■ Other factors that increase venous pressure, such as compression of the infant's skull during vaginal delivery, application of forceps, and use of constricting headbands (tight bilirubin masks).

■ Rapid administration of hypertonic solutions (e.g., sodium bicarbonate and glucose), rapid volume expansion, hypernatremia, hypercarbia, caregiving interventions, and environmental stress can increase cerebral blood flow and pressure.

■ Repeated or prolonged seizures raise the blood pressure and can lead to hypoxia.

(Bissinger & Annibale, 2014; Ditzenberger & Blackburn, 2014; Inder & Volpe, 2011; Levene & deVries, 2009; Pettorini et al., 2014; Volpe, 2008)

CLINICAL MANIFESTATIONS/DIAGNOSIS

■ Over 90% bleed within the first 72 hours after birth; 50% of the bleeding occurs in the first 24 hours.

■ Late hemorrhages are seen after a few days or weeks in about 10% of infants, primarily preterm infants with severe, prolonged respiratory problems; new hemorrhage or an extension of a previous one may develop.

■ Full anterior fontanelle; changes in activity level; decreased/ increased tone.

■ Other: impaired visual tracking; altered lower extremity tone, hypotonia of the neck, brisk tendon reflexes.

■ Catastrophic deterioration usually involves major hemorrhages that evolve rapidly over several minutes or hours.

  ▓ Present with stupor progressing to coma, respiratory distress progressing to apnea, generalized tonic seizures, decerebrate posturing, and fixation of pupils to light and flaccid quadriparesis.

  ▓ Associated with a declining hematocrit value, bulging fontanelle, hypotension, bradycardia, temperature alterations, hypoglycemia, syndrome of inappropriate antidiuretic hormone.

■ Diagnosis by cranial ultrasonography to determine the presence, severity, and progression of the hemorrhage; monitor later complications (PVL, progressive ventricular dilation and posthemorrhagic hydrocephalus).

■ Laboratory findings: declining hematocrit; failure of the hematocrit to increase after transfusion, and spinal fluid findings: increased red blood cell levels, increased protein levels, decreased glucose levels, and xanthochromia.

(Bassan, 2009; Ditzenberger & Blackburn, 2014; McCrea & Ment, 2008; Pettorini et al., 2014; Takenouchi & Perlman, 2012; Volpe, 2008)

TREATMENT

■ Acute treatment of infants with IVH:

  ▓ Provide physiologic support.

  ▓ Minimize physical manipulations, handling, and environmental stressors to reduce the risk of hypoxia and of fluctuations in arterial blood pressure and cerebral blood flow.

■ Position head in the midline or to the side, without flexing the neck. The head of the bed can be elevated slightly; avoid the Trendelenburg position.

■ Monitor vital signs, blood pressure, tone, activity, and level of consciousness.

■ Routine ultrasonographic screening of infants at risk for IVH to identify infants with silent bleeding or bleeding with nonspecific symptoms

■ Prevention or risk reduction in the perinatal period, with the prevention of preterm birth, perinatal hypoxic–ischemic injury, and birth trauma

■ Antenatal steroids associated with decreased incidence of IVH

■ Postbirth prevention and risk-reduction activities

■ Prompt resuscitation by a trained neonatal intensive care unit (NICU) team and interventions to prevent or reduce hypoxic or ischemic events

■ Prevent rapid changes in cerebral blood flow, fluctuations in systemic blood pressure, and hyperosmolarity; prevent or minimize fluctuations in ICP

■ Management of progressive ventricular dilation

■ Initial treatment is observation since ventricular growth often arrests spontaneously without therapy (Whitelaw & Aquilina, 2009).

■ Progressive ventricular dilation with increasing ICP is managed with a VP shunt or, if the infant cannot tolerate surgery, with temporary ventricular drainage.

SPECIFIC NURSING CARE (IN ADDITION TO GENERALIZED NURSING CARE)

■ Avoid or minimize activities that can increase ICP or cause wide swings in arterial or venous pressure, especially during the first 72 hours of life

■ Provide interventions, such as containment or swaddling, during aversive procedures such as endotracheal suctioning to promote greater physiologic stability and a more rapid return to baseline

■ Monitor for signs of progressive posthemorrhagic ventricular dilation

■ Assess head size: head size can increase without increases in ICP (normopressive hydrocephalus)

■ Assess fontanelles (tense fontanelle may only be noted when the infant is placed in an upright position)

■ Observe for signs of increased ICP (bulging anterior fontanelle, setting-sun sign, dilated scalp veins, and widely separated sutures)

■ Administer hypertonic solutions and volume expanders slowly, with careful monitoring of vital signs and color

■ Position head in the midline and raise head of bed slightly to reduce ICP

■ Avoid turning head sharply; turn body as a unit

■ Keep head of bed flat, avoid raising the feet above the head, such as with a diaper change

■ Minimize handling and stimuli

■ Family support and teaching include how to interact with and care for the infant at risk for IVH in a developmentally appropriate manner, promoting opportunities for interaction while minimizing stressful events

(Bassan, 2009; Bissinger & Annibale, 2014; Ditzenberger & Blackburn, 2014; Levene & deVries, 2009; McCrea & Ment, 2008; Takenouchi & Perlman, 2012; Volpe, 2008; Wang, Wang, Gong, & Zhao, 2014)

Care of an infant with a VP shunt

■ Position after surgery on the side opposite the shunt, with the head of the bed flat or slightly elevated to prevent rapid loss of CSF and decompression

- Position can be rotated to supine every few hours to prevent skin breakdown
- Keep the skin around the shunt clean and dry
- Observe for signs of localized or systemic infection
    - Shunt infection may appear as localized redness or drainage around the incision, temperature instability, altered activity, poor feeding
    - Observe for shunt obstruction (accumulation of CSF, enlargement of the head, and signs of increased ICP)
    - Monitor fluid status and intake and output; observe for signs of dehydration from too rapid loss of CSF (sunken fontanelle, agitation or restlessness, increased urine output, and electrolyte abnormalities)
    - Provide parent teaching: care of the infant and shunt, including positioning and skin care, signs of shunt malfunction, increased ICP, infection, and dehydration

(Bissinger & Annibale, 2014; Ditzenberger & Blackburn, 2014; Solanki & Hockley, 2009)

PROGNOSIS

- Severity and extent of hemorrhage and the presence of associated problems influence mortality and morbidity
- The milder or smaller the hemorrhage, the lower the mortality and the incidence of major neurologic sequelae and posthemorrhagic ventricular dilation
- Incidence of neurologic sequelae ranges from 15% in infants with moderate hemorrhage to 35% to 90% in infants with severe hemorrhages
- Sequelae include cerebral palsy, developmental delay, sensory and attention problems, learning disorders, and hydrocephalus

(Bassan, 2009; Ditzenberger & Blackburn, 2014; Inder & Volpe, 2011; Levene & deVries, 2009; Myers & Ment, 2009; Takenouchi & Perlman, 2012; Volpe, 2008)

WMI IN PRETERM INFANTS

INCIDENCE

■ WMI is the most common severe neurologic insult seen in preterm infants.

■ Focal cystic necrotic lesions are seen in 3% to 15% of surviving very-low-birth-weight infants; the more common diffuse noncystic lesions associated with disturbances in myelinization are seen in up to 50% of survivors.

■ Time of onset is variable.

(Bonifacio et al., 2012; deVries, Counsell, S. J., & Levene, 2009; Ditzenberger & Blackburn, 2014; Vandertak, 2009; Verney, Monier, Fallet-Bianco, & Gressens, 2010; Volpe et al., 2011)

PHYSIOLOGY/PATHOPHYSIOLOGY

WMI involves both cystic and noncystic focal necrotic lesions as well as diffuse WMI with damage to the premyelinating oligodendrocytes, astrogliosis, and microglial infiltration. This injury is referred to as PVL. PVL is a symmetric, nonhemorrhagic, usually bilateral lesion caused by ischemia from alterations in arterial circulation. Leukomalacia refers to change in the brain's white matter reflective of softening. WMI often is associated with IVH, but it is a separate lesion that may also occur in the absence of IVH.

(Bonifacio et al., 2012; deVries et al., 2009; Deng, Pleasure, & Pleasure, 2008; Ditzenberger & Blackburn, 2014; Inder & Volpe, 2011; Vandertak, 2009; Verklan, 2009; Verney, Monier, Fallet-Bianco, & Gressens, 2010; Verney et al., 2012; Volpe et al., 2009)

PVL begins with ischemic necrosis of the white matter dorsal and lateral to the external angles of the lateral ventricles. Pathologic changes begin with patchy areas of focal ischemic coagulation that may occur as early as 5 to 8 hours after the initial hypoxic–ischemic insult. This is followed within a few days by proliferation of macrophages and astrocytes, along with endothelial and glial infiltration. Later changes include thinning of the white matter and liquefaction in the central portion of the necrotic area, as well as cavitation, cystic changes, and decreased myelinization. Cerebral atrophy leads to expansion of the lateral ventricles and hydrocephalus.

The pathogenesis of WMI involves an interaction between three maturation-dependent factors: (a) immature vascular supply to the WM (reducing oxygen delivery to vulnerable areas of the brain); (b) impairments in cerebral autoregulation; and (c) vulnerability of premyelinating oligodendrites to damage from reactive oxygen and nitrogen species (free radicals), glutamate, adenosine, and cytokines. Damage to the premyelinating oligodendrites leads to further release of cytokines (indicating an inflammatory process), glutamate, and free radicals. Oligodendrocyte development and survival are impaired, leading to hypomyelinization with subsequent motor, cognitive, and behavioral neurodevelopmental problems. Axonal damage and disruption also occur. Perinatal infection and an immune-mediated inflammatory response with release of proinflammatory cytokines are thought to play a prominent role in the pathogenesis of PVL (Deng et al., 2008; deVries et al., 2009; Ditzenberger & Blackburn, 2014; Vandertak, 2009; Verklan, 2009; Verney et al., 2012; Volpe, 2008; Volpe et al., 2011).

ASSESSMENT

- Risk factors include any event during the prenatal, intrapartal, or postbirth periods that results in cerebral ischemia; this includes asphyxia, IVH, hypoxia, hypercarbia, hypotension, cardiac arrest, and infection (in which blood flow is diminished by the action of endotoxins).

- The major risk factors are IVH, asphyxia, and chorioamnionitis (deVries et al., 2009; Ditzenberger & Blackburn, 2014).

CLINICAL MANIFESTATIONS/DIAGNOSIS

■ Often no clinical findings are specific to PVL during the first weeks of life unless the damage is severe.

■ Identify signs of hypoxia and ischemia and institute interventions to prevent further ischemic damage.

■ Cranial ultrasonography can identify infants at risk for, or who have early signs of, PVL.

■ MRI can identify changes early and is especially useful with diffuse WMI (Ditzenberger & Blackburn, 2014; El-Dib et al., 2010; Lodygensky, Menache, & Huppi, 2012).

TREATMENT

■ Initial treatment focuses on treating the primary insult and its attendant complications and preventing further hypoxic–ischemic damage, including preventing or minimizing hypotension, hypoxia, acidosis, and severe apneic and bradycardic episodes.

■ Head ultrasound and MRI are used serially to diagnose PVL and to follow its progression in infants at risk.

■ Infants at risk for WMI should undergo serial cranial ultrasonographic examinations with later follow-up.

SPECIFIC NURSING CARE (IN ADDITION TO GENERALIZED NURSING CARE)

■ Reduce environmental stressors (see section on IVH)

■ Provide developmental and environmental interventions (see section on IVH)

■ Parent teaching on promoting an understanding of the infant's health status and care, providing anticipatory guidance, and discussing how to interact with and care for their infant in a developmentally appropriate manner

PROGNOSIS

- Infants are at higher risk for later problems that affect motor, cognitive, and visual function.

- The most prominent sequelae in survivors: spastic diplegia with or without hydrocephalus.

- Infants with diffuse WMI are more likely to develop visual, cognitive, and neurobehavioral impairments.

(Ditzenberger & Blackburn, 2014; Inder & Volpe, 2011; Mwaniki, Atieno, Lawn, & Newton, 2012; Myers & Ment, 2009; Takenouchi & Perlman, 2012; Vople, 2008)

REFERENCES

Ballabh, P. (2010). Intraventricular hemorrhage in premature infants: Mechanism of disease. *Pediatric Research*, 67(1), 1–8.

Bassan, H. (2009). Intracranial hemorrhage in the preterm infants: Understanding it, preventing it. *Clinics in Perinatology*, 36(4), 737–762.

Bissinger, R. L., & Annibale, D. J. (2014). *Golden hours: Care of the very low birth weight infant*. Chicago, IL: The National Certification Corporation (NCC).

Bonifacio, S. L., Gonzalez, F., & Ferriero, D. M. (2012). Central nervous system injury and neuroprotection. In C. A. Gleason & S. Devaskar (Eds.), *Avery's diseases of the newborn* (9th ed., pp. 869–891). Philadelphia, PA: Saunders/Elsevier.

deVries, L. S., Counsell, S. J., & Levene, M. (2009). Cerebral ischemic lesions. In M. Levene & F. A. Chervenak (Eds.), *Fetal and neonatal neurology and neurosurgery* (4th ed., pp. 431–471). Edinburgh, Scotland: Churchill Livingstone/ Elsevier.

Deng, W., Pleasure, J., & Pleasure, D. (2008). Progress in periventricular leukomalacia. *Archives of Neurology*, 65(10), 1291–1295.

Ditzenberger, G. R., & Blackburn, S. T. (2014). Neurologic system. In C. Kenner & J. W. Lott (Eds.), *Comprehensive neonatal nursing care* (5th ed., pp. 393–437). New York, NY: Springer Publishing Company.

El-Dib, M., Massaro, A. N., Bulas, D., & Aly, H. (2010). Neuroimaging and neurodevelopmental outcome of premature infants. *American Journal of Perinatology*, 27(10), 803–818.

Inder, T. E., & Volpe, J. J. (2011). Intraventricular hemorrhage in the neonate. In R. A. Polin, W. W. Fox, & S. H. Abman (Eds.), *Fetal and neonatal physiology* (4th ed., Vol. 2, pp. 1830–1847). Philadelphia, PA: Saunders/Elsevier.

Levene, M., & deVries, L. S. (2009). Neonatal intracranial hemorrhage. In M. Levene & F. A. Chervenak (Eds.), *Fetal and neonatal neurology and neurosurgery* (4th ed., pp. 395–430). Edinburgh, Scotland: Churchill Livingstone/Elsevier.

Lodygensky, G. A., Menache, C. C., & Huppi, P. S. (2012). Magnetic resonance imaging's role in the care of the infant at risk for brain injury. In J. M. Perlman (Ed.), *Neonatology* (2nd ed., pp. 285–324). Philadelphia, PA: Saunders/Elsevier.

McCrea, H., & Ment, L. R. (2008). The diagnosis, management, and postnatal prevention of intraventricular hemorrhage in the preterm neonate. *Clinics in Perinatology, 35*(4), 777–792.

Mwaniki, M. K., Atieno, M., Lawn, J. E., & Newton, C. R. (2012). Long-term neurodevelopmental outcomes after intrauterine and neonatal insults: A systematic review. *The Lancet, 379*, 445–452.

Myers, E., & Ment, L. R. (2009). Long-term outcome of preterm infants and the role of neuroimaging. *Clinics in Perinatology, 36*(4), 773–790.

Perlman, J. (2011). Cerebral blood flow in premature infants: Regulation, measurement, and pathophysiology of intraventricular hemorrhage. In R. A. Polin, W. W. Fox, & S. H. Abman (Eds.), *Fetal and neonatal physiology* (4th ed., Vol. 2, pp. 1820–1829). Philadelphia, PA: Saunders/Elsevier.

Pettorini, B., Keh, R., Ellenbogen, J., Williams, D., & Zebian, B. (2014). Intraventricular haemorrhage in prematurity. *Infant, 10*(6), 186–190.

Solanki, G. A., & Hockley, A. D. (2009). Neurosurgical management of hydrocephalus. In M. Levene & F. A. Chervenak (Eds.), *Fetal and neonatal neurology and neurosurgery* (4th ed., pp. 834–846). Edinburgh, Scotland: Churchill Livingstone/Elsevier.

Takenouchi, T., & Perlman, J. M. (2012). Intraventricular hemorrhage and white matter injury in the preterm infant. In J. Perlman (Ed.), *Neurology* (2nd ed., pp. 27–46). Philadelphia, PA: Saunders/Elsevier.

Vandertak, K. (2009). Cool competence. The nursing challenges of therapeutic hypothermia. *Journal of Neonatal Nursing, 15*(6), 200–203.

Verklan, M. T. (2009). The chilling details: Hypoxic-ischemic encephalopathy. *Journal of Perinatal & Neonatal Nursing, 23*(1), 59–68.

Verney, C., Monier, A., Fallet-Bianco, C., & Gressens, P. (2010). Early microglial colonization of the human forebrain and possible involvement in periventricular white-matter injury of preterm infants. *Journal of Anatomy*, *217*(4), 436–448.

Verney, C., Pogledic, I., Biran, V., Adle-Baissette, H., Fallet-Bianco, C., & Gressens, P. (2012). Microglial reaction in axonal crossroads is a hallmark of noncystic periventricular white matter injury in very preterm infants. *Journal of Neuropathology and Experimental Neurology*, *71*(3), 251–264.

Volpe, J. J. (2008). *Neurology of the newborn* (5th ed.). Philadephia, PA: Saunders/ Elsevier.

Volpe, J. J., Kinney, H. C., Jensen, F. E., & Rosenberg, P. A. (2011). The developing oligodendrocyte: Key cellular target in brain injury in the premature infant. *International Journal of Developmental Neuroscience*, *29*(4), 423–440.

Volpe, P., Campobasso, G., De Robertis, V., & Rembouskos, G. (2009). Disorders of prosencephalic development. *Prenatal Diagnosis*, *29*(4), 340–354.

Wang, M., Wang, Z.-P., Gong, R., & Zhao, Z.-T. (2014). Maternal smoking during pregnancy and neural tube defects in offspring: A meta-analysis. *Child's Nervous System*, *30*(1), 83–89.

Whitelaw, A., & Aquilina, K. (2009). Neonatal hydrocephalus-clinical assessment and non-surgical treatment. In M. Levene & F. A. Chervenak (Eds.), *Fetal and neonatal neurology and neurosurgery* (4th ed., pp. 819–833). Edinburgh, Scotland: Churchill Livingstone/Elsevier.

BRAIN INJURY IN TERM INFANTS

HYPOXIC–ISCHEMIC ENCEPHALOPATHY

Hypoxic-ischemic encephalopathy (HIE) is an injury to the brain caused by oxygen deficit resulting from either systemic hypoxemia (decreased oxygen in the blood supply) or ischemia (diminished cerebral blood perfusion) or a combination of the two conditions. The hypoxemia and ischemia may occur simultaneously or sequentially, and it appears from recent evidence that ischemia is the more important of the two oxygen deprivation states in causing the brain injury. In addition, the subsequent reperfusion of the affected brain area has been shown to be the time at which the majority of the injury to the brain occurs. Glucose deprivation also plays a part in the severity of the brain injury (Ditzenberger & Blackburn, 2014; Sorem, Smith, & Druzin, 2009; Volpe, 2008).

HIE may occur secondary to prenatal, intrapartum, or postnatal insults in both preterm and term infants. The site of injury varies with maturational changes in the vascular anatomy and metabolic activity of the brain (Bonifacio et al., 2012; deVries & Jongmans, 2010; Dickey, Long, & Hunt, 2011; Ditzenberger & Blackburn, 2014; Douglas-Escobar & Weiss, 2015; Simbruner et al., 2010; Wachtel & Hendricks-Muñoz, 2011).

INCIDENCE

■ Between four to eight per 1,000 live births

■ Mortality and morbidity: one per 1,000

PHYSIOLOGY/PATHOPHYSIOLOGY

■ Five types of lesions

　▪ Selective neuronal necrosis

　▪ Status marmoratus of the neurons of the basal ganglia and thalamus, with loss of neurons in these areas

　▪ Parasagittal cerebral injury

　▪ PVL (primarily in preterm infants)

　▪ Focal or multifocal ischemic brain necrosis (Ditzenberger & Blackburn, 2014; Volpe, 2008)

■ Primary hypoxic injury: neuronal necrosis in cerebrum and cerebellum, with damage to the gray matter at the depths of the sulci

■ Primary ischemic injury: posterior portion of the parasagittal region secondary to watershed or border zone infarcts

■ After a hypoxic–ischemic insult, the entire cortex initially may be edematous, and further ischemic damage may occur as a result of compression of the cortex against the skull

(Dickey et al., 2011; Ditzenberger & Blackburn, 2014; Johnston, Fatemi, Wilson, & Northington, 2011; Sorem et al., 2009; Stola & Perlman, 2008; Volpe, 2008)

ASSESSMENT/DIAGNOSIS

■ Characteristic pattern of neurologic findings over the first 72 hours of life: seizures, altered level of consciousness, altered tone, altered activity, irregular respirations, apnea, poor or absent Moro reflex, abnormal cry, poor suck, and altered pupillary responses and eye movements

■ Clinical signs categorizing the severity of HIE classified in three stages (Sarnat & Sarnat, 1976):

■ Stage 1 (mild): mild depression or hyperalertness, irritability, and sympathetic nervous system excitation (tachycardia, dilated pupils)

• Good Moro reflex and deep tendon reflexes; generally are symptomatic for less than 24 hours

■ Stage 2 (moderate): lethargy interspersed with brief arousal, decreased tone, altered primary reflexes, and increased parasympathetic tone (bradycardia, decreased pupil size, and blood pressure) and may develop seizures

■ Stage 3 (severe): varying levels of consciousness initially; then become stuporous or comatose

• Depressed deep tendon and Moro reflexes, hypotonia, and most develop seizures

■ Seizures occur in up to 60% infants with HIE

■ Onset at 12 to 14 hours of age

■ Most often seen are multifocal clonic seizures in term infants

■ Occasionally, myoclonic, clonic, and subtle seizures

■ Extensive workup to define the type, extent, and location of the injury may include cranial ultrasonography, brainstem auditory evoked potentials, MRI, EEG, and measurements of cerebral blood flow, ICP, and the creatinine kinase level

■ Labs: glucose, calcium, magnesium, serum and urinary electrolyte levels and osmolality; blood urea nitrogen, serum creatinine levels; fluid and electrolyte balance

■ At risk for hypocalcemia and hypoglycemia

(Ditzenberger & Blackburn, 2014; Johnston et al., 2011; Volpe, 2008)

TREATMENT

Infants with HIE have multiorgan and multisystem problems that arise from the original hypoxic–ischemic insult (Sarkar, Barks, Bhagat, & Donn, 2009; Tagin, Woolcott, Vincer, Whyte, & Stinson, 2012; Zanelli, Buck, & Fairchild, 2011). As a result, management of these infants is complex and requires a coordinated team effort, preferably within a NICU/tertiary care center.

■ Acute management

  ■ Delivery room resuscitation and stabilization

  ■ Management of the primary problem and related alterations in the cardiovascular, pulmonary, gastrointestinal, and renal systems

  ■ Prompt identification and treatment of seizures to prevent further alterations in ICP and cerebral blood flow

  ■ Focuses on elimination of the cause of the original hypoxia, alleviation of tissue hypoxia, and promotion of adequate cerebral perfusion and brain oxygenation with maintenance of an adequate glucose supply

(Ditzenberger & Blackburn, 2014; Stola & Perlman, 2008; Volpe, 2008; Wachtel & Hendricks-Muñoz, 2011)

■ NICU treatment

  ■ Establish ventilation and adequate perfusion

  ■ Prevent/minimize hypotension, hypoxia and acidosis, rapid alterations in cerebral blood flow and systemic blood pressure, and severe apneic and bradycardic episodes

■ Avoid hyperoxia: can result in cerebral vasoconstriction and diminished perfusion

■ Monitor and document neurologic status

■ Must be differentiated from other neurologic dysfunctions caused by trauma, infection, or CNS anomalies

(Ditzenberger & Blackburn, 2014; Gunny & Lin, 2012; Stola & Perlman, 2008; Tao & Mathur, 2010; Toet & deVries, 2012; Toet & Lemmers, 2009; Wachtel & Hendricks-Muñoz, 2011; Walsh, Murray, & Boylan et al., 2011)

■ Fluid management is critical not only for treating the cerebral edema but also for managing the alterations in renal function.

■ Induced mild hypothermia has been shown to provide neuroprotection and reduce the extent of tissue injury and is increasingly the treatment of choice for infants ≥ 36 weeks gestation with moderate to severe HIE (refer to whole body cooling protocol).

■ For use only in NICU/high acuity nurseries:

• Infants undergoing a cooling regimen, either selective head cooling or whole body cooling, require optimal care and attention at the bedside; this intervention is only being done in tertiary NICU settings.

• Induced hypothermia is not recommended either prior to or during transport.

■ Care should be taken that the infants not become hyperthermic with core temperatures greater than 37°C

(Barks, 2008; Ditzenberger & Blackburn, 2014; Glass, 2010; Hoehn et al., 2008; Pfister & Soll, 2010; Reynolds & Talmage, 2011; Selway, 2010; Zanelli et al., 2011)

■ Therapeutic window: must begin within 6 hours of birth for neuroprotective interventions; early hypothermia studies indicate that cooling may be less effective if started after onset of seizures or in infants with most severe EEG changes before therapy.

■ The cooling regimen continues for 72 hours.

■ Infants are assessed by a neonatologist team and/or pediatric neurologist to determine whether hypothermia criteria are met before the cooling regimen is initiated.

　▤ Current criteria used to determine if a newborn is a candidate for hypothermia are:

　　• Term infants ≥ 36 weeks gestation without major congenital anomalies, IUGR (≤ 1,800 g), or known chromosomal anomaly

　　• Admitted to NICU at ≤ 6 hours of age

　　• Assessed to be in Stage 2 moderate HIE, or Stage 3, severe HIE

(Bonifacio et al., 2011, 2012; Ditzenberger & Blackburn, 2014; Hoehn et al., 2008; Gancia & Pomero, 2011; Gluckman et al., 2005; Gunn et al., 2008; Hoehn et al., 2008; Laptook, 2012; Stola & Perlman, 2008; Volpe, 2008)

SPECIFIC NURSING CARE (IN ADDITION TO GENERALIZED NURSING CARE)

■ During acute phase and cooling phase:

　▤ Fluctuations in systemic blood pressure with increased ICP and altered cerebral hemodynamics can occur as a result of caregiving or environmental stress, potentially worsening HIE complications

　▤ Developmentally supportive care of these infants to reduce stress is essential

　▤ Maintain minimal handling, as well as decreased auditory, visual, and sensory input

　▤ Positioning and skin care are important, especially for hypoactive, obtunded, or comatose infants

　▤ Monitor vital signs, neurologic status, seizures

■ During recovery

　▤ Gradually introduce sensory experiences as tolerated

　　• Will be easily overwhelmed; monitor response closely

　▤ Continue monitoring physiologic and neurologic status

■ Observe for changes in level of consciousness, tone, and activity and seizures

■ Parental support

   ■ Teach reasons for lack of infant responsiveness if the infant is sedated, hypoactive, stuporous, or comatose

   ■ Prepare for possibility of death; consider the implications for later neurologic deficits

   ■ Focus on promoting an understanding of the infant's health status and care and providing anticipatory guidance regarding changes in the infant's state, as well as the outcome

   ■ Demonstrate how to interact with and care for their infant in a developmentally appropriate manner, with the goal of promoting opportunities for interaction while minimizing stressful events

(Ditzenberger & Blackburn, 2014; Gudsnuk & Champagne, 2011; Long & Brandon, 2007; Selway, 2010; Sullivan et al., 2011)

PROGNOSIS

■ Varies with the extent and severity of the insult and the resulting brain injury

   ■ Ranges from perinatal death to severe neurologic impairment to minimal or no sequelae

   ■ Specific sequelae not apparent for several months or longer

   ■ Some infants make a significant recovery, although the rate and degree of recovery vary

   ■ MRI or CT can be used to assess the location, degree, and extent of the injury

   ■ Sequelae of HIE in term infants are related to the site of injury (e.g., the cortex) and include mental retardation, microcephaly, cortical blindness, hearing deficits, and epilepsy

   ■ Generally, infants with mild HIE do well

   ■ Moderate HIE or severe HIE have a higher mortality rate and later cognitive and motor problems

(deVries & Jongmans, 2010; Ditzenberger & Blackburn, 2014; Epelman, Daneman, Chauvin, & Hirsch, 2012; Gunn et al., 2008; Gunny & Lin, 2012; Lodygensky et al., 2012; Lori et al., 2011)

REFERENCES

Barks, J. (2008). Technical aspects of starting a neonatal cooling program. *Clinics in Perinatology, 35*(4), 765–776.

Bonifacio, S. L., Glass, H. C., Peloquin, S., & Ferriero, D. M. (2011). A new neurological focus in neonatal intensive care. *Nature Review Neurology, 7*(9), 485–494.

Bonifacio, S. L., Gonzalez, F., & Ferriero, D. M. (2012). Central nervous system injury and neuroprotection. In C. A. Gleason & S. Devaskar (Eds.), *Avery's diseases of the newborn* (9th ed., pp. 869–891). Philadelphia, PA: Saunders/Elsevier.

deVries, L. S., & Jongmans, M. J. (2010). Long-term outcome after neonatal hypoxic-ischaemic encephalopathy. *Archives of Disease in Childhood—Fetal and Neonatal Edition, 95*(3), F220–F224.

Dickey, E. J., Long, S. N., & Hunt, R. W. (2011). Hypoxic ischemic encephalopathy—What can we learn from humans? *Journal of Veterinary Internal Medicine, 25*(6), 1231–1240.

Ditzenberger, G. R., & Blackburn, S. T. (2014). Neurologic system. In C. Kenner & J. W. Lott (Eds.), *Comprehensive neonatal nursing care* (5th ed., pp. 393–437). New York, NY: Springer Publishing Company.

Douglas-Escobar, M., & Weiss, M. D. (2015). Hypoxic-ischemic encephalopathy: A review for the clinician. *JAMA Pediatrics, 169*(4), 397–403. doi:10.1001/jamapediatrics.2014.3269

Epelman, M., Daneman, A., Chauvin, N., & Hirsch, W. (2012). Head ultrasound and MR imaging in the evaluation of neonatal encephalopathy: Competitive or complementary imaging studies? *Magnetic Resonance Imaging Clinics of North America, 20*(1), 93–115.

Gancia, P., & Pomero, G. (2011). Brain cooling and eligible newborns: Should we extend the indications? *Journal of Maternal-Fetal and Neonatal Medicine, 24*(S1), 53–55.

Glass, H. C. (2010). Neurocritical care for neonates. *Neurocritical Care, 12*(3), 421–429.

Gluckman, P. D., Wyatt, J. S., Azzopardi, D., Ballard, R., Edwards, A. D., Ferriero, D. M., ... Gunn, A. J. (2005). Selective head cooling with mild systemic hypothermia after neonatal encephalopathy: Multicentre randomised trial. *The Lancet, 365*(9460), 663–670.

Gudsnuk, K. M., & Champagne, F. A. (2011). Epigenetic effects of early developmental experiences. *Clinics in Perinatology, 38*(4), 703–718.

Gunn, A. J., Wyatt, J. S., Whitelaw, A., Barks, J., Azzopardi, D., Ballard, R., ... Thoresen, M. (2008). Therapeutic hypothermia changes the prognostic value of clinical evaluation of neonatal encephalopathy. *Journal of Pediatrics, 152*(1), 55–58.e51.

Gunny, R. S., & Lin, D. (2012). Imaging of perinatal stroke. *Magnetic Resonance Imaging Clinics of North America, 20*(1), 1–33.

Hoehn, T., Hansmann, G., Bührer, C., Simbruner, G., Gunn, A. J., Yager, J., ... Thoresen, M. (2008). Therapeutic hypothermia in neonates. Review of current clinical data, ILCOR recommendations and suggestions for implementation in neonatal intensive care units. *Resuscitation, 78*(1), 7–12.

Johnston, M. V., Fatemi, A., Wilson, M. A., & Northington, F. (2011). Treatment advances in neonatal neuroprotection and neurointensive care. *The Lancet Neurology, 10*(4), 372–382.

Laptook, A. R. (2012). The use of hypothermia to provide neuroprotection for neonatal hypoxic-ischemic brain injury. In J. Perlman (Ed.), *Neurology* (2nd ed., pp. 63–76). Philadelphia, PA: Saunders/Elsevier.

Lodygensky, G. A., Menache, C. C., & Huppi, P. S. (2012). Magnetic resonance imaging's role in the care of the infant at risk for brain injury. In J. M. Perlman (Ed.), *Neonatology* (2nd ed., pp. 285–324). Philadelphia, PA: Saunders/Elsevier.

Long, M., & Brandon, D. H. (2007). Induced hypothermia for neonates with hypoxic-ischemic encephalopathy. *Journal of Obstetric, Gynecologic, & Neonatal Nursing, 36*(3), 293–298.

Lori, S., Bertini, G., Molesti, E., Gualandi, D., Gabbanini, S., Bastianelli, M. E., ... Dani, C. (2011). The prognostic role of evoked potentials in neonatal hypoxic-ischemic insult. *Journal of Maternal-Fetal and Neonatal Medicine, 24*(S1), 69–71.

Pfister, R., & Soll, R. (2010). Hypothermia for the treatment of infants with hypoxic–ischemic encephalopathy. *Journal of Perinatology, 30*, S82–S87.

Reynolds, R., & Talmage, S. (2011). "Caution! Contents should be cold": Developing a whole-body hypothermia program. *Neonatal Network: Journal of Neonatal Nursing, 30*(4), 225–230.

Sarkar, S., Barks, J., Bhagat, I., & Donn, S. (2009). Effects of therapeutic hypothermia on multiorgan dysfunction in asphyxiated newborns: Whole-body cooling versus selective head cooling. *Journal of Perinatology, 29,* 558–563.

Sarnat, H., & Sarnat, M. (1976). A clinical and electroencephalographic study. *Archives of Neurology, 33,* 696–795.

Selway, L. D. (2010). State of the science: Hypoxic ischemic encephalopathy and hypothermic intervention for neonates. *Advances in Neonatal Care, 10*(2), 60–66.

Simbruner, G., Mittal, R. A., Rohlmann, F., Muche, R., & neo.nEURO.network Trial Participants. (2010). Systemic hypothermia after neonatal encephalopathy: Outcomes of neo.nEURO.network RCT. *Pediatrics, 126*(4), e771–e778.

Sorem, K., Smith, J. F., & Druzin, M. L. (2009). Antenatal prediction of asphyxia (pp. 491–505). In M. Levene & F. A. Chervenak (Eds.), *Fetal and neonatal neurology and neurosurgery.* Edinburgh, Scotland: Churchill Livingstone/Elsevier.

Stola, A., & Perlman, J. (2008). Post-resuscitation strategies to avoid ongoing injury following intrapartum hypoxia–ischemia. *Seminars in Fetal and Neonatal Medicine, 13*(6), 424–431.

Sullivan, R., Perry, R., Sloan, A., Kleinhaus, K., & Burtchen, N. (2011). Infant bonding and attachment to the caregiver: Insights from basic and clinical science. *Clinics in Perinatology, 38,* 643–656.

Tagin, M. A., Woolcott, C. G., Vincer, M. J., Whyte, R. K., & Stinson, D. A. (2012). Hypothermia for neonatal hypoxic ischemic encephalopathy: An updated systematic review and meta-analysis. *Archives of Pediatrics and Adolescent Medicine, 166*(6), 558–566.

Tao, J. D., & Mathur, A. M. (2010). Using amplitude-integrated EEG in neonatal intensive care. *Journal of Perinatology, 30*(S1), S73-S81.

Toet, M. C., & deVries, L. S. (2012). Amplitude-integrated EEG and its potential role in augmenting management within the NICU. In J. M. Perlman (Ed.), *Neurology* (2nd ed., pp. 263–284). Philadelphia, PA: Saunders/Elsevier.

Toet, M. C., & Lemmers, P. M. A. (2009). Brain monitoring in neonates. *Early Human Development, 85*(2), 77–84.

Volpe, J. J. (2008). *Neurology of the newborn* (5th ed.). Philadephia, PA: Saunders/Elsevier.

Wachtel, E. V., & Hendricks-Muñoz, K. D. (2011). Current management of the infant who presents with neonatal encephalopathy. *Current Problems in Pediatric and Adolescent Health Care, 41*(5), 132–153.

Walsh, B. H., Murray, D. M., & Boylan, G. B. (2011). The use of conventional EEG for the assessment of hypoxic ischaemic encephalopathy in the newborn: A review. *Clinical Neurophysiology*, *122*(7), 1284–1294.

Zanelli, S., Buck, M., & Fairchild, K. (2011). Physiologic and pharmacologic considerations for hypothermia therapy in neonates. *Journal of Perinatology*, *31*(6), 377–386.

BIRTH INJURIES

Traumatic injury to the central or peripheral nervous system can occur during the perinatal or postnatal period. Most of these injuries happen during the intrapartum period and may occur with perinatal hypoxic–ischemic events. Perinatal events most frequently associated with birth injury include mid-forceps delivery, shoulder dystocia, low-forceps delivery, birth weight exceeding 3,500 g, and second stage of labor lasting longer than 60 minutes. The incidence of injury has declined markedly in recent years as a result of improvement in obstetrical care and increased use of cesarean sections for abnormal presentations. However, birth injuries can also arise from trauma during a cesarean section or resuscitation. Injuries that occur before the intrapartum period usually are caused by compression or pressure injuries from an unusual fetal position. The risk of injury to the central or peripheral nervous system is greater with malpresentation (especially breech), prolonged or precipitate labor, prematurity, multiple gestation, shoulder dystocia, macrosomia, and instrumental delivery.

The most prevalent types of injury to the nervous system are extracranial hemorrhage, intracranial hemorrhage, skull fractures, spinal cord injury, and peripheral nerve injury (Bonifacio et al., 2012; Ditzenberger & Blackburn, 2014).

EXTRACRANIAL HEMORRHAGE

- Caput succedaneum and cephalohematoma: most common types, most benign of birth injury
  - Caput succedaneum: soft, pitting, superficial edema several millimeters thick; overlies presenting part in a vertex delivery; crosses suture lines

■ Edematous area above the periosteum

- Edema consists of serum, blood, or both

■ Infants with caput succedaneum may also have ecchymosis, petechiae, or purpura over the presenting part

■ Occurs after a spontaneous vertex delivery or after use of a vacuum extractor

■ Resolves within a few days after birth with no sequelae

■ Cephalohematoma: firm, fluctuant mass; does not cross the suture lines

■ Occurs in 1.5% to 2.5% of newborns; most often in males

■ Subperiosteal bleeding, usually over the parietal bone but possibly over other cranial bones

- Mass often enlarges slightly by 2 to 3 days of age

■ Occurs after the use of forceps; after a prolonged, difficult delivery; and in infants born to primiparas

■ Usually unilateral, can be bilateral

- Approximately 5% of infants with unilateral and 18% with bilateral have a linear skull fracture underlying the mass

■ Generally asymptomatic

■ Observe for symptoms of intracranial hemorrhage or skull fracture; hyperbilirubinemia

■ Occasionally anemia develops with a large cephalohematoma

■ Resolve between 2 weeks and 6 months of age; most by 8 weeks

- Calcium deposits occasionally develop

- Swelling may remain for the first year

(Bonifacio et al., 2012; Ditzenberger & Blackburn, 2014; Fenichel, 2007; Waller, Gopalani, & Benedetti, 2012; Watchko, 2009)

■ Subgaleal hemorrhage

Subgaleal or subaponeurotic hemorrhage is the most serious form of extracranial hemorrhage in newborns (Schierholz & Walker, 2014; Waller et al., 2012).

- Incidence
- Spontaneous vaginal deliveries: four per 10,000
- Vacuum-assisted deliveries: 59 per 10,000
- Increased with precipitous deliveries, macrosomia, and severe dystocia, and with failed vacuum deliveries requiring forceps
- Mortality: 17% to 25%

(Ditzenberger & Blackburn, 2014; Fenichel, 2007; Volpe, 2008)

PHYSIOLOGY/PATHOPHYSIOLOGY

- Traction or application of intense shearing forces to the scalp pull the aponeurosis from the vault and rupture large emissary veins. Blood collects in a large potential space between the galea aponeurotica and the periosteum of the skull through which the large emissary veins pass.
- The area is called a potential space because it is not present until blood separates the galea aponeurotica from the periosteum of the skull. This space can quickly expand to accommodate 260 to 280 mL of blood.
- Total newborn blood volume is 80 to 100 mL/kg. The amount of blood entering the subgalial space may be more than the entire blood volume of some newborns.
- Subgaleal hemorrhage is a clinical emergency. These infants usually present at birth or within a few hours.

(Bonifacio et al., 2012; Ditzenberger & Blackburn, 2014; Fenichel, 2007; Schierholz & Walker, 2010, 2014; Volpe, 2008)

ASSESSMENT

- Birth history
- Observation during first hours of life

CLINICAL MANIFESTATIONS/DIAGNOSIS

- Firm, ballotable head mass crossing sutures and fontanelles
  - Often extends from the orbital ridge, around the ears to the neck
- Develops after birth and increases in size quickly within first 1 to 3 hours of life
- Each centimeter of enlargement is estimated to be equivalent to 40 mL of blood loss
- Mimics edema; shifts with head repositioning
- Usually accompanied by pain on manipulation of the scalp or head
- Symptoms: anemia, hypovolemia, pallor, hypotension, tachycardia, tachypnea, hypotonia, and other signs of shock
- Laboratory results: rapidly falling hematocrit, platelets, clotting factors

TREATMENT

- Rapid recognition
- Monitor cardiovascular (HR, BP), respiratory status
- Check hematocrit/hemoglobin results at minimum every hour; d-dimers, fibrinogen levels every 2 to 4 hours during acute phase
- Administer blood and volume expanders
- Control bleeding with fresh frozen plasma and cryoprecipitate
- Supportive care:
  - Fluids, electrolytes, glucose
  - Oxygen, ventilator support
- Central lines (umbilical arterial and venous catheters) for immediate access, blood samples, cardiovascular support, blood products

(Bonifacio et al., 2012; Ditzenberger & Blackburn, 2014; Fenichel, 2007; Schierholz & Walker, 2010, 2014; Volpe, 2008)

PROGNOSIS

■ If infant survives initial acute hemorrhagic event and HIE does not develop, usually resolves in 2 to 3 weeks

■ Morbidity related to neurologic deficits associated with HIE (Volpe, 2008)

INTRACRANIAL HEMORRHAGE

Several clinically important types of intracranial bleeding can occur in the neonate, including IVH (described earlier), primary SAH, subdural hemorrhage, and intracerebellar hemorrhage. These latter three types of hemorrhage arise from trauma or hypoxia during the perinatal period.

PRIMARY SAH

INCIDENCE

■ Rare; often is associated with severe asphyxial event and birth trauma

■ Most prevalent form of intracranial hemorrhage in neonates

PHYSIOLOGY/PATHOPHYSIOLOGY

■ Hemorrhage into the subarachnoid space
  ▪ Newborns: venous blood; older children and adults: arterial blood
  ▪ Blood leaks from the leptomeningeal plexus, bridging veins, or ruptured vessels in the subarachnoid space
  ▪ Associated with trauma or asphyxia

(Ditzenberger & Blackburn, 2014; Levene & deVries, 2009; Volpe, 2008)

ASSESSMENT

- Perinatal: birth trauma, prolonged labor, difficult delivery, fetal distress, perinatal hypoxic–ischemic events
- Hemorrhage is discovered accidentally with "bloody" lumbar puncture

CLINICAL MANIFESTATIONS/DIAGNOSIS

- Can be asymptomatic
- May present at day 2 to 3 with isolated seizure for term; apnea for preterm
  - Between seizures, infant appears and acts healthy
- Massive SAH: rapid and fatal course
- MRI and CT confirm the diagnosis; ultrasonography is unreliable

TREATMENT

- Prevent or reduce the risk of trauma and hypoxia during the perinatal period
- Observe at-risk infants for seizures and other neurologic signs
- General nursing care

(Ditzenberger & Blackburn, 2014; Levene & deVries, 2009; Volpe, 2008)

PROGNOSIS

- Most survive
- Asymptomatic/isolated seizure on day 2 to 3: usually do well developmentally
- Symptomatic with severe SAH: up to one half of infants with severe traumatic or hypoxic injury: neurologic sequelae; occasional hydrocephalus

(Ditzenberger & Blackburn, 2014; Levene & deVries, 2009; Volpe, 2008)

SUBDURAL HEMORRHAGE

INCIDENCE

- Uncommon among the hemorrhages seen in newborns
- Incidence has declined markedly due to improvements in obstetrical care

(Ditzenberger & Blackburn, 2014; Levene & deVries, 2009)

PATHOPHYSIOLOGY

- Unilateral or bilateral bleeding between dura and arachnoid with rupture of superficial cerebral veins or of "bridging" veins between superomedial aspect of the cerebrum and superior sagittal sinus

(Ditzenberger & Blackburn, 2014; Fenichel, 2007; Levene & deVries, 2009; Volpe, 2008)

ASSESSMENT

- Perinatal history: precipitous, prolonged, or difficult delivery, use of midforceps or high forceps, prematurity, cephalopelvic disproportion, macrosomia, breech presentation
- Recognition important for immediate intervention for large subdural hemorrhage
- Associated with cephalohematoma; subgaleal, subconjunctival, and retinal hemorrhages; skull fractures; and brachial plexus or facial palsies

(Ditzenberger & Blackburn, 2014; Fenichel, 2007; Levene & deVries, 2009; Volpe, 2008; Waller et al., 2012)

CLINICAL MANIFESTATIONS/DIAGNOSIS

■ Most common: minor hemorrhage

  ■ Asymptomatic or have signs such as irritability and hyperalertness

■ Second pattern: primarily focal seizures in first 2 to 3 days of life; occasional hemiparesis; unequal pupils with sluggish response to light; full or tense fontanelle; bradycardia; irregular respirations

■ Third pattern (rare): symptoms appear at 4 weeks to 6 months of age: increasing head size due to continued hematoma formation, poor feeding, failure to thrive, altered level of consciousness, and occasionally, seizures caused by the chronic subdural effusion

■ MRI or CT confirm diagnosis

(Ditzenberger & Blackburn, 2014; Fenichel, 2007; Volpe, 2008)

TREATMENT

■ Observe for seizures and other neurologic signs

■ Massive posterior fossa hemorrhage requires craniotomy and surgical aspiration of the clot

(Ditzenberger & Blackburn, 2014; Fenichel, 2007; Levene & deVries, 2009)

PROGNOSIS

■ Varies with the location and severity of the hemorrhage

■ Asymptomatic/transient neonatal seizures: do well

■ Most infants with bleeding over the tentorium or falx cerebri die; severe hydrocephalus and neurologic sequelae usually develop in those that survive (Ditzenberger & Blackburn, 2014; Volpe, 2008)

PERINATAL STROKE

Ischemic strokes are more common in the perinatal period than at any other time of life and are the leading cause of hemiplegic cerebral palsy, yet until recently they have been poorly understood and oftentimes not diagnosed in the neonatal period.

INCIDENCE

■ Estimated to be from fairly rare (17–93 per 100,000 live births) to relatively common (one in 2,300–5,000 live births)

(Benders, Groenendaal, F., & deVries, 2009; Chabrier, Husson, Dinomais, Landrieu, & Nguyen The Tich, 2011; Cheong & Cowan, 2009; Ditzenberger & Blackburn, 2014; Kirton & deVeber, 2009; Mineyko & Kirton, 2011; Murias, 2014; Myers & Ment, 2012)

PHYSIOLOGY/PATHOPHYSIOLOGY

■ Result of a focal disruption of cerebral blood flow secondary to an arterial or venous thrombosis or embolism occurring between 20 weeks gestation and the 28th postnatal day of life (National Institute of Neurological Disorders and Stroke, 2006)

(Ditzenberger & Blackburn, 2014; Kirton & deVeber, 2009; Mineyko & Kirton, 2011; Myers & Ment, 2012)

■ Perinatal strokes classified as fetal, neonatal, presumed perinatal ischemic

■ Fetal stroke: occurred between 20 weeks gestation and the onset of labor or cesarean section

■ Neonatal stroke: occurred between the onset of labor and actual delivery

■ Presumed perinatal ischemic strokes: identified by neuroimaging in infants greater than 28 days of life as having had a focal infarction at some point between 20 weeks gestation and postnatal day 28

(Chabrier et al., 2011; Ditzenberger & Blackburn, 2014; Kirton & deVeber, 2009; Lynch, 2009; Myers & Ment, 2012)

ASSESSMENT

■ Maternal, pregnancy/labor, fetal, and neonatal history
■ Multifactorial, still being identified
   ■ Maternal: thrombophilias (factor V Leiden, factor VIII, protein S deficiency, protein C deficiency, prothrombin mutation, and antiphospholipid antibodies) and/or preexisting conditions such as thyroid disease, diabetes mellitus, or gestational diabetes or history of infertility
   ■ Pregnancy/labor-related: significant maternal trauma, primiparity, placental abnormalities, oligohydramnios, decreased fetal movement, prolonged rupture of membranes, chorioamnionitis, prolonged second stage of labor, or assisted delivery
   ■ Fetal or neonatal: fetal distress during labor, cord abnormalities (tight nuchal or body cord, true cord knot), thrombophilias, congenital cardiac defects, and corrective surgery
■ May be a gender effect, occurs more frequently in males

(Chabrier et al., 2011; Cheong & Cowan, 2009; Ditzenberger & Blackburn, 2014; Kirton & deVeber, 2009; Lynch, 2009; Mineyko & Kirton, 2011; Myers & Ment, 2012)

CLINICAL MANIFESTATIONS/DIAGNOSIS

■ Determined by the timing of the initial insult
■ Bulging and/or pulsatile fontanelle, dilated head and neck veins, papilledema, asymmetrical movements, primitive reflexes, or seizure-like activity (Kirton & deVeber, 2009)
■ Transient hemiparesis or generalized tone anomalies in early newborn phase

■ Seizures occur in 85% to 92% of affected newborns

    ■ Often the earliest manifestation for healthy appearing newborns

    ■ Most occur within the first 72 hours of life

    ■ Approximately 50% focal motor, 33% generalized motor, 17% subtle

■ If not diagnosed during the newborn stage, identified ~ 6 months

    ■ Asymmetry of reach and grasp

    ■ Seizures occurring after 28 days of life; language delay also reported

(Ditzenberger & Blackburn, 2014; Kirton & deVeber, 2009; Myers & Ment, 2012)

■ EEG and neuroimaging to evaluate for diagnosis

■ Echocardiogram and electrocardiogram may be indicated to assess for cardiac dysfunction or rhythm disorders

(Cheong & Cowan, 2009; Ditzenberger & Blackburn, 2014; Kirton & deVeber, 2009; Myers & Ment, 2012)

TREATMENT

■ Supportive; directed at minimizing secondary brain injury

■ Avoid hyperthermia and hyperthermic environment

■ Document and aggressively treat seizures

(Ditzenberger & Blackburn, 2014; Kirton & deVeber, 2009; Myers & Ment, 2012)

PROGNOSIS

■ Varies with area of original insult

■ Estimated 20% to 70% of hemiplegic cerebral palsy associated with perinatal stroke, with spasticity more marked in upper extremities

- Intelligence is within normal parameters for two thirds of affected infants
- Neurologic deficits usually associated with cerebral injury from original trauma and/or hypoxic event

(Ditzenberger & Blackburn, 2014; Myers & Ment, 2012)

SPINAL CORD INJURY

INCIDENCE

- Uncommon

PHYSIOLOGY/PATHOPHYSIOLOGY

- Injury can occur at any point along the cord
- Caused by excessive traction, rotation, and torsion of the vertebral column and neck
- Occurs from stretching of spinal cord; damage ranges from complete transection to laceration, edema, hemorrhage, and hematoma formation (Bonifacio et al., 2012; Ditzenberger & Blackburn, 2014; Fenichel, 2007; Madsen, Frim, & Hansen, 2005; Volpe, 2008)

ASSESSMENT

- Birth history: breech delivery, dystocia, macrosomia, cephalopelvic disproportion

CLINICAL MANIFESTATIONS/DIAGNOSIS

- Spinal cord shock: hypotonia, weakness, flaccid extremities, sensory deficits, relaxed abdominal muscles, diaphragmatic breathing, Horner syndrome (ipsilateral ptosis, anhidrosis, and miosis), distended bladder
- Low cervical lesions: shallow, paradoxical respirations

■ Degree of neurologic insult often cannot be accurately evaluated until the infant has recovered from the initial period of spinal shock and any edema or hemorrhage has been reabsorbed

■ Spinal ultrasonography, CT, or MRI to determine level and extent of injury

TREATMENT

■ Stabilize

■ Treat associated problems (e.g., asphyxia, hemorrhage, shock)

■ Maintain respiratory status

  ■ Midcervical to upper cervical or brainstem lesions require assisted ventilation

■ Monitor for signs of respiratory infection and pneumonia

■ Maintain skin integrity over the paralyzed area

■ Require meticulous bowel, bladder care; regular glycerin suppositories, urinary catheterization

■ Follow-up care: multidisciplinary team: nursing, medicine, neurology, neurosurgery, physical therapy, orthopedics, urology, social work, and psychology

PROGNOSIS

■ Depends on the level and severity of the injury; generally, poor

■ Many are stillborn or die shortly after birth

■ Survivors have varying degrees of residual paralysis, respiratory problems, and bowel and bladder dysfunction, depending on the level of the injury

(Bonifacio et al., 2012; Ditzenberger & Blackburn, 2014; Fenichel, 2007; Madsen et al., 2005; Volpe, 2008)

PERIPHERAL NERVE INJURIES

Peripheral nerve injuries result from stretching, compression, twisting, hyperextension, or separation of nerve tissue. Injury can occur before, during, or after birth and is seen predominantly in term and large for gestational age (LGA) infants.

The more common sites affected are the radial, median, sciatic, and phrenic nerves and the brachial plexus. Damage can range from swelling of the nerve to complete peripheral degeneration (with later total recovery) to complete division of all structures (Bonifacio et al., 2012; Ditzenberger & Blackburn, 2014; Fenichel, 2007; Levene, 2009; Volpe, 2008).

RADIAL NERVE INJURY

■ Usually results from compression of the nerve caused by fracture of the humerus during a breech delivery or by intrauterine compression of the arm

■ Symptoms: wrist drop with a normal grasp reflex

■ Recovery: over the first few weeks to months

MEDIAN AND SCIATIC NERVE INJURIES

■ Typically, postnatal iatrogenic events

■ Median nerve injury can be a complication of brachial or radial arterial punctures

■ Symptoms: diminished pincer grasp and thumb strength; flexed fourth finger

■ Recovery is variable

■ Sciatic nerve injuries: often permanent

■ Trauma from a misplaced intramuscular injection or from ischemia from an injection of hypertonic solutions into the gluteal muscle

■ Symptoms: diminished abduction and distal joint movement

(Bonifacio et al., 2012; Ditzenberger & Blackburn, 2014; Levene, 2009; Missios, Bekelis, K., & Spinner, 2014; Volpe, 2008)

FACIAL NERVE PALSY

Facial nerve palsy must be differentiated from nuclear agenesis (Möebius syndrome), a significant disorder characterized by congenital facial muscle paralysis (Ditzenberger & Blackburn, 2014; Levene, 2009; Terzis & Anesti, 2011; Volpe, 2008).

- ◼ Incidence: 0.23%
- ◼ Caused by trauma from oblique application of forceps, prolonged pressure on the nerve during labor from the maternal sacral promontory, or pressure from an abnormal fetal posture
- ◼ Most common on the left
- ◼ Clinical manifestations vary, depending on whether the injury is to the central nerve, the peripheral nerve, or the peripheral nerve branch
  - ◼ Complete peripheral nerve injury: unilateral inability to close the eye or open the mouth; lower lip on the affected side does not depress during crying, forehead does not wrinkle; affected side appears full and smooth, with obliteration of the nasolabial fold; dribble milk while feeding
  - ◼ Central injury: spastic paralysis of the lower portion of the face contralateral to the side of CNS injury without involvement of eyes or forehead
  - ◼ Peripheral injury: varying degrees of paralysis of the forehead, eye, or lower face, depending on the branch involved; paralysis is apparent at birth or within 1 to 2 days after birth

PROGNOSIS

- ◼ Almost all infants recover completely by 1 to 4 weeks

(Ditzenberger & Blackburn, 2014; Fenichel, 2007; Levene, 2009; Terzis & Anesti, 2011)

PHRENIC NERVE PALSY

Phrenic nerve palsy must be differentiated from CNS, cardiac, and pulmonary problems.

INCIDENCE

■ Rare

PHYSIOLOGY/PATHOPHYSIOLOGY

■ Paralysis of the diaphragm due to phrenic nerve damage

■ Usually unilateral, on the right side

■ Caused by injury of the cervical nerve roots at C3 to C5

■ Results from tearing of the nerve sheath, accompanied by edema and hemorrhage

■ May occur as an isolated event or in association with brachial nerve palsy

ASSESSMENT

■ Birth history: vaginal delivery of LGA infants, shoulder dystocia, breech presentations, prolonged labor, or difficult delivery

CLINICAL MANIFESTATIONS/DIAGNOSIS

■ Respiratory difficulty

■ Recurrent episodes of cyanosis and dyspnea

■ Primarily thoracic movement with minimal or no abdominal excursions, opposite of the normal newborn breathing pattern

■ If complete avulsion or bilateral injury: severe respiratory distress from birth

TREATMENT

■ Promote ventilation and oxygenation

■ If severe distress: positive pressure ventilation or constant positive airway pressure for support until recovery occurs

■ Position on affected side

■ No enteral feeds until respiratory status improves; gavage; advance as tolerated to oral feeds

■ Surgical plication of the diaphragm may be needed if no improvement is noted or if the infant is still ventilator dependent at 4 to 6 weeks of age

PROGNOSIS

■ Recovery 6 to 12 months of age

■ Some infants recover clinically but have residual abnormalities of diaphragmatic movement on radiography (Fenichel, 2007; Volpe, 2008).

BRACHIAL PLEXUS INJURY

INCIDENCE

■ 0.5% to 2%; almost exclusively in term infant

PHYSIOLOGY/PATHOPHYSIOLOGY

■ Injury of the C5 to T1 nerve roots

■ Degree of injury varies, ranging from edema and hemorrhage of the nerve sheath to avulsion of the nerve root from the spinal cord

ASSESSMENT

■ Birth history: vaginal delivery of LGA infants, shoulder dystocia, breech presentations, prolonged labor, or difficult delivery

■ Can occur in uncomplicated deliveries; after cesarean birth

■ Usually unilateral, on left side; clavicle fracture may occur

CLINICAL MANIFESTATIONS/DIAGNOSIS

■ Vary with the location and severity of the injury

■ Usually apparent from birth; may be delayed for several days to a few weeks

■ Can be heredity; autosomal dominant inheritance (mapped to 17q25); should be considered with uncomplicated delivery and positive family history

Erb (Erb-Duchenne) palsy (most common)

■ Upper plexus injury involving C5 to C7; shoulder and upper arm; denervation of the deltoid, supraspinous, biceps, and brachioradialis muscles

  ■ Passive arm, abducted and internally rotated; pronated forearm; flexed wrist and fingers; absent Moro reflex; biceps, radial reflexes diminished, or absent; normal grasp reflex

Klumpke palsy

■ Lower plexus injury at C5 to T1; seen primarily in breech infants whose arm has been hyperabducted and delivered with the head affecting the flexors of the wrist and hand

  ■ Affected hand and arm without sensation; held passively to side; claw hand position; absent Moro, grasp reflexes; triceps reflex diminished or absent; biceps and radial reflexes present

Erb-Klumpke (total) palsy

■ Injury to the nerve roots of the brachial plexus from C5 to T1

■ Complete paralysis of the upper and lower arm and hand; flaccid; no sensation; absent deep tendon, Moro reflexes

■ MRI or CT: visualize the degree of injury

■ If improvement is not noted within the first few months, electromyography and nerve conduction studies to determine the extent of the damage, to follow recovery, and to determine whether surgical intervention is needed

TREATMENT

■ Protect arm until localized edema and pain subsides

■ Support arm in position of relaxation; no splints; do not immobilize

■ Provide comfort measures to reduce pain

■ Evaluate for associated problems: fractures; respiratory difficulty secondary to phrenic nerve paralysis

■ After edema subsides, 7 to 10 days: physical therapy

■ Continue massage and exercise over the first months until total or partial recovery occurs

PROGNOSIS

■ Depends on the level and severity of the injury

■ Approximately 65% to 95%: full recovery by 4 months to 3 years of age

■ Infants with total paralysis most likely for ongoing residual functional deficits: alterations in shoulder abduction and external rotation; restricted movement of the elbow, forearm; hand weakness; potential for abnormal muscle development and arm growth

(Alfonso, 2011; Ditzenberger & Blackburn, 2014; Doumouchtsis & Arulkumaran, 2009; Fenichel, 2007; Levene, 2009; Volpe, 2008)

CONCLUSION

Infants with neurologic dysfunction present a significant challenge to the neonatal nurse. The nurse must respond to infants with life-threatening conditions, such as perinatal hypoxic–ischemic injury and intracranial hemorrhage; to those with transient problems, such as an isolated seizure; and to those with chronic problems, such as NTDs. Nurses must also deal with their own responses and those of the families of infants who may die during the neonatal or early infancy periods or whose short-term and long-term outcome may be altered by the extent of neurologic insult. Nurses must understand the basis for and the implications of specific types of neurologic dysfunction; recognize the clinical manifestations of these types of dysfunction; and respond appropriately in concert with other health care professionals.

Nursing management of the infant involves activities to address alteration in level of consciousness, potential for injury related to trauma or infection, impairment of skin integrity, alterations in comfort, impaired mobility, alterations in thermoregulation, alterations in nutrition and fluid and electrolyte status, and promotion of neurobehavioral organization and development. Nurses must also assess family coping, interactive processes, knowledge, and grieving to assist the family in coping with the birth of an ill infant and, for many families, with the uncertainty or certainty of long-term neurologic deficits in their infant.

REFERENCES

Alfonso, D. T. (2011). Causes of neonatal brachial plexus palsy. *Bulletin of the NYU Hospital for Joint Diseases, 69*(1), 11–16.

Benders, M. J. N. L., Groenendaal, F., & deVries, L. S. (2009). Preterm arterial ischemic stroke. *Seminars in Fetal and Neonatal Medicine, 14*(5), 272–277.

Bonifacio, S. L., Gonzalez, F., & Ferriero, D. M. (2012). Central nervous system injury and neuroprotection. In C. A. Gleason & S. Devaskar (Eds.), *Avery's diseases of the newborn* (9th ed., pp. 869–891). Philadelphia, PA: Saunders/Elsevier.

Chabrier, S., Husson, B., Dinomais, M., Landrieu, P., & Nguyen The Tich, S. (2011). New insights (and new interrogations) in perinatal arterial ischemic stroke. *Thrombosis Research, 127*(1), 13–22.

Cheong, J. L. Y., & Cowan, F. M. (2009). Neonatal arterial ischaemic stroke: Obstetric issues. *Seminars in Fetal and Neonatal Medicine, 14*(5), 267–271.

Ditzenberger, G. R., & Blackburn, S. T. (2014). Neurologic system. In C. Kenner & J. W. Lott (Eds.), *Comprehensive neonatal nursing care* (5th ed., pp. 393–437). New York, NY: Springer Publishing Company.

Doumouchtsis, S., & Arulkumaran, S. (2009). Are all brachial plexus injuries caused by shoulder dystocia? *Obstetrical and Gynecological Survey, 64*(9), 615–623.

Fenichel, G. M. (2007). *Neonatal neurology* (4th ed.). Philadelphia, PA: Churchill/Livingstone/Elsevier.

Kirton, A., & deVeber, G. (2009). Advances in perinatal ischemic stroke. *Pediatric Neurology, 40*(3), 205–214.

Levene, M. (2009). Disorders of the spinal cord, cranial and peripheral nerves. In M. Levene & F. A. Chervenak (Eds.), *Fetal and neonatal neurology and neurosurgery* (4th ed., pp. 778–791). Edinburgh, Scotland: Churchill Livingstone/Elsevier.

Levene, M., & deVries, L. S. (2009). Neonatal intracranial hemorrhage. In M. Levene & F. A. Chervenak (Eds.), *Fetal and neonatal neurology and neurosurgery* (4th ed., pp. 395–430). Edinburgh, Scotland: Churchill Livingstone/Elsevier.

Lynch, J. K. (2009). Epidemiology and classification of perinatal stroke. *Seminars in Fetal and Neonatal Medicine, 14*(5), 245–249.

Madsen, J. R., Frim, D. M., & Hansen, A. R. (2005). Neurosurgery of the newborn In M. G. McDonald, M. D. Mullett, & M. M. Seshia (Eds.), *Avrey's neonatology: Pathophysiology and management of the newborn* (6th ed., pp. 1410–1427). Philadelphia, PA: Lippincott, Williams and Wilkins.

Mineyko, A., & Kirton, A. (2011). The black box of perinatal ischemic stroke pathogenesis. *Journal of Child Neurology, 26*(9), 1154–1162.

Missios, S., Bekelis, K., & Spinner, R. J. (2014). Traumatic peripheral nerve injuries in children: Epidemiology and socioeconomics. *Journal of Neurosurgery: Pediatrics, 14*(6), 688–694 (7p.). doi:10.3171/2014.8.PEDS14112

Murias, K. G. (2014). A review of cognitive outcomes in children following perinatal stroke. *Developmental Neuropsychology, 39*(2), 131–157.

Myers, E., & Ment, L. R. (2012). Perinatal stroke. In J. Perlman (Ed.), *Neurology* (2nd ed., pp. 91–108). Philadelphia, PA: Saunders/Elsevier.

National Institute of Neurological Disorders and Stroke. (2006). Report and workshop on perinatal and childhood stroke. *Journal of Child Neurology, 21*, 415–418.

Schierholz, E., & Walker, S. R. (2010). Responding to traumatic birth: Subgaleal hemorrhage, asssessment, and management during transport. *Advances in Neonatal Care, 10*(6), 311–315.

Schierholz, E., & Walker, S. R. (2014). Responding to traumatic birth: Subgaleal hemorrhage, assessment, and management during transport. *Advances in Neonatal Care: Official Journal of the National Association of Neonatal Nurses,* 14(Suppl. 5), S11–S15. doi:10.1097/ANC.0b013e3181fe9a49

Terzis, J. K., & Anesti, K. (2011). Developmental facial paralysis: A review. *Journal of Plastic, Reconstructive & Aesthetic Surgery,* 64(10), 1318–1333.

Volpe, J. J. (2008). *Neurology of the newborn* (5th ed.). Philadephia, PA: Saunders/Elsevier.

Waller, S. A., Gopalani, S., & Benedetti, T. (2012). Complicated deliveries: Overview. In C. A. Gleason & S. Devaskar (Eds.), *Avery's diseases of the newborn* (9th ed., pp. 146–158). Philadelphia, PA: Saunders/Elsevier.

Watchko, J. F. (2009). Identification of neonates at risk for hazardous hyperbilirubinemia: Emerging clinical insights. *Pediatric Clinics of North America,* 56(3), 671–687.

ADDITIONAL CHAPTER REFERENCES

Ayres, A. (1987). *Sensory integration and the child* (8th Print ed.). Torrance, CA: Western Psychological Services.

Bruner, J. P. (2007). Intrauterine surgery in myelomeningocele. *Seminars in Fetal and Neonatal Medicine,* 12(6), 471–476.

Bui, B., Rees, S., Loeliger, M., Caddy, J., Rehn, A. H., Armitage, J. A., & Vingrys, A. J. (2002). Altered retinal function and structure after chronic placental insufficiency. *Investigative Ophthalmology & Visual Science,* 43(3), 805–812.

Chambers C. D. (2006). Risks of hyperthermia associated with hot tub or spa use by pregnant women. *Birth Defects Research Part A: Clinical and Molecular Teratology,* 76(8), 569–573.

Chan, W. Y., Lorke, D. E., Tiu, S. C., & Yew, D. T. (2002). Proliferation and apoptosis in the developing human neocortex. *The Anatomical Record,* 267(4), 261–276.

Cohen, A. R. (2014). Chapter 65: Myelomeningocele and related neural tube disorders. In R. J. Martin, A. A. Fanaroff, & M. C. Walsh (Eds.), *Neonatal–perinatal medicine: Diseases of the fetus and newborn* (10th ed.). Philadelphia, PA: Mosby/Elsevier.

Correa, A., & Marcinkevage, J. (2013). Prepregnancy obesity and the risk of birth defects: An update. *Nutrition Reviews, 71,* S68–S77. doi:10.1111/nure.12058

Demir, S., Demir, B., Demir, F., Bingöl, G., Kaya, E., Balsak, D., & Sakar, M. N. (2014). Encephalocele: A case report. *Perinatal Journal/Perinatoloji Dergisi, 22,* SE18. doi:10.2399/prn.14.SE001058

Dreier, J. W., Andersen, A.-M. N., & Berg-Beckhoff, G. (2014). Systematic review and meta-analyses: Fever in pregnancy and health impacts in the offspring. *Pediatrics, 133*(3), e674–688.

DuPlessis, A. J. (2008). Cerebrovascular injury in premature infants: Current understanding and challenges for future prevention. *Clinics in Perinatology, 35*(4), 609–642.

Eliot, L. (1999). *What's going on here? How the brain and mind develop in the first five years of life.* New York, NY: Bantam Books.

Feil, R., Waterland, R. A., Fraga, M. F., & Jirtle, R. L. (2012). Epigenetics and the environment: Emerging patterns and implications. *Nature Reviews Genetics, 13*(2), 97–109.

Gomella, T. L., & Cunningham, M. D. (2013). *Neonatology: Management, procedures, on-call problems, diseases, and drugs* (7th ed.). New York, NY: McGraw Hill/Lange.

Graven, S. N., & Browne, J. V. (2008). Sleep and brain development: The critical role of sleep in fetal and early neonatal brain development. *Newborn & Infant Nursing Reviews, 8*(4), 173–179.

Kenner, C., & McGrath, J. (Eds.). (2010). *Developmental care of newborns and infants* (2nd ed.). Glenview, IL: National Association of Neonatal Nurses.

Kranowitz, C. A. (1998). *The out-of-sync child.* New York, NY: The Berkley Publishing Group.

Lickliter, R. (2011). The integrated development of sensory organization. [Review Article]. *Clinics in Perinatology, 38,* 591–603. doi:10.1016/j.clp.2011.08.007

Lynam, L., & Verklan, T. (2010). Neurologic disorders. In M. T. Verklan & M. Walden (Eds.), *Core curriculum for neonatal intensive care nursing* (4th ed.). St. Louis, MO: Elsevier.

Munch, T. N., Rasmussen, M. H., Wohlfahrt, J., Juhler, M., & Melbye, M. (2014). Risk factors for congenital hydrocephalus: A nationwide, register-based, cohort study. *Journal of Neurology, Neurosurgery, and Psychiatry, 85*(11), 1253–1259. doi:10.1136/jnnp-2013-306941

National Perinatal Association (NPA). (2010). *Position paper: NICU developmental care.* Lonedell, MO: NPA.

Padmanabhan, R. (2006). Etiology, pathogenesis and prevention of neural tube defects. *Congenital Anomalies, 46*(2), 55–67.

Pitcher, J. B., Schneider, L. A., Drysdale, J. L., Ridding, M. C., & Owens, J. A. (2011). Motor system development of the preterm and low birthweight infant. *Clinics in Perinatology, 38*(4), 605–625.

Rees, S., Harding, R., & Walker, D. (2011). The biological basis of injury and neuroprotection in the fetal and neonatal brain. *International Journal of Developmental Neuroscience, 29*(6), 551–563. doi:10.1016/j.ijdevneu.2011.04.004

Rehn, A. E., Loeliger, M., Hardie, N. A., Rees, S. M., Dieni, S., & Shepherd, R. K. (2002). Chronic placental insufficiency has long-term effects on auditory function in the guinea pig. *Hearing Research, 166*(1–2), 159–165.

Rehn, A. E., Van Den Buuse, M., Copolov, D., Briscoe, T., Lambert, G., & Rees, S. (2004). An animal model of chronic placental insufficiency: Relevance to neurodevelopmental disorders including schizophrenia. *Neuroscience, 129*(2), 381–391.

Rhawn, J. (1999). Fetal brain and cognitive development. *Developmental Reviews, 20*, 81–98.

Thoerner, A., Warner, B., & Kallapur, S. (2007). Neurologic system. In L. Altimier (Ed.), *Mosby's neonatal nursing online course.* St. Louis, MO: Mosby.

Thompson, D. K., Inder, T. E., Faggian, N., Johnston, L., Warfield, S. K., Anderson, P. J., … Egan, G. F. (2011). Characterization of the corpus callosum in very preterm and full-term infants utilizing MRI. *NeuroImage, 55*(2), 479–490.

Waterland, R. A., & Jirtle, R. L. (2003). Transposable elements: Targets for early nutritional effects on epigenetic gene regulation. *Molecular & Cell Biology, 23*(15), 5293–5300.

Wilson, R. D., SOGC Genetics Committee, Wilson, R. D., Audibert, F., Brock, J., Campagnolo, C., … Popa, V. (2014). Prenatal screening, diagnosis, and pregnancy management of fetal neural tube defects. *Journal of Obstetrics and Gynaecology Canada: JOGC [Journal D'obstétrique Et Gynécologie Du Canada: JOGC], 36*(10), 927–993.

Zabihi, S., & Loeken, M. R. (2010). Understanding diabetic teratogenesis: Where are we now and where are we going? *Birth Defects Research. Part A, Clinical and Molecular Teratology, 88*(10), 779–790.

Gastrointestinal System

Ann Gibbons Phalen

OVERVIEW

The primary functions of the gastrointestinal (GI) system are ingestion, absorption, and digestion of nutrients and elimination of waste products. These processes are dependent on a patent, structurally intact, and adequately functioning GI tract.

ANATOMY AND PHYSIOLOGY OF THE GASTROINTESTINAL SYSTEM

ANATOMIC DEVELOPMENT OF THE GI TRACT

The development of the human GI tract begins between the third and fourth fetal week and is essentially complete by the 20th fetal week. The GI tract develops in a cranial-to-caudal and ventral direction. The horseshoe-shaped tube that rises from the embryonic neural plate is divided into three distinct regions of the GI tract: the foregut, midgut, and hindgut.

The foregut forms the pharynx, esophagus, stomach, liver, gallbladder, pancreas, and the proximal duodenum, and blood is supplied to the foregut by the celiac artery. Common anomalies associated with a disruption in foregut development include:

- Atresia of the esophagus
- Tracheoesophageal fistula (TEF)
- Pyloric stenosis

■ Duodenal atresia or stenosis

■ Biliary atresia

■ Annular pancreas

The midgut forms the lower (caudal) portion of the duodenum, jejunum, ileum, appendix, ascending colon, and first two thirds of the transverse colon, and blood is supplied to the midgut by the superior mesenteric artery. Midgut development is characterized by rapid elongation of the gut and associate mesentery. Midgut development involves four stages:

■ Herniation—loops of intestines protrude into the umbilical cord (around the 7th fetal week)

■ Rotation—rotates in a counterclockwise fashion about 90° at the same time of herniation

■ Retraction—after sufficient expansion of the abdominal cavity, the loops of intestines retract back into the abdomen and rotate again in a counterclockwise fashion another 180° (around the 10th fetal week)

■ Fixation—once in proper placement, the mesentery attaches to the posterior abdominal wall

Common anomalies associated with a disruption in midgut development include:

■ Omphalocele, gastroschisis, umbilical hernia, intestinal stenosis atresia malrotation.

The hindgut is the precursor of the distal one third of the transverse colon, the descending colon, the rectum, and the urogenital sinus. Blood is supplied to the hindgut by the inferior mesenteric artery. Common anomalies associated with a disruption in hindgut development include:

■ Urorectal septal defects—when the descent of the urorectal septum is arrested and the cloaca persists

■ Lower anorectal defects such as imperforate anus

■ Anal agenesis

■ Hirschsprung disease

PHYSIOLOGIC DEVELOPMENT OF THE GI SYSTEM

Development of the digestive and liver enzyme systems as well as the absorptive surfaces of the intestines begin in fetal life and mature during the postnatal period. By 33 to 34 weeks gestation processes needed for adequate enteral nutrition are in place.

During postnatal maturation of GI development and function, certain factors can influence GI development, which include:

- Genetic factors
- Intrinsic timing mechanisms
- Initiation of feeding
- Type of feeding
- Composition of diet
- Hormonal regulatory mechanisms
- Gut trophic factors such as nutrients, hormones, and peptides

Meconium

Meconium is first seen around 10 to 12 fetal weeks and moves into the colon around the 16th fetal week. It is found in amniotic fluid in small amounts during the second trimester until development of the anal sphincter function around 20 to 22 fetal weeks. In the postnatal period, meconium is an essential step in initiation of intestinal function. It consists of vernix, lanugo, squamous epithelial cells, occult blood, bile, and other intestinal secretions. It is initially sterile, but within 24 hours bacteria is present. Most healthy full-term newborns will pass meconium within 48 hours of delivery, although premature infants without GI disease may not pass meconium for several days. In premature infants who are ill and not receiving enteral feedings, passage of meconium may be further delayed.

Swallowing

Swallowing begins around 10 to 14 fetal weeks; by the 16th fetal week, the fetus swallows 2 to 6 mL of amniotic fluid/day and increases to approximately 500 to 1,000 mL/day by term. Twenty percent of fluid swallowed during this period is lung fluid. Failure to adequately swallow amniotic fluid is associated with polyhydramnios and GI obstruction.

Swallowing is typically well developed by 28 to 30 weeks; however, premature infants born between 30 and 35 weeks do not have the endurance of the term infant. The gag reflex presents by 18 weeks but is not complete until around 34 weeks. Air and milk swallowed compete for space in the neonate's stomach, leading to regurgitation.

Sucking

All components of suck–swallow–breathe are present by 28 weeks; however, coordination of these activities is warranted for safe enteral feedings to occur. Maturation of sucking is related to gestational age and not postnatal age.

There are two types of sucking, nonnutritive sucking (NNS) and nutritive sucking (NS), which is most efficient after 32 to 34 weeks. Sucking stimulates secretion of GI regulatory peptides and enhances gastric emptying.

There are three stages of the suck–swallow pattern:

■ Mouthing—no effective suck
■ Immature pattern—short burst and not synchronized with swallowing
■ Mature pattern—long burst, coordinated swallowing, and propulsive peristaltic waves in the esophagus

Esophageal motility

In the esophagus, food is moved by peristaltic waves initiated by impulses from autonomic nerves (enteric nervous system [ENS]) and coordinated by the swallowing center in the medulla. Esophageal motility and muscle tone are decreased during the first 3 postnatal days.

When the contractions begin, the lower esophageal sphincter (LES) relaxes, allowing food to pass from the esophagus into the stomach. The LES forms a pressure barrier between the esophagus and stomach to prevent reflux. In neonates, the length of the LES is reduced (located primarily above the diaphragm) increasing the chance of reflux. LES tone develops rapidly during the first week of life, though the sphincter remains immature for 6 to 12 months.

Gastric emptying

Gastric emptying is delayed in neonates, especially during the first 3 postnatal days. Factors that influence gastric emptying include:

■ Muscle tone—low tone delays emptying

■ Mucus—delays emptying

■ Pyloric sphincter tone

■ Presence of amniotic fluid

■ Gastrin level—an elevated level leads to delayed emptying

■ Hormones

Types of nutrients can also influence gastric emptying time as follows:

■ Carbohydrates—increase emptying time

■ Fats—decrease emptying time

■ Medium-chain triglycerides (MCT) empty faster than long-chain triglycerides (LCT)

■ Human milk empties twice as fast as formula

■ High caloric formula—take longer to empty than regular formula

Intestinal motility

In the intestines, peristaltic waves continue to propel food from the stomach toward the small intestines. Once in the small intestines, contractions become more oscillatory to promote the absorptive and digestive processes.

In the premature neonate, both the intestinal musculature and motor mechanisms are immature, which result in irregular peristaltic activity and disorganized patterns. Disorganized movements of this nature lead to:

■ Decreased ability to clear upper gut

■ Decreased absorptive function

■ Prolonged transit time in upper intestine

■ More rapid emptying of the ileum and colon

The immature surface of small intestines of the premature infant reduces absorption of important nutrients; however, as gestational age increases, so does the number of intestinal villi and epithelial cells, thereby improving absorption. Enteral feedings after birth promote epithelial hyperplasia, increase cell turnover, and stimulate production of pancreatic lipase, amylase, and trypsin. Colostrum and human milk also contain factors that stimulate cell turnover and maturation, whereas ischemia, anoxia, and infection have a negative impact on the surface area of small intestines.

THE GI SYSTEM AND IMMUNITY

The neonate's gut is exposed to bacteria and antigens, and complex immune and nonimmune host defenses are present that serve to enhance the neonate's immune response. Factors that enhance GI immunity include:

■ Efficient motility prevents colonization of bacteria in the lumen of the gut

■ Early enteral nutrition stimulates the release of gastric acid and pancreaticobiliary secretions that inhibit bacterial growth and activate proteolysis

■ Mucus lining of the gut provides a protective barrier to larger bacterial molecules

■ Epithelial cells, goblet cells, M cells, and subepithelial cells retard cellular penetration of large macromolecules and the delivery of micro-organisms to lymphoid tissue

■ Cytokines stimulate chemotaxis of neutrophils and promotion of IgA expression after mucosal injury

■ Human milk contains substances that protect the gut from infection as well as enhance maturation of the system

■ Certain cells, immunonutrients, probiotics, and prebiotics also play a role in the immune defense of the neonatal gut

ASSESSMENT OF THE GI TRACT

PRENATAL ASSESSMENT OF THE GI TRACT

In prenatal assessment of the GI tract, it is important to review family history for genetic or congenital anomalies. Some GI disorders are related to chromosomal and single-gene defects or exist as part of a multisystem syndrome. Examples include:

■ Apert syndrome—cleft palate, pyloric stenosis

■ Trisomy 13—cleft lip and/or palate, omphalocele, malrotation

■ Trisomy 18—cleft lip and/or palate, omphalocele, malrotation, pyloric stenosis

■ Trisomy 21—VACTERL VATER (vertebral defects, anal atresia, tracheoesophageal fistula with esophageal atresia, and radial and renal dysplasia) association, duodenal atresia, TEF, Hirschsprung disease

■ Cystic fibrosis—occurs in 95% of cases of meconium ileus

In prenatal assessment of the GI tract, ultrasonography is best performed during the second and third trimester. Ultrasonography is of particular value in the following assessments:

■ To survey the abdominal wall

■ To observe insertion of the umbilical cord

■ To visualize the fluid-filled stomach

■ To observe for bowel dilation

■ To survey for abnormal echolucencies that resemble cysts but are abnormal collections of fluid within the bowel, secondary to obstruction

■ To visualize, if possible, facial features—noting clefts or other abnormalities

■ To evaluate for the presence of polyhydramnios—indicative of a high defect in the GI tract

POSTNATAL ASSESSMENT OF THE GI TRACT

In postnatal assessment of the GI tract, it is particularly important to note three cardinal signs indicating a possible GI obstruction: persistent vomiting, abdominal distention, and failure to pass meconium.

With persistent vomiting, the following should be noted:

■ Bile-stained vomiting can indicate the point of obstruction is distal to the ampulla of VATER.

■ Nonbilious vomiting can indicate the point of obstruction is proximal to the ampulla of VATER.

Failure to pass meconium within the first 48 hours after birth can indicate obstruction of the large intestines.

PHYSICAL ASSESSMENT OF THE GI TRACT

In physical assessment of the GI tract, direct visualization is a hallmark, as many GI defects are evident in the following:

■ Oral-facial structures: Inspect position, size, shape, symmetry, integrity of the mouth, lips, palate, and uvula.

■ Abdomen: Inspect the overall abdomen for contour, symmetry, and integrity as well as distention and surface color, as the presence of visible peristalsis accompanied by vomiting or distention can be a sign of obstruction. Inspect the umbilical cord for size, shape, and the insertion site.

■ Anus: Examine the anus for presence and position and inspect the perineal area for fistulas. Do not insert a rectal thermometer to assess rectal patency, as this increases the risk of perforating the rectum. If indicated, a digital examination is performed using a gloved small finger.

- Bowel sounds: Bowel sounds are initially absent; however, as the neonate swallows air and peristaltic activity is initiated, bowel sounds become audible within the first 30 minutes of life. In assessing bowel sounds, note the following:

  - Bowel sounds have a metallic tinkling quality and occur two to five times per minute.

  - Bowel sounds can be hyperdynamic or absent in a normal examination.

  - Hyperdynamic sounds along with distention and vomiting should be concerning signs and require further evaluation.

Palpation of the abdomen is best performed on a quiet infant lying in the supine position and within the first 24 hours. The abdominal musculature is most lax at this time. Holding an infant's knees and hips in a flexed position helps facilitate relaxation of the musculature.

Palpation is best done gently with a warmed hand using the pads of the fingers; this helps to avoid stressing the infant, resulting in a transient elevation of systolic and diastolic pressures.

- Liver: Palpate the liver by placing the index finger in the area of the right groin and advancing slowly upward until the liver edge is felt. Note normal/abnormal findings:

  - Normal findings—the organ is firm, but not hard, and the sharp edge is 1 to 2 cm below the right costal margin and can be followed across the abdomen into the left upper quadrant.

  - Abnormal findings—the organ is hard and enlarged. When the liver edge is greater than 3.5 cm in a newborn, this is considered hepatomegaly (Wolf & Lavine, 2000). In infants, the most common causes of hepatomegaly are infection and biliary obstruction.

- Spleen: Palpate the spleen using the same technique as that used for the liver. In most instances, the spleen cannot be palpated. If palpable, one should feel only the size of a small fingertip.

- Kidneys: Locate the kidneys in the flank areas above the level of the umbilicus; normally 4.5 to 5 cm in length in the term infant. Palpate the kidneys as follows:
  - Bimanual palpation—one hand is placed posterior, supporting the flank area, while the thumb or a finger of the free hand moves anterior over the same area
  - Single-hand palpation—the fingers of one hand support the flank posterior, while the thumb of the same hand moves anterior over the same area

RELATED FINDINGS IN ASSESSMENT OF THE GI TRACT

- Respiratory difficulties:
  - Can occur secondary to the infant's inability to handle excessive oral secretions or aspiration of gastric content associated with a TEF.
  - Abdominal distention can compromise diaphragmatic excursion, resulting in respiratory distress.
  - Frank airway obstruction can occur in an infant with a cleft palate as inspiratory pressures pull the tongue into the hypopharynx, causing obstruction.
- Jaundice: Occurs when the excretion of bilirubin is impeded from such problems as biliary atresia, Hirschsprung disease, intestinal atresias, and meconium ileus.
- Systemic hypertension: Rare, but occurs when a mass or significant distention increases intra-abdominal pressure.

REFERENCE

Wolf, A. D., & Lavine, J. E. (2000). Hepatomegaly in neonates and children. *Pediatrics in Review, 21*(9), 303–310.

DIAGNOSTIC PROCEDURES FOR EVALUATION OF THE GI TRACT

A number of various diagnostic tools are used to evaluate a neonate when a GI problem is suspected, including various radiographic studies, ultrasonography, testing of various bodily substances, and others.

■ Radiography: Includes x-ray, upper GI series, and contrast enema.

■ X-ray: Useful in the diagnosis of an obstruction, since air serves as a naturally occurring contrast medium. Within 30 minutes of birth, air should be seen in the stomach; within 3 to 4 hours, air is seen in the small bowel; and by 6 to 8 hours, the entire colon and rectum should be filled with air. When an obstruction is present, air is not seen in the intestine distal to the obstruction. However, the infant continues to swallow air; therefore, the area proximal to the obstruction becomes distended and is seen as dramatic radiolucent (black) bubbles on x-ray.

  ▨ Esophageal and intestinal atresias, often diagnosed with flat and upright radiographic views of the chest and abdomen.

  ▨ Cross-table lateral views are helpful in identifying air in the rectum of infants with intestinal obstructions.

  ▨ A left lateral decubitus view assists in determining the presence of free air in the peritoneal cavity, for example, in the case of necrotizing enterocolitis (NEC).

■ Upper GI series (radiographic study): Assists in the diagnosis of pyloric stenosis and malrotation, although it is not reliable in the diagnosis of gastroesophageal reflux (GER) as it only measures a brief window of time. In the upper GI series procedure, the following occurs:

  ▨ The infant receives nothing by mouth (NPO) for 4 to 6 hours prior to the study.

  ▨ The study uses contrast material, such as barium or Gastrografin. This is swallowed or administered via a naso/orogastric (NG/OG) tube and observed by fluoroscopy as it travels through the digestive tract (Gastrografin is preferred when perforation is suspected since it is a water-soluble solution [Kee, 2001]).

▣ The procedure can take as long as 4 hours, depending on the motility of the small intestine.

■ Contrast enema (radiographic study): Assists in the diagnosis of malrotation, Hirschsprung disease, meconium ileus, and meconium plug syndrome. In the contrast enema procedure, the following occurs:

▣ The study uses contrast material, such as barium or Gastrografin, and is instilled through the rectum.

▣ No specific preparation is necessary.

▣ Gentle saline enemas postprocedure may be used to help clear the barium and trapped air. If barium is allowed to harden, resulting in impaction, then more aggressive procedures are warranted for evacuation.

■ Ultrasonography: Used in the diagnosis of pyloric stenosis, enteric duplication, and biliary atresia, if the intrahepatic or proximal extrahepatic tract are dilated. Ultrasonography uses sound waves from the tissues and transforms them into scans, graphs, or audible sounds. In the ultrasonography procedure, conducting gel and a transducer are placed on the abdomen to identify the sound waves.

■ Gastric aspirate: Gastric aspirate is a point of care testing procedure that measures the pH of gastric content, which is obtained by inserting a premeasured feeding tube into the stomach. At least 1 mL of gastric content is withdrawn and sent to the laboratory for analysis.

■ Apt test: Differentiates neonatal blood loss from swallowed maternal blood. In this procedure, the following occurs:

▣ Bloody aspirate or bloody stool is collected and sent to the laboratory for analysis.

■ The bloody aspirate or stool is centrifuged in 5 mL of water. One part 0.25% sodium hydroxide is added to five parts supernatant.

■ If the fluid turns pink, it indicates fetal blood; if the fluid turns brown, it indicates maternal blood.

■ Stool culture: Used in cases of bloody diarrhea, where a stool culture helps to differentiate between an intestinal lining insult and an infection. In this procedure, a stool specimen is taken from a diaper, placed in a container, labeled, and sent to a laboratory for testing.

■ Stool hematest: The stool hematest is a rapid and convenient test to detect fecal occult blood. In this procedure, the following occurs:

■ Thin smear of stool is placed on guaiac paper and developer is applied over the smear. Results are read in 60 seconds.

■ Any blue colorization on or at the edge of the smear indicates a positive occult blood result.

■ Certain drugs can cause a false positive result, such as iron preparations, indomethacin, potassium preparations, salicylates, and steroids.

■ Large amounts of ascorbic acid may cause a false negative result.

■ Stool-reducing substances: Stool-reducing substances help in the detection of carbohydrate intolerance. In this procedure, the following occurs:

■ Stool specimen is taken from a diaper, placed in a container, labeled, and sent to a laboratory for testing.

■ A Clinitest tablet is added to the test tube containing the prepared supernatant; after 15 seconds it is gently shook. The color of the liquid is compared with the color chart on the Clinitest bottle.

▦ More than 0.5% glucose in the stool indicates an abnormal amount of sugar and carbohydrate intolerance should be suspected.

■ 24-hour pH monitoring: This diagnostic tool represents the gold standard used to diagnose gastroesophageal reflux disease (GERD). In this procedure, the following occurs:

▦ A thin, flexible pH probe is inserted into the distal esophagus for a 24-hour period.

▦ The test records the amount of time the esophagus is exposed to an acidic pH level. It measures the time, duration (should be < 4 minutes of exposure), frequency of reflux, time of longest episode, and the percentage of time the infant was having reflux during the 24-hour period.

▦ Formula feedings may obscure episodes of reflux by buffering the gastric acid.

▦ Results can be compromised by such factors as infant position during the study, activity, frequency, and composition of feedings and medications.

▦ The nursing role is to document time of feedings, feeding composition, and medications administered during the study, as well as the position and activity of the infant throughout the study.

■ Scintigraphy: Used to measure gastric emptying, aspiration with swallowing, and reflux with aspiration. In this procedure, the infant is fed a radionucleotide-tagged formula—a technetium radioisotope is added to formula and has relatively low radiation.

■ Endoscopy: Assists in the diagnosis of esophagitis. In this procedure, flexible endoscopy with biopsy of the distal esophagus can detect basal cell hyperplasia, increased stromal papillary length, and the presence of intraepithelial eosinophils.

■ Fecal fat: Used to screen for the presence of malabsorption. Fecal fat content greater than 6 g/24 hours is predictive of malabsorption syndrome. It should be noted that small stool samples can cause false test results.

■ Chromosomal studies: Such studies may be indicated if a GI anomaly is found with other multisystem abnormalities.

REFERENCE

Kee, J. L. (2001). *Laboratory and diagnostic tests with nursing implications* (4th ed.). Upper Saddle River, NJ: Prentice Hall.

COMMON NURSING MANAGEMENT INTERVENTIONS RELATED TO GI SYSTEM ALTERATIONS

A variety of nursing procedures and interventions are used in the management and treatment of GI system alterations and include the following:

■ Gastric decompression: Prevents aspiration, respiratory compromise, and perforation. In this procedure, the following occurs:

   ▪ OG/NG tube is connected to low intermittent suction.

   ▪ Tube patency should be maintained to ensure proper tube functioning.

   ▪ Tube should be irrigated with 2 mL of air every 2 to 4 hours.

   ▪ There are several types of OG/NG tubes including the 8 or 10 French red rubber tube and the 10 French soft vinyl, double-lumen gastric sump tube.

■ Fluid and electrolytes balance: Vomiting, diarrhea, gastric drainage, and the shifting of fluids from the vascular bed into the interstitial compartment can lead to dehydration, hypovolemia, hypoperfusion, and electrolyte abnormalities. The treatment goal is to maintain fluid and electrolyte balance; this includes the following:

   ▪ Maintenance fluids: 60 to 80 mL/kg for the first 24 hours

   ▪ Increase daily by 10 mL/kg/day or as needed to 120 to 160 mL/kg/day

■ Monitor urine output: 1 to 2 mL/kg/hr; adjust fluids to maintain urine output

In patients at risk for increased sodium and potassium losses, it is important to:

■ Provide sodium at a rate of 2 to 3 mEq/kg/day

■ Provide potassium at a rate of 2 mEq/kg/day

Increased gastric losses via NG/OG tube require replacement. In this procedure, the following occurs:

■ Measure drainage every 4 to 8 hours.

■ Replace the total volume of gastric output with one half normal saline with potassium chloride 10 to 20 mEq/L every 4 to 8 hours. Replacement fluids are in addition to maintenance fluids.

■ Metabolic alkalosis, metabolic acidosis, and respiratory acidosis can occur with gastric losses.

■ Metabolic alkalosis is associated with pyloric stenosis or high jejunal obstruction due to a loss of acidic gastric juice.

■ Metabolic acidosis occurs with obstructions in the distal segment of the small intestines because large quantities of alkaline fluids are lost.

■ Respiratory acidosis develops when there is abdominal distention because of carbon dioxide retention from hypoventilation.

■ Thermoregulation: In this procedure for patients with abdominal wall defects, the following should occur:

■ Monitor for heat loss, especially with abdominal wall defects due to exposed bowel.

■ Treatment should include providing an external heat source, covering the head, and monitoring temperature hourly.

■ In defects with exposed bowel, apply sterile warm saline soaks over the defect and use a bowel bag or plastic wrap from the feet to axilla.

■ Positioning: The heads-up position assists in reducing reflux of gastric content as follows:

■ In neonates with a tracheal esophageal fistula, this position reduces reflux of gastric content into the trachea via the distal fistula.

■ In neonates with GER, this position may reduce the reflux of gastric content.

In neonates with isolated esophageal atresia, the flat or head-down position assists in the gravity drainage of the esophageal pouch.

■ Prevention of infection: Note increased susceptibility for infection; use broad spectrum antibiotics for presumed infections.

■ Pain management: Pain is considered the fifth vital sign and needs to be monitored, particularly pre- and postoperative pain. It is important to use a valid pain assessment tool that assesses physiologic and behavioral cues of pain; pain should be assessed at regular intervals and interventions evaluated for effective relief.

■ Nonpharmacologic pain measures include the following:

- Containment when possible

- Positioning strategies

- Pacifier

- Skin-to-skin care when possible

■ Pharmacologic measures include opioids, such as morphine and fentanyl.

■ Nutrition: Meeting the nutritional needs of neonates preoperatively and postoperatively is challenging. Enteral feeding is not ordered in the preoperative period and then may be delayed by days or weeks in the postoperative period. Parenteral nutrition with hyperalimentation is ordered to meet the caloric and metabolic needs and is administered via a peripherally inserted central catheter (PICC) or a surgically inserted central catheter. Once enteral feeds are introduced, gradual advancement is warranted, as follows:

■ Start with elemental formula, such as Pregestimil, or human milk complemented with parenteral nutrition.

- Introduce small, frequent feedings or continuous feedings, and gradually advance as tolerated.
- The extent of bowel loss or severity of the defect will influence tolerance.
- Signs of intolerance include vomiting, diarrhea, abdominal distention, or presence of reducing substances in the stool.

■ General preoperative management: Principles of preoperative management include the following:

- Replacement of fluid losses
- Decompression of the distended bowel
- Support failing organ systems
- Maintain thermoregulation to prevent cold stress
- Maintain adequate oxygenation, ventilation, and acid–base balance
- Provide nutrition with parenteral nutrition
- Prevent infection through antibiotic therapy, covering both aerobic and anaerobic infections
- Pain management

■ General postoperative management: Includes the same principles as preoperative management as well as the following:

- Maintaining skin integrity postoperatively
- Providing ostomy care for infants with ostomies
- Monitoring for complications such as infections, respiratory distress, fluid and electrolyte imbalance, third spacing of fluids, skin breakdown, pain, short bowel syndrome, peritonitis, and intestinal obstructions related to adhesions, strictures, or volvulus

■ Ethical issues: Congenital malformations often have associated organ defects. Advice, treatment, and support require individual patient/family consideration and evaluation. In such instances, wishes of parents and the opinions of each member of the interprofessional team must be considered.

■ Family support: Family members of a neonate with a GI system disorder/anomaly experience grief, feelings of loss, guilt, and confusion. In these occurrences, communication is most important, in order to:

  ▨ Provide factual information about the disorder, prognosis, and plan of care

  ▨ Ensure communication with family members is frequent and reinforced

  ▨ Provide a supportive environment for parents to express their concerns

  ▨ Encourage parents to participate in care activities such as skin-to-skin holding, diapering, and feedings

  ▨ Prepare families for their infant's discharge early in the transition period and connect them with support services when indicated

SELECTED GASTROINTESTINAL PROBLEMS IN THE NEONATE

Two significant GI problems in the neonate are (a) cleft lip and palate and (b) GER/GERD.

CLEFT LIP AND PALATE

A cleft lip is a congenital fissure in the upper lip, whereas a cleft palate is a congenital fissure in either the soft palate alone or in both the hard and soft palate. The two conditions can occur as separate defects or together. They can be unilateral or bilateral. The most severe form is bilateral cleft lip and palate occurring together.

INCIDENCE

Cleft lip with or without an associated cleft palate reportedly occurs at a rate of one in 700 in different populations, depending on geographic location (Vieira, 2008). The occurrence is higher in males and in Asians. Isolated cleft palate has a lower incidence rate and occurs more frequently in females. Seventy percent of neonates with unilateral cleft lip and 85% of neonates with bilateral cleft lip will also have a cleft palate (Merritt, 2005). Ten percent of neonates with cleft lip and cleft palate will have an associated syndrome. In parents with a cleft lip/palate, the offspring has a 3% to 5% risk of being born with a cleft lip/palate. No single gene has been identified to explain clefts, but various mutations of at least 14 genes have been associated. Environmental factors also contribute to the development of clefts.

PATHOPHYSIOLOGY

Cleft lip and cleft palate are considered distinct embryologic disorders. Cleft lip occurs when the maxillary process fails to merge with the medial nasal elevation on one or both sides; cleft palate occurs when the lateral palatine processes fail to meet and fuse with each other, the primary palate, or the nasal septum. When both cleft lip and palate occur together, the failure of the secondary palate to close may be a developmental consequence of the abnormalities in the primary palate associated with the cleft lip rather than an intrinsic defect in the secondary palate.

Maternal conditions associated with clefting include smoking, alcohol use, diabetes, hypo/hypervitaminosis, and influenza and fever (Spritz, 2001). Antenatal exposure to certain medications are associated with clefting; these include benzodiazepines, phenytoin, opiates, penicillin, salicylates, cortisone, and high doses of vitamin A. Mothers taking folic acid reduce the risk of orofacial clefts by one third (Wilcox et al., 2007).

TREATMENT

Treatment of clefts includes an interprofessional team of health care providers and incorporates emotional support for parents, thorough history to identify etiology, and surgical repair.

Goals of surgical repair include minimizing maxillary growth retardation, limiting dental deformity, and allowing normal speech development. Cleft lip repair can occur around 3 months of age, although cleft palate repair is delayed to allow for medial movement of the palatal shelves. The hard palate is repaired around 14 to 16 months; soft palate repair occurs later, around 18 months. If further cosmetic repair of the lip is required, this occurs around 12 years of age.

Oral feedings require patience and attention to technique, as infants with a cleft are unable to create a vacuum for adequate sucking. In such instances, several techniques are identified to be successful.

■ Infant's cheeks are grasped to close the cleft.

■ Frequent burping occurs due to excessive amounts of air being swallowed.

■ Infant is positioned in an upright or semi-upright position to avoid choking.

■ The flow of milk is directed to the side of the mouth.

■ Use of a "squeeze" bottle, "preemie" nipple, or a special cleft palate nipple have been helpful.

■ Small volume and frequent feedings are used to prevent exhaustion and frustration.

■ Breastfeeding is possible and requires the support of a lactation counselor.

■ Some prosthetic devices are available to occlude the cleft; they are molded to the shape of the infant's mouth. The device is rinsed with water after feedings.

■ Milk does collect around the cleft. To prevent infection and excoriation, offer a small amount of sterile water after oral feedings.

PROGNOSIS

An excellent prognosis for survival is expected, although infants with clefts are at risk for and require close follow-up for language and speech delays, an associated hearing impairment, and dental problems such as malocclusions, irregularity of teeth, and dental caries.

Over 300 syndromes include cleft lip, cleft palate, or both, and may not be recognized in the early neonatal period. The prognosis can vary for infants with an associated anomaly.

In providing emotional support for parents, the informational website "About Face USA" (http://www.aboutfaceUSA.org) can be useful.

GER AND GERD

GER is defined as the physiologic retrograde of stomach content into the esophagus (Hibbs, 2015, p. 1371), whereas GERD is defined as the pathologic condition where this retrograde of fluid from the stomach into the esophagus causes medical complications (Hibbs, 2015, p. 1371).

INCIDENCE

Incidence is higher in premature infants born at less than 32 weeks of age, although 50% of healthy term infants will have symptomatic reflux at 2 months of age.

Incidence is higher in infants diagnosed with a neurologic disorder or inborn errors of metabolism, small bowel obstruction, or other intestinal anomalies.

PATHOPHYSIOLOGY

The esophagus enters the stomach at the angle of HIS (Montrowl, 2014, p. 203).

In premature neonates, the angle is decreased, thereby increasing the chance for reflux of gastric content into the esophagus. The distal portion of the esophagus has higher pressure than the proximal esophagus and stomach. The pressure helps prevent reflux of gastric content into the esophagus. However,

■ Lower esophageal pressure below gastric pressure allows for the retrograde of gastric content. This is often seen in the immature neonate.

■ Transient LES relaxations are often seen in the premature neonate, leading to reflux.

Poor gastric motility or emptying time contributes to GER (Hibbs, 2015, p. 1372). Neonates born with structural abnormalities can cause malposition of the esophagus or stomach and an increase of intra-abdominal pressure (Montrowl, 2014, p. 203).

CLINICAL PRESENTATION

The most common presentation with GER is vomiting. Regurgitation occurs with burping during a feeding or occurs 2 to 3 hours after feeding. The vomiting can be forceful.

Symptoms seen in infants with GERD include regurgitation, irritable behavior such as crying, arching or aversion to feeding, stridor, worsening lung disease, apnea, and bradycardia.

Insufficient evidence exists to confirm that GER causes apnea (Finer, Higgins, Kattwinkel, & Martin, 2006; Sherman et al., 2009). Insufficient evidence also exists to support the causality between GERD and bronchopulmonary dysplasia (BPD) (Sherman et al., 2009).

DIFFERENTIAL DIAGNOSIS

GER should be suspected in an otherwise healthy infant with post-prandial regurgitation.

Evaluate the neonate for other problems that cause reflux, such as sepsis, urea cycle defects, formula intolerance, increased intracranial pressure, drug toxicity, and hydronephrosis.

Consider an upper GI series to rule out other anatomic causes, such as esophageal stricture, esophageal webs, volvulus, meconium ileus/plug, peptic stricture, and esophageal dysmotility.

Diagnostic procedures include (Hibbs, 2015, p. 1373) contrast studies, esophageal pH studies, and nuclear medicine scintigraphy.

- Contrast studies: In general, these are not reliable and only measure a brief window of time, although they can be useful in ruling out anatomic abnormalities that mimic GERD.

- Esophageal pH studies: These require monitoring for 12 to 24 hours to provide data on the timing and frequency of GER events.

Esophageal pH probes measure acid reflux, and a pH < 4 indicates GER. Esophageal multichannel intraluminal impedance (MII-pH) detects the presence of fluid in the esophagus regardless of pH and assesses the direction of flow and the distance from the LES of each GER event. This can help determine the association between GER events and symptoms (Shin et al., 2012).

■ Nuclear medicine scintigraphy: Identifies postprandial reflux and aspiration and quantifies gastric emptying time. Age-specific norms have not been established in infants and therefore are not recommended as routine testing.

TREATMENT

Treatment for GER and GERD includes noninvasive/nonpharmacologic treatment options, pharmacologic options, and surgical options.

Noninvasive/nonpharmacologic treatment options: 75% of GERD can be treated using a medical management approach (Montrowl, 2014, p. 203) that includes small volume, frequent feedings, and positioning by elevating the head of the bed. Prone positioning is contraindicated because of the increased risk of sudden infant death (SID).

Thickening of feeding reduces clinical vomiting but not necessarily the physiologic measures of GER (Carroll, Garrison, & Christakis, 2002; Horvath, Dziechciarz, & Szajewska, 2008). Efficacy and safety of thickened feeds have not been well studied in the premature infant.

Thickening agents include rice, carob, cornstarch, locust-bean gum, and commercially prepared formulas. Risks associated with thickening agents include diarrhea, increased cough, poor growth, and malabsorption (Horvath et al., 2008).

Pharmacologic options (Hibbs, 2015, pp. 1374 to 1375): Drug therapy may be considered in neonates with chronic irritability or failure to thrive. Presently, insufficient evidence exists for either the efficacy or safety of pharmacologic interventions in the treatment of GERD in the neonatal population.

Histamine-2 (H_2) receptor antagonists suppress HCL production and therefore decrease gastric acidity. This action protects the esophageal mucosa from acid injury and the development of esophagitis. Examples include ranitidine, cimetidine, and famotidine. Risks include late-onset sepsis, NEC, and bradyarrhythmias.

Proton pump inhibitors (PPIs) inhibit the action of the acid pump. Examples are omeprazole, lansoprazole, dexlansoprazole, esomeprazole, pantoprazole, and rabeprazole. No PPIs are currently labeled for use in infants younger than 1 year of age, though their use in infants has increased exponentially.

Drugs to improve GI motility—the idea is if gastric emptying is increased or esophageal motility and LES are improved, then there is a decrease in GER. Examples are metoclopramide and erythromycin. Cisapride and domperidone can cause serious cardiac arrhythmias and QT prolongation (Djeddi et al., 2008) and should not be used in infants.

Surgical options (Montrowl, 2014, pp. 204–205): Several gastric fundoplication techniques can be considered for neonates with life-threatening GERD when other management therapies have failed. These include:

- Nissen's fundoplication—stomach is wrapped 360° around the distal esophagus.

- Thal's fundoplication—stomach is wrapped 270°, which may decrease gastric distention of the stomach.

The wrap increases the pressure in the lower esophagus and acts as a one-way valve. Often a gastrostomy tube is inserted to ensure adequate nutrition and provide a vent for gas. Procedures are performed laparoscopically, allowing for better recovery during the postoperative period and decrease in the length of hospitalization. Postoperative complications include:

- Bleeding and irritation at the site of the gastrostomy tube
- Leaking around the site
- Gaseous distention of the stomach
- Retching and difficulty swallowing

- Failure or overtightness of the wrap
- Delayed gastric emptying
- Hiatal herniation
- Revision of the fundoplication may be indicated, especially in cases of infants with TEF, congenital diaphragmatic hernia, and neurologic disorders

Postoperative care: In most cases, enteral feedings can be reestablished within 24 hours.

Proper fit of the gatrostomy tube and intragastric and transabdominal seals must be provided as follows:

- Tube must fit closely against the stomach wall.
- If a balloon is present, the volume of water used to inflate the balloon is documented.
- Regularly measure the length of the tube that is visible on the outside.
- Evaluate for leaking—common causes are either evaporation of water from the balloon or failure of the transabdominal seal.
- Family education is important in care of the postoperative patient.

PROGNOSIS ASSOCIATED WITH GERD

There are some risks associated with the prognosis of GERD, most notably the aspiration of gastric content into the lungs, which can cause pneumonia. Severe GERD can lead to failure to thrive, esophagitis, anemia, esophageal strictures, and inflammatory esophageal polyps.

Seventy-five percent of GERD patients will recover with medical treatment (Montrowl, 2014, p. 203), although 10% to 15% will require long-term medical treatment. When symptoms are controlled by medical management, reflux ceases by 15 months of age and therapy can be discontinued. Between 10% and 15% will require surgery; however, long-term surgical results are good (Salminen, Hurme, & Ovaska, 2012).

REFERENCES

Carroll, A. E., Garrison, M. M., & Christakis, D. A. (2002). A systematic review of nonpharmacological and nonsurgical therapies for gastroesophageal reflux in infants. *Archives of Pediatrics and Adolescent Medicine, 156*(2), 109–113.

Djeddi, D., Kongolo, G., Lefaix, C., Mounard, J., & Leke, A. (2008). Effect of domperidone on QT interval in neonates. *Journal of Pediatrics, 153*(5), 663–666.

Finer, N. N., Higgins, R., Kattwinkel, J., & Martin, R. J. (2006). Summary proceedings from the apnea-of-prematurity group. *Pediatrics, 117*(Pt 2), S47–S51.

Hibbs, A. M. (2015). Gastroesophageal reflux and gastroesophageal reflux disease in the neonate. In R. J. Martin, A. A. Fanaroff, & M. C. Walsh (Eds.), *Fanaroff and Martin's neonatal-perinatal medicine* (10th ed., pp. 1371–1378). Philadelphia, PA: Elsevier/Saunders.

Horvath, A., Dziechciarz, P., & Szajewska, H. (2008). The effect of thickened-feed interventions on gastroesophageal reflux in infants. *Pediatrics, 122*(6), e1268–e1277.

Merritt, L. (2005). Part 1: Understanding the embryology and genetics of cleft lip and palate. *Advances in Neonatal Care, 5*(2), 64–71.

Montrowl, S. (2014). Gastrointestinal system. In C. Kenner & J. W. Lott (Eds.), *Comprehensive neonatal nursing care* (5th ed., pp. 189–228). New York, NY: Springer Publishing Company.

Salminen, P., Hurme, S., & Ovaska, J. (2012). Fifteen-year outcome of laparoscopic and open nissen fundoplication: A randomized clinical trial. *Annals of Thoracic Surgery, 93*(1), 228–233.

Sherman, P. M., Hassall, E., Fagundes-Neto, U., Gold, B. D., Kato, S., Koletzko, S., Orenstein, S., … Vandenplas, Y. (2009). A global evidence-based consensus on the definition of gastroesophageal reflux disease in the pediatric population. *American Journal of Gastroenterology, 104*(5), 1278–1295.

Shin, M. S., Shim, J. O., Moon, J. S., Kim, H. S., Ko, J. S., Choi, J. H., & Seo, J. K. (2012). *Journal of Maternal-Fetal and Neonatal Medicine, 25*(11), 2406–2410.

Spritz, R. (2001). The genetics and epigenetics of orofacial clefts. *Current Opinions in Pediatrics, 13*(6), 556–560.

Vieira, A. R. (2008). Unraveling human cleft lip and palate research. *Journal of Dental Research, 87*(2), 119–125.

Wilcox, A. J., Lie, R. T., Solvoll, K., Taylor, J., McConnaughey, D. R., Abyholm, F., … Drevon, C. A. (2007). Folic acid supplements and risk of facial clefts: National population based case-control study. *British Medical Journal*, *25*(3), 334–464.

ADDITIONAL CHAPTER REFERENCE

Blackburn, S. T. (2013). Gastrointestinal and hepatic systems and perinatal nutrition. In S. T. Blackburn (Ed.), *Maternal, fetal and neonatal physiology: A clinical perspective* (4th ed., pp. 408–423). Maryland Heights, MO: Elsevier/ Saunders.

Renal System

Leslie A. Parker

OVERVIEW

The renal and urinary system consists of the kidneys, ureters, urinary bladder, and the urethra. The kidney regulates fluid and electrolyte balance, maintains arterial blood pressure, and excretes toxic and waste substances. These regulatory mechanisms are intimately tied to the formation of urine that involves three basic processes: ultrafiltration of plasma by the glomerulus, reabsorption of water and solutes from the ultrafiltrate, and secretion of certain solutes into the tubular fluid.

ANATOMY AND PHYSIOLOGY

The nephron, the functional unit of the kidney, is the site of urine formation. It consists of a glomerulus (Bowman's capsule and glomerular capillaries) and a renal tubule that has three sections: a proximal convoluted tubule, the loop of Henle, and a distal convoluted tubule. After urine is produced by the nephron, it drains into the minor and major calyces, then into the renal pelvis, out through the ureter, and into the bladder.

As blood flows into the kidney via the renal artery, it is directed into the afferent arteriole and carried into the glomerulus. Plasma driven through the glomerular capillaries is filtered and the protein-free plasma (ultrafiltrate) is forced into the Bowman's capsule or leaves via the efferent arteriole and enters into the renal vein. To produce ultrafiltrate, the glomerulus functions as a filtering site.

The glomerular filtration rate (GFR) is the rate at which fluid is filtered through the glomerulus and reflects kidney function. Oncotic and hydrostatic pressures (Starling forces) drive the ultrafiltration process. Oncotic pressure is osmotic pressure generated by large proteins or colloids. Hydrostatic pressure is pressure exerted by fluids in equilibrium and depends on arterial pressure and vascular resistance. GFR is, therefore, affected by changes in arterial blood pressure, vascular resistance, concentration of plasma proteins, and glomerular capillary permeability.

The kidneys control fluid and electrolyte balance by reabsorption and secretion of sodium and water. The four segments of the nephron, the proximal tubule, loop of Henle, distal tubule, and the collecting duct, determine the composition and volume of urine.

Tubular reabsorption, secretion, and excretion are closely tied together and function in maintenance of internal homeostasis and regulation of fluids and electrolytes. Tubular reabsorption is the process where substances from the tubular lumen move into the capillary system through simple diffusion and active transport. Many of the body's nutrients, electrolytes, and 99% of the filtered water are reabsorbed. Tubular secretion moves substances such as potassium and hydrogen from the epithelial lining of the tubules' capillaries into the interstitial fluid and finally into the tubular lumen. Tubular excretion is the process where substances enter the filtrate that will eventually exit the body as urine. Ions such as potassium, which are secreted in the distal tubule (a portion is also reabsorbed in the proximal tubule), find their way into the urine when the body has no need for higher concentration levels.

URINARY TRACT INFECTION

INCIDENCE

- 0.1% to 2% in all newborns
- 20% in preterm and high-risk infants

- More common in males, potentially due to an increased risk in uncircumcised males
- Increased risk in infants with a neurogenic bladder

PHYSIOLOGY

Urinary tract infections (UTIs) are defined as an infection of the kidney and/or bladder. Infection occurring in the kidney is called pyelonephritis, while infection of the bladder is cystitis. If not properly treated, UTIs can result in long-term sequelae including decreased renal function, renal scarring, and hypertension.

PATHOPHYSIOLOGY

The bacteria most commonly responsible for UTIs include *Escherichia coli, Klebsiella, Pseudomonas, Proteus, Enterococcus, Staphylococcus*, and *Candida*. UTIs commonly occur in conjunction with systemic sepsis.

ASSESSMENT

While a UTI can be an isolated occurrence, it can also be associated with systemic infection or an underlying abnormality of the urinary tract system.

CLINICAL MANIFESTATIONS/DIAGNOSIS

The diagnosis of a UTI is based on history, physical exam, and laboratory findings, as well as urine Gram stain and culture.

Physical exam

- Symptoms may be nonspecific, especially during the first 1 to 2 months of life
- Temperature instability, poor feeding, cyanosis, abdominal distention, poor weight gain, hepatomegaly, jaundice, and fever
- Protein, blood, nitrites, or leukocytes on urine dipstick

Diagnostic procedures/tests

- Elevated or decreased white blood cell count with a left shift
- Elevated C-reactive protein (CRP)
- Positive leukocytes or nitrites on urinalysis
- Bacteria present on Gram stain and/or culture obtained by suprapubic aspiration or sterile bladder catheterization prior to initiation of antibiotics
  - Never use a bagged urine specimen because of contamination risk
  - Any bacteria obtained from a suprapubic aspiration is diagnostic
  - More than 10^5 colony-forming units (CFUs) obtained from a catheterization is diagnostic
- Obtain a blood culture due to high risk of systemic infection

TREATMENT

- Antibiotic therapy:
  - Empiric broad-spectrum intravenous (IV) antibiotic therapy
  - Adjust antibiotics as needed following identification of infective organisms on culture and specification of sensitivities
  - Continue antibiotic therapy for 7 to 14 days IV
  - Obtain repeat urine culture 48 to 72 hours following initiation of treatment
- Renal ultrasound is used to assess for hydronephrosis, renal scarring, severe vesico-urethral reflux, or obstructive uropathy.
- A voiding cystourethrogram (VCUG) is performed after the first UTI if the ultrasound is abnormal.
- VCUG is performed for any subsequent UTIs.
- Nonpharmacologic interventions including sucrose nipples, swaddling, and nonnutritive sucking may be helpful for associated pain and discomfort.

■ Symptoms of a UTI should be included in the discharge instructions and parents should be instructed to seek medical care immediately if symptoms occur.

PROGNOSIS

Prompt treatment is imperative to prevent complications including renal scarring that can lead to hypertension or permanent kidney failure. With prompt diagnosis and treatment, the prognosis is generally excellent for isolated UTIs. The prognosis of UTIs associated with renal abnormalities is dependent on the severity and type of underlying abnormality.

ACUTE RENAL FAILURE

INCIDENCE

■ 24% of neonates admitted to the neonatal intensive care unit (NICU)
■ May be underestimated
■ Associated with significant mortality and morbidity

PHYSIOLOGY

Acute renal failure (ARF) occurs when the GFR abruptly decreases or completely ceases, leading to impairment in fluid and electrolyte regulation and acid–base homeostasis. Any condition that interferes with normal kidney function can cause acute kidney injury.

PATHOPHYSIOLOGY

ARF can be classified as prerenal, intrinsic, or postrenal. Prerenal failure, the most common type, accounts for 75% to 80% of cases and is due to inadequate perfusion to a normal kidney. Failure to adequately treat prerenal failure can result in permanent kidney damage.

Intrinsic renal failure (IRF) results from damage to the renal parenchyma and can occur due to progression of either prerenal or postrenal failure, infection, renal vein thrombosis, and nephrotoxicity from medications. Acute tubular necrosis (ATN) is the most common cause of IRF and results from renal tubular cellular injury due to severe hypoxia, dehydration, sepsis, or blood loss. Other causes of IRF include structural abnormalities of the kidney such as renal dysplasia and polycystic or multicystic kidney disease.

Postrenal failure is caused by obstruction of the urinary tract. Obstruction can be caused by posturethral valves, ureteropelvic and ureterovesical junction obstruction, prune-belly syndrome, and neurogenic bladder. Backflow of urine into the kidney pelvis can cause damage to the renal parenchyma.

ASSESSMENT

Any infant with a history of asphyxia and those born prematurely should be considered at high risk for ARF and should undergo a thorough assessment. The severity of ARF is related to the underlying etiology.

CLINICAL MANIFESTATIONS/DIAGNOSIS

The diagnosis of ARF is based upon history, physical exam, and laboratory analysis.

Physical exam findings

■ Urine output less than 1 mL/kg/hr, which is a cardinal sign

■ Infants with nonoliguric renal failure, who may have a normal or high urine output

■ Edema

■ Hypertension

■ Possible flank mass, abnormal genitalia, or other genitourinary (GU) abnormalities

Laboratory findings

- Elevated blood urea nitrogen (BUN) and creatinine levels
- Hyperphosphatemia, hyponatremia, metabolic acidosis, and hypocalcemia
- Hematuria and proteinuria on urine dipstick and urinalysis
- A urine-to-plasma osmolality ratio ≤ 1:1

Diagnostic procedures/tests

- Family, prenatal, perinatal, and postnatal history
  - Prenatal ultrasound results
  - Amniotic fluid measurements
  - History of perinatal depression, conditions associated with decreased renal blood flow, and administration of nephrotoxic medications
- Administration of 10 to 20 mg/kg of an IV isotonic solution may be used to differentiate between prerenal and IRF
  - Urine output of at least 1 mL/kg/hr within 2 hours suggests prerenal failure.
  - Diuretic administration following the fluid challenge may be necessary.
- A FeNa (fractional excretion of sodium) greater than 3% and a renal failure index less than 3% suggest prerenal failure
  - Only accurate after 48 hours following delivery
- Placement of a urinary catheter can diagnose postrenal failure
- Renal ultrasound to evaluate the etiology of intrinsic and postrenal failure

TREATMENT

Prerenal failure

- Increase renal perfusion through administration of intravascular fluids and possibly low-dose dopamine.

Intrinsic renal failure

- Limit fluid administration to replacement of insensible water losses, other fluid losses, and urine output
- Carefully calculate fluid intake, electrolytes, and urine output
- Monitor for signs of infection
- Assess vital signs, including blood pressure
- Monitor for complications related to electrolyte abnormalities
- Treat hyponatremia with additional sodium administration
- Treat hyperphosphatemia
    - Phosphorus restriction
    - Oral calcium carbonate which binds phosphate and prevents absorption
- Treat hypocalcemia with calcium supplementation
- Treat hyperkalemia
    - Eliminate or severely limit potassium intake
    - Use sodium bicarbonate and a combination of insulin and dextrose
        - Drives potassium from the intracellular into the extracellular space
    - Use IV calcium for cardiac protection
    - Use kayexalate to increase elimination
- Treat metabolic acidosis
    - IV sodium acetate
    - Oral or IV sodium bicarbonate
- Treat anemia due to decreased production and release of erythropoietin
- Treat hypertension with sodium/fluid restriction and antihypertensives
- Limit renally excreted medication and monitor levels carefully

■ Promote adequate nutrition

    ■ Limit protein to 1 to 2 g/kg/d

    ■ Restrict fluid administration

    ■ Consider Similac PM 60/40 (Ross Laboratories, Columbus, OH), SMA (Wyeth, Madison, NJ), or breast milk to limit sodium, potassium, and phosphorous

■ Dialysis may be indicated in the following situations:

    ■ Continued clinical deterioration

    ■ High BUN, creatinine, and ammonia levels

    ■ Severe hyperkalemia, metabolic acidosis, hypocalcemia, and hyperphosphatemia

    ■ Volume overload and malnutrition

Postrenal failure

■ Relief of urinary obstruction

■ Correction of underlying condition

PROGNOSIS

Early recognition and treatment of ARF may prevent further renal failure and improve outcome. Prognosis is related to severity of the underlying disease and the ability to treat the underlying problem. ARF increases mortality and is associated with short- and long-term complications including renal dysfunction and hypertension.

HYDRONEPHROSIS

INCIDENCE

■ The most common renal abnormality detected prenatally

■ Present in 2.3% of all pregnancies

PATHOPHYSIOLOGY

Hydronephrosis is the accumulation of urine within the renal pelvis and calices, causing overdistention that can cause irreversible kidney damage. It can be caused by obstruction of urine flow at the junction of the ureteropelvis, the ureterovesical valve, or the urethrovesical valve. Nonobstructive abnormalities such as vesicourethral reflux and prune-belly syndrome as well as obstruction from kidney stones or tumors can also result in hydronephrosis. Severity is classified from grade I to grade V depending on the diameter of the renal pelvis.

ASSESSMENT

The severity of the hydronephrosis is determined by the degree of hydronephrosis and whether renal failure is present. Severe hydronephrosis may cause signs of Potter's syndrome from severe antenatal oligohydramnios. Following delivery, infants with severe hydronephrosis can have signs of ARF including oliguria, hypertension, and fluid/electrolyte disturbances.

CLINICAL MANIFESTATIONS/DIAGNOSIS

The diagnosis of hydronephrosis is based on history and physical exam, as well as renal ultrasound and VCUG findings.

Physical findings

- Decreased urine output and signs of ARF if hydronephrosis is bilateral and severe
- Features of Potter's syndrome from oligohydramnios
- Symptoms of a UTI
    - Hematuria, proteinuria, and white blood cells on urinalysis
    - Positive urine culture
- Large, smooth, solid, palpable abdominal mass
- Hypertension

Diagnostic procedures and tests

- Presence of a dilated renal pelvis on prenatal ultrasound
- Postnatal renal ultrasound
  - Determines presence, severity, and etiology of the hydronephrosis
  - Often delayed until 24 to 72 hours of age, since the newborn's dehydration may mask hydronephrosis
- VCUG to assess for reflux of urine into the kidney

TREATMENT

- The goal is preservation of renal function.
- It is dependent upon severity.
- If mild to moderate, management is usually conservative with close ultrasound monitoring.
- Severe cases are initially managed conservatively but may require pyeloplasty if renal function deteriorates.
- Prophylactic antibiotics are used to prevent UTI if urinary reflux is present.
- If severe, a prenatal vesicoamniotic shunt (catheter to drain urine from bladder) may be indicated.
  - Reduces oligohydramnios and its associated complications
  - Sustains kidney function
- Careful assessment of vital signs including blood pressure is performed.
- Monitoring of fluid and electrolyte status including serum creatinine and BUN is also utilized.
- After birth, definitive surgery is necessary to correct the obstructive defect or to provide a diversion for urine flow.

PROGNOSIS

Prognosis depends on the underlying cause, severity, and presence of permanent renal damage. Outcome ranges from complete resolution to end-stage renal disease. Complications include hypertension, UTI, and progressive renal damage. Hydronephrosis secondary to vesicoureteral reflux (VUR) generally spontaneously resolves. Antenatally diagnosed hydronephrosis can indicate obstruction or other serious abnormalities but can also represent a transient developmental change that resolves prior to birth.

CHAPTER RESOURCES

American Academy of Pediatrics. (2011). Urinary tract infection: Clinical practice guidelines for the diagnosis and management of the initial UTI in febrile infants and children 2 to 24 months. *Pediatrics, 128*(3), 595–610.

Andreoli, S. P. (2004). Acute renal failure in the newborn. *Seminars in Perinatology, 28,* 112–123.

Barrantes, F., Tian, J., Vazquiz, R., Amoatenq-Adjepong, Y., & Manthous, C. A. (2008). Acute kidney injury criteria predict outcomes of critically ill patients. *Critical Care Medicine, 36,* 1397–1403.

Basu, R. K., Devarajan, P., Wong, H., & Wheeler, D. S. (2011). An update and review of acute kidney injury in pediatrics. *Pediatric Critical Care, 12*(3), 339–347.

Biyikli, N. K., Alpay, H., Ozek, E., Akman, I., & Bilgen, H. (2004). Neonatal urinary tract infections: Analysis of the patients and recurrences. *Pediatrics International, 46,* 21–25.

Cataldi, L., Mussap, M., & Fanos, V. (2006). Urinary tract infections in infants and children. *Journal of Chemotherapy, 18,* 5–84.

Cataldi, L., Zaffanello, M., Gnarra, M., & Fanos, V. (2010). Urinary tract infection in the newborn and the infant: State of the art. *Journal of Maternal-Fetal and Neonatal Medicine, 23*(S3), 90–93.

Chandler, J. C., & Gauderer, M. W. (2004). The neonate with an abdominal mass. *Pediatric Clinics of North America, 51,* 979–997.

Goldstein, S. L. (2011). Continuous renal replacement therapy: Mechanism of clearance, fluid removal, indications and outcomes. *Current Opinions in Pediatrics, 23,* 181–185.

Haycock, G. B. (2003). Management of acute and chronic renal failure in the newborn. *Seminars in Neonatology, 8,* 325–334.

Ismaili, K., Lolin, K., Damry, N., Alexander, M., Lepage, P., & Hall, M. (2011). Febrile urinary tract infections in 0- to 3-month-old infants: Prospective follow-up study. *Journal of Pediatrics, 158,* 91–94.

Jelton, J. G., & Askenazi, D. J. (2012). Update on acute kidney injury in the neonate. *Current Opinions in Pediatrics, 24*(2), 191–196.

Karlowicz, M. G., & Adelman, R. D. (2005). Acute renal failure. In A. R. Spitzer (Ed.), *Intensive care of the fetus and neonate.* Philadelphia, PA: Mosby.

Koeppen, B., & Stanton, B. (2006). *Renal physiology.* St. Louis, MO: Mosby.

Maayan-Metzger, A., Lotan, D., Jacobson, J. M., Raviv-Zilka, L., Ben-Shlush, A., Kuint, J., & Mor, Y. (2011). The yield of early postnatal ultrasound scan in neonates with documented antenatal hydronephrosis. *American Journal of Perinatology, 28*(8), 613–617.

Mesrobian, H. G., & Mirza, S. P. (2013). Hydronephrosis: A view from the inside. *Pediatric Clinics of North America, 59*(4), 839–851.

Penido Silva, J. M., Oliveira, E. A., Diniz, J. S., Bouzada, M. C., Bergara, R. M., & Souza, B. C. (2006). Clinical course of prenatally detected primary vesicoureteral reflux. *Pediatric Nephrology, 21,* 86–91.

Riccabona, M. (2004). Assessment and management of newborn hydronephrosis. *World Journal of Urology, 22,* 73–78.

Sairam, S., Al-Habib, A., Sasson, S., & Thilaganathan, B. (2001). Natural history of fetal hydronephrosis diagnosed on mid-trimester ultrasound. *Ultrasound in Obstetrics and Gynecology, 17,* 191–196.

Shaikh, N., Monroe, N. E., Bost, J. E., & Farrell, M. H. (2008). Prevalence of urinary tract infection in childhood: A meta-analysis. *Pediatric Infectious Disease Journal, 27,* 302–308.

Subramanian, S., Agarwal, R., Deorari, A. K., Paul, V. K., & Bagga, A. (2008). Acute renal failure in neonates. *Indian Journal of Pediatrics, 73,* 385–391.

Sweetman, D. U., Riordan, M., & Molloy, E. J. (2013). Management of renal dysfunction following term perinatal hypoxia-ischaemia. *Acta Paediatrics, 102*(3), 233–241.

Wald, E. (2004). Urinary tract infections in infants and children: A comprehensive overview. *Current Opinions in Pediatrics, 16,* 85–88.

Wedekin, M., Ehrich, J. H. H., Offner, G., & Pape, L. (2010). Renal replacement therapy in infants with chronic renal failure in the first year of life. *Clinical Journal of American Society of Nephrology, 5,* 18–23.

Weems, M. F., Wei, D., Rananatha, R., Barton, L., Vachon, L., & Sardesai, S. (2015). Urinary tract infections in a neonatal intensive care unit. *American Journal of Perinatology, 32*(7), 695–702.

Yang, Y., Hou, Y., Niu, Z. B., & Wany, C. L. (2010). Long-term follow-up and management of prenatally detected, isolated hydronephrosis. *Journal of Pediatric Surgery, 45,* 1701–1706.

Hematologic and Immune System

Carole Kenner

OVERVIEW

The hematologic system is very complex as it involves the development of the body's blood cells and regulates the hemostatic system. The hematopoietic system is characterized by the presence of pluripotent stem cells that differentiate into three types of circulating blood cells: red blood cells (RBCs), white blood cells (WBCs), and thrombocytes (platelets). Hematopoiesis is an ongoing process of cell development and death. The liver is the main site of this activity (Bagwell, 2014). The maturation of the cells is dependent on gestational and postnatal age.

Hemostasis is dependent on blood coalition and fibrinolysis or the breakdown of a clot. The three components of the hemostatic system are procoagulants or clotting factors, anticoagulants or inhibitors, and fibrinolytics or clot dissolvers. The initial steps in hemostasis are: vascular spasm, platelet plug formation, and coagulation (Bagwell, 2014).

BLOOD GROUP INCOMPATIBILITIES

Blood group incompatibilities were first recognized in the 1940s with the discovery of the Rh grouping and the first test for detection of antibody-coated RBCs, which was devised by Coombs in 1946. Before the introduction of Rh immune globulin in 1964 and its release for general use in 1968, Rh incompatibility accounted for one third of all blood group incompatibilities. With the use of RhIgG, the frequency or Rh incompatibility dropped significantly. ABO has become the main blood group incompatibility, with sensitization occurring in 3% of all infants. Both of these conditions are related to maternal antibodies released in response to fetal antigens and passed to the fetus. The Rh antibody is only released upon an exposure to the antigen (Bagwell, 2014).

ABO INCOMPATIBILITY

Antigens or agglutinogens present on the RBC surface of each blood type (A, B, O, and AB) react with antibodies or agglutinins found in the plasma of opposing blood types. If the antibodies conflict, then RBCs can be destroyed or they can clump together due to an antibody binding to more than one RBC. This clump or agglutination can cause vessel blockage and impair circulation and tissue oxygenation (Bagwell, 2014). Hemolysis can also occur if there are high antibody titers (hemolysins) that stimulate release of proteolytic enzymes that cause the cell's membrane to rupture (Bagwell, 2014).

In a transfusion reaction, when opposing blood types are mixed, the donor's RBCs are agglutinated, whereas the recipient's blood cells tend to be protected. The plasma portion of the donor blood that contains antibodies becomes diluted by the recipient's blood volume, thus reducing donor antibody titers in the recipient's circulation. However, recipient antibody titers are adequate to destroy the donor RBCs by agglutination and hemolysis or by hemolysis alone. This is the situation in ABO incompatibility. In such cases, the maternal blood type usually is O, containing anti-A and anti-B antibodies in the serum, whereas the fetus or newborn is type A or B. Although incompatibility can occur between A and B types, it is not as frequent as AO or BO because of the globulin composition of the antibodies. When transplacental hemorrhage (TPH) occurs between an ABO-incompatible mother and fetus, fetal blood entering the maternal circulation undergoes agglutination and hemolysis by maternal antibodies (Bagwell, 2014).

INCIDENCE

- 40% to 50% of the occurrences are in a first pregnancy; however, only about 3% to 20% of the infants ever show symptoms.
- A 1.5% to 2% risk is present with each pregnancy.

ASSESSMENT

Jaundice is the primary manifestation seen in the first 24 hours of life.

Peripheral blood smear may show spherocytes or RBCs that appear to lack the normal central pallor and biconcave disk-like shape that is expected.

- Hepatosplenomegaly
- Labs
- Positive direct Coombs
- Positive indirect Coombs

TREATMENT

In the fetus:

- Amniocentesis and monitoring of amniotic fluid bilirubin levels
- Intrauterine transfusions
- Early delivery

In the newborn:

- Phototherapy
- Exchange transfusions (Bagwell, 2014)

Rh INCOMPATIBILITY

INCIDENCE

- There is a 16% chance with each pregnancy of Rh incompatibility problems when there is an Rh difference between the mother and fetus/newborn.

■ The maternal Rh antibody is slow to develop and initially may consist exclusively of IgM, which cannot cross the placenta due to its size. This is followed by the production of IgG, which can cross the placenta and enter fetal circulation. The maximum concentration of the IgG form of antibody occurs within 2 to 4 months after termination of the first pregnancy that sensitizes the mother's system. This sensitization can also occur from a small fetal bleed, often undetectable, or from an aminocentesis, or an abortion, ectopic pregnancy, or during labor. Whatever the cause there is a release of fetal RBCs that trigger the mother's immune response producing antibodies against the fetal blood that is not compatible (Hall, 2011). If the initial immunization occurs shortly before or at the time of delivery, the first Rh-positive infant born to such a mother may trigger the initial antibody response, with no effect on that infant. However, each subsequent pregnancy will carry a risk for the fetus/infant.

ERYTHROBLASTOSIS FETALIS

Erythroblastosis fetalis is caused by the hemolysis in the fetus due to Rh incompatibility.

ASSESSMENT

The assessment is based on the expected clinical signs of incompatibility related to immature RBCs and hemolysis.

■ Clinical manifestations

  ■ Anemia

  ■ Hyperbilirubinemia

  ■ Jaundice

  ■ Hepatosplenomegaly

  ■ Hydrops (Hydrops fetalis is a severe, total body edema often accompanied by ascites and pleural effusions. This only occurs in 25% of the affected infants.)

  ■ Altered hepatic synthesis, which can impair vitamin K and vitamin K–dependent clotting factors, leading to hemorrhage

▓ Petechiae or prolonged bleeding from the cord or blood sampling sites

▓ Hypoglycemia related to hyperplasia of the pancreatic islet cells (Bagwell, 2014)

TREATMENT

Antenatally

■ Screening for incompatibilities

■ Coombs testing

■ Blood typing

■ Unsensitized Rh-negative mothers should receive RhIgG (use Kleihauer–Betke test for fetal cells to determine if this treatment should be used)

Postnatally

Assessment of cardiorespiratory status is important as ascites, pleural effusions, and circulatory collapse can occur, often requiring airway stabilization and mechanical ventilation.

Paracentesis or thoracentesis is recommended if there is peritoneal or pleural fluid that is compromising the infant.

Delivery of an infant shortly after intraperitoneal transfusion may not allow adequate time for absorption of blood from the peritoneal cavity. Lung expansion can be compromised and result in respiratory failure. Mechanical ventilation may be necessary. Blood may need to be removed via paracentesis.

COLLABORATIVE MANAGEMENT

■ Assess for adequacy of circulating blood volume.

■ If hydrops is present, anemia is treated with transfusion of packed RBCs. O-negative or type-specific Rh-negative blood cross-matched against the maternal blood should be used.

■ Single-volume or partial exchange may be needed.

■ Congestive heart failure (CHF) may occur during transfusion.

■ Damage to the liver can result in coagulation problems and hyperbilirubinemia.

■ Liver function tests need to be followed along with hematocrit and coagulation studies.

■ Position to reduce abdominal pressure to allow lung expansion.

■ Watch vital signs closely for cardiorespiratory changes.

■ Maintain PaO_2 without overexpansion of the lungs; lungs may be hypoplastic.

■ Administer intravenous immunoglobulin (IVIG) if there is a rapid rising bilirubin level.

■ Perform phototherapy as needed.

■ If bilirubin levels do not require immediate exchange, check levels every 4 to 8 hours, depending on the initial cord blood levels and subsequent rate of rise (Bagwell, 2014). In Rh incompatibility, exchange is imminent if the rate of rise exceeds 1 mg per hour for the first 6 hours of life. The interval of blood sampling may be increased to 6 to 12 hours after the infant is 48 hours old (Bagwell, 2014).

REFERENCES

Bagwell, G. A. (2014). Hematologic system. In C. Kenner & J. W. Lott (Eds.), *Comprehensive neonatal nursing care* (5th ed., pp. 334–375). New York, NY: Springer Publishing Company.

Hall, J. E. (2011). *Guyton and Hall textbook of medical physiology* (12th ed.). Philadelphia, PA: Saunders/Elsevier.

BILIRUBIN

Ann Schwoebel

OVERVIEW

Neonatal hyperbilirubinemia is manifested by jaundice, the yellow-orange tint found in the sclera and skin of infants with a total serum bilirubin (TSB) level greater than 5 mg/dL (86 mcmol/L). It is estimated that 60% of term infants and 80% of preterm newborns will appear clinically jaundiced during the first weeks of life. Although this condition is generally a benign, transitional phenomenon, unconjugated bilirubin levels that can pose a direct threat of serious brain injury develop in a small proportion of neonates.

BILIRUBIN METABOLISM

Bilirubin is the final by-product from the breakdown of RBCs. This "unbound" bilirubin will rapidly bind to the carrier protein albumin for transport to the liver, where it is conjugated. The binding of unconjugated bilirubin can be influenced by decreases in albumin, changes in binding capacity, or competition for binding sites by certain drugs (e.g., sulfisoxazole, salicylates, and sodium benzoate) or free fatty acids. A harmful effect can occur when there is insufficient binding that results in increased amounts of unbound or "free" bilirubin. Unconjugated bilirubin can be troublesome because it is not water soluble, it is difficult to excrete, and it can cross the intact blood–brain barrier causing acute bilirubin encephalopathy (ABE). Conjugated bilirubin is water soluble and is excreted via the biliary system to the small intestine and excreted into the stool.

Conjugated bilirubin is an unstable substance in the newborn's intestines. In the presence of an enzyme in the intestine called beta-glucuronidase, which is 10 times the adult concentration, conjugated bilirubin can be hydrolyzed back into unconjugated bilirubin. This unconjugated bilirubin reenters the bloodstream via enterohepatic circulation. Delayed stooling, decreased intestinal motility, and starvation potentially increase exposure of conjugated bilirubin to beta-glucuronidase, necessitating repetition of the entire conjugation process.

RISK FACTORS FOR HYPERBILIRUBINEMIA

Risk factors that place an infant at increased risk of hyperbilirubinemia are as follows:

- Exclusively breastfed
- Infant known hemolytic disease (e.g., glucose-6-phosphate dehydrogenase [G6PD] deficiency)
- Gestational age 35 to 37 weeks 6 days out of 7

■ Infant of diabetic mother

■ Previous sibling received phototherapy

■ Weight loss greater than 10% of birth weight

■ Cephalohematoma or significant bruising at birth

■ Discharge less than 24 hours of age

■ Jaundice observed before discharge

■ ABO incompatibility with positive Coombs or direct antiglobulin test (DAT)

Two tools that can be used to identify the risk toward the development of hyperbilirubinemia in newborns over 35 weeks gestational age are the Bhutani nomogram and the BiliTool™.

CLINICAL PATTERNS OF NEONATAL HYPERBILIRUBINEMIA

Physiologic jaundice is a term to describe transient, mild unconjugated hyperbilirubinemia that occurs between 24 and 72 hours of life. The patient's TSB usually rises to a peak level of 12 to 15 mg/dL (204–257 mcmol/L) by day 3 and then falls. In preterm infants, the TSB peak level occurs on day 3 to 7 of age and can rise over 15 mg/dL. It can last up to 1 to 2 weeks in both term and preterm newborns.

Pathologic jaundice

Elevated bilirubin levels within the first 24 hours of life and exceeding 15 mg/dL should be considered pathologic and deserve investigation. These pathologic conditions can be classified as follows:

1. Increase in RBC breakdown (e.g., Rh, ABO incompatibility, G6PD, sepsis, drug reactions, extravascular blood, and polycythemia)

2. A decrease in bilirubin clearance (e.g., bowel obstructions, hypoxia or asphyxia, inborn error of metabolism such as congenital hypothyroidism, and galactosemia)

3. Those that interfere with bilirubin conjugation (e.g., breast milk jaundice, drug interactions, hypothyroidism, acidosis, and hypoxia)

Premature infants develop more significant jaundice due to two factors: decreased oral intake and immaturity of the liver's conjugating system.

Jaundice and the breastfed neonate

Inadequate breastfeeding contributes to an increased incidence of newborn jaundice because of a decreased amount of breast milk along with a weight loss (> 6% by the third postnatal day) and a slow intestinal peristalsis, as well as an increase in the enterohepatic circulation of bilirubin. This type of early-onset jaundice is termed "breast-milk jaundice" since it is not breastfeeding itself that determines jaundice but breastfeeding inadequacy. Successful breastfeeding will decrease the risk of hyperbilirubinemia. Newborns need to be fed at least 8 to 12 times in the first days after birth to improve mother's milk supply. Monitoring urine output, stool output, and weight are the best ways to judge successful breastfeeding. Newborns should have four to six wet diapers and three to four yellow seedy stools per day by the fourth day after birth. Formula supplementation or intravenous (IV) fluids may be necessary if the newborn has significant weight loss, poor urine output, poor caloric intake, and lethargy.

Late-onset breast-milk jaundice will typically appear between days 4 and 7 of life, reaching a peak around 2 to 3 weeks, and can take up to 3 months to resolve completely. The newborn will have a regular weight gain and a normal production of urine and stool. Although the exact mechanism is not completely clear, it is believed that certain substances present in breast milk cause a reduced intestinal motility and increased reabsorption of bilirubin. It is no longer recommended to stop breastfeeding for a brief time to identify breast-milk jaundice. Even if breastfeeding withdrawal is short, it places the newborn at risk to return to exclusive breastfeeding and becomes a source of worry for the mother such as to discourage breastfeeding.

BILIRUBIN ENCEPHALOPATHY

When the blood–brain barrier is intact, the rate of bilirubin uptake by the brain is determined by the following:

■ Concentration of unbound bilirubin
■ Vulnerability of the brain

- Duration of exposure
- Ability of bilirubin to bind to albumin
- Local cerebral blood perfusion

The exact level of when unconjugated serum bilirubin becomes neurotoxic is unclear but the effects can lead to ABE. The classic signs of ABE are increased hypertonia, varying degrees of drowsiness, poor feeding, hypotonia, alternating tone, and high-pitched cry. Prompt and effective interventions when ABE symptoms appear can usually prevent the chronic kernicteric sequelae. The classic clinical features of kernicterus are athetoid cerebral palsy, impairment of upward gaze, hearing loss, and enamel dysplasia of the teeth. Approximately one third of infants with kernicterus develop intellectual impairment.

NURSING ASSESSMENT AND ACTIONS

Reviewing the neonate's family and birth history can indicate which neonates may have an increased risk for severe hyperbilirubinemia.

Visual assessment can be a noninvasive and easy way to identify jaundice. Jaundice is assessed by placing the neonate in a well-lit area, preferably in natural daylight. Apply gentle pressure to the skin, blanching it to reveal the underlying color of the skin and subcutaneous tissue. Mucous membranes should also be assessed. Jaundice progresses in a cephalocaudal direction from the face to the trunk and then to the lower extremities. The assessments should be made at least every 8 to 12 hours, preferably each time vital signs are measured. When jaundice is present in the first 24 hours or if jaundice seems excessive for the newborn's age in hours, a TSB or transcutaneous bilirubin (TcB) should be measured. It is difficult to accurately predict the TSB concentration based on caudal progression alone due to interobserver variability.

TSB is a diagnostic blood test that most accurately measures bilirubin levels. All bilirubin levels are to be interpreted according to the infant's age in hours.

TcB measurements are a noninvasive method of assessing bilirubin levels and may be used as a screening tool when the bilirubin level is less than 15 mg/dL (257 mcmol/L).

TREATMENT

In addition to nutritional support to ensure adequate hydration, milk intake, and gastrointestinal motility, common treatment strategies for severe hyperbilirubinemia include phototherapy, exchange transfusion, and drug therapy.

Phototherapy remains the mainstay of treating hyperbilirubinemia. It acts by converting insoluble unconjugated bilirubin into soluble isomers that can be excreted in urine and stool. It is typically used either prophylactically in preterm newborns or those with a known hemolytic process to prevent a significant rapid rise and therapeutically to reduce excessive bilirubin levels. It is important to be familiar with institutional policies, procedures, and manufacturer recommendations regarding care and use because of the wide range of phototherapy lighting equipment available. Nursing care of the infant receiving phototherapy should include the following:

- Check the irradiance of the bulbs prior to use and then daily.

- Place light sources as close to the infant as possible, with the exception of halogen-lamp phototherapy units.

- Avoid assessing an infant's well-being solely by skin color because of the "blue hue" effect of the phototherapy lights.

- Use opaque eye shields at all times; inspect the eyes for drainage, edema, and abrasions when the lights are turned off and eye shields are removed for infant feedings and parent visits.

- Assess the infant's skin integrity with every diaper change to prevent breakdown due to loose stools, urinary excretion of bilirubin, and exposure to the phototherapy lights. In most cases, it is not necessary to remove the diaper or boundary materials while providing phototherapy unless the bilirubin levels are approaching the exchange transfusion range.

■ Monitor the infant's temperature every 4 hours for hypothermia and hyperthermia.

■ Maintain adequate hydration.

■ Promote parent–infant interactions. Phototherapy can be interrupted at feeding times to allow for breastfeeding, parental visits, and skin-to-skin care unless the bilirubin level is approaching the exchange level.

■ Monitor bilirubin levels every 6 to 24 hours depending on the rate of rise. Phototherapy lights must be turned off while drawing the blood samples for serum bilirubin testing.

Exchange transfusion is considered if the bilirubin levels start to approach those associated with kernicterus despite intensive phototherapy or signs of ABE (even if TSB is falling). A double-volume exchange transfusion (170 mL/kg) removes 85% to 90% of circulating RBC; however, because most of the infant's total bilirubin is in the extravascular compartment, only 25% of the total bilirubin is removed. This procedure may need to be repeated more than once before stabilization of the bilirubin level occurs. Significant morbidities include apnea, anemia, thrombocytopenia, electrolyte and calcium imbalance, necrotizing enterocolitis, hemorrhage, infection, and catheter-related complications.

Pharmacologic agents

For infants with severe hyperbilirubinemia due to blood group incompatibilities, administration of IVIG (0.5–1 g/kg over 2 hours) is used if the TSB is rising despite intensive phototherapy, or if the TSB is within 2 to 3 mg/mL of the exchange level. There is no proven evidence regarding the benefits of other drugs such as phenobarbital, steroids, or tin-mesoporphyrin to prevent or treat hyperbilirubinemia.

Sunlight is not a recommended source of light for phototherapy. The effect of heat and water loss/dehydration, risk to skin and eyes, and the effect of exposure to unnecessary ultraviolet light from direct sunlight are potential side effects and complications of sunbathing.

NEONATAL INFECTION

Tamara Wallace

OVERVIEW

The neonate, although born with an immature immune system, is still capable of responding to foreign antigens from the environment. This immaturity, however, does make the neonate—term and especially preterm—vulnerable to infections. These infections can be acquired in utero, intrapartally, or postnatally. The latter can be due to invasive procedures and exposure to pathogens in the neonatal intensive care units, resulting in nosocomial or hospital-acquired infections. Globally, infections in the form of pneumonia, sepsis, tetanus, meningitis, and diarrhea are the major causes of neonatal death. Most of these deaths are preventable (Healthy Newborn Network, 2015; Liu et al., 2014). Therefore, awareness of risk factors, early identification, and appropriate timely treatment are essential if infectious diseases are to be prevented or at least minimized.

INCIDENCE

- On a global scale, incidence varies widely according to the region of the world (Bodin, 2014; Liu et al., 2014). However, global data suggest that 23% of the neonatal deaths are due to severe infections (5% pneumonia; 17% sepsis, meningitis, tetanus; and 1% diarrhea) (Healthy Newborn Network, 2015).

- In the United States, the incidence in term newborns two to four per 1,000 live births.

- Incidence occurs more frequently in male and low-birth-weight infants.

■ Maternal group B strep colonization, prolonged rupture of membranes, chorioamnionitis, and preterm delivery increase the risk of infection.

PHYSIOLOGY

During pregnancy, the infant is protected from many sources of infection by the uterus and the fetal membranes. The fetal immune system is immature and easily overwhelmed even when delivery occurs at term. Preterm infants are at an even greater risk of infection due to immaturity, the interruption in the passage of maternal antibodies, and the need for instrumentation. Rupture of membranes, exposure to the vaginal canal, and the external environment introduce a variety of microorganisms and put the newborn at risk for infection.

PATHOPHYSIOLOGY

Neonatal infections can be categorized in several ways. These categories may help guide evaluation and management of infection in the newborn. Sepsis can be classified as early onset or late onset. Early-onset infections are generally recognized as those occurring in the first 7 days of life. Late-onset infections occur from day 7 to day 30. Late-onset infections can be further categorized as nosocomial or hospital acquired if the infection is related to care in a hospital. Infections can also be categorized by the site of the infection, such as pneumonia, bacteremia, or meningitis. The patterns of infection seen and outcomes are different for each of these categories.

The most frequent causes of early-onset neonatal infection are bacteria, including group B strep, *E. coli*, and *Listeria*, but neonates can also develop infections due to viruses, such as herpes.

Late-onset infections can be caused by these organisms, but also by staph species and a broad spectrum of gram negatives. Hospital-acquired infections may also be caused by *Pseudomonas*, *Klebsiella*, *Serratia*, *Escherichia coli*, and unit-specific species.

ASSESSMENT

The nurse must maintain a high index of suspicion for any newborn with an abnormal exam or behaviors. The neonate's immature immune system frequently can only provide nonspecific symptoms of infection.

Nursing assessment should include a complete maternal and neonatal history, a complete physical exam, glucose screening, and vital signs at frequent intervals. Any infant with even subtle signs of possible infection should be medically evaluated and receive increased nursing surveillance. Complications of infection may include signs of shock, problems with coagulation, and abnormalities in neurologic status. Nursing surveillance should include ongoing assessment for hypotension, bleeding, glucose, and changes in the patient's neurologic exams, including seizures.

Box 6.1.   Signs and Symptoms of Neonatal Infection

Clinical
- General
- Poor feeding
- Irritability
- Lethargy
- Temperature instability

Skin
- Petechiae
- Pustulosis
- Sclerema
- Edema
- Jaundice

(continued)

Box 6.1. Signs and Symptoms of Neonatal Infection (*continued*)

Respiratory
- Grunting
- Nasal flaring
- Intercostal retractions
- Tachypnea/apnea

Gastrointestinal
- Diarrhea
- Hematochezia
- Abdominal distention
- Emesis
- Aspirates

Central Nervous System
- Hypotonia
- Seizures
- Poor spontaneous movement

Circulatory
- Bradycardia/tachycardia
- Hypotension
- Cyanosis
- Decreased perfusion

  Laboratory Values:

White Blood Cell Count
- Neutrophils
  - < 5,000 cells/mm^3, neutropenia
  - > 25,000 cells/mm^3, neutrophilia
- Absolute neutrophil count (neutrophil and bands)
  - < 1,800 cells/mm^3 (during first week)

(*continued*)

Box 6.1.   Signs and Symptoms of Neonatal Infection (*continued*)

- Immature: total neutrophil ratio
  - 0:2
- Platelet count
  - < 100,000, thrombocytopenia

Cerebrospinal Fluid

- Protein
  - 150–200 mg/L (term)
  - 300 mg/L (preterm)
- Glucose
  - 50%–60% or more of blood glucose level

Adapted with permission from Lott and Kilb (1992).

CLINICAL MANIFESTATIONS AND DIAGNOSIS

Evaluation may include:

- Blood cultures
- Complete blood count, with platelet count and differential
- Lumbar puncture with culture and chemistries performed on cerebrospinal fluid if infant believed to be at risk for meningitis
- Urine cultures (for late-onset infections)
- Screening for acidosis
- In the hospitalized patient, screening of any indwelling tubes should be considered if the infant is older than 7 days.
- More specific testing may be required if the infant is suspected of an atypical infection or viral infection.
- Other screens for inflammation: C-reactive protein (CRP), many other screening labs (IL-6, procalcitonin, Neutrophil CD 64,

RNA markers, etc.) are being developed and tested to identify the body's response to infection and monitor response to antimicrobial treatment. Availability of these screens is variable and site dependent.

An evaluation for coagulopathy should be performed if the infant has multisystem involvement or signs of bleeding (peripheral blood smear, prothrombin time, activated partial thromboplastin time, fibrinogen, fibrinogen split products, or d-dimer) (Gallagher, 2014).

Some screening can be performed on the placenta when possible; when infection is suspected, the placenta should be sent for pathologic evaluation.

Culture-negative sepsis may be diagnosed in the infant whose mother received antibiotics prior to delivery. Even if all cultures are negative, the infant may appear to have clinical signs and symptoms of infection and respond to the use of antimicrobials.

TREATMENT

Treatment of infection includes the support of airway, breathing, and circulation as needed; evaluation for complications; and the administration of appropriate antimicrobials. Newborn antimicrobials ideally should be provided by the IV route. There are a few very specific instances in low-resource environments where the use of intramuscular or even oral antibiotics are acceptable (World Health Organization [WHO], 2013a). The newborn should also be screened for the complications of infection, including shock and bleeding abnormalities.

Initial treatment of early-onset infection: Broad spectrum antibiotics should be started before confirmatory testing is complete. The choice of antibiotics should be based on the most frequent pathogens seen in infants born in the specific region. For most infants, in most places, a combination of ampicillin and gentamicin is preferred (WHO, 2013a). These antibiotics provide coverage for frequently seen bacterial pathogens and are synergistic against meningitis. A third generation cephalosporin may be considered rather than gentamicin. Acyclovir should be added if herpes is suspected.

Initial treatment of late-onset infection: Broad spectrum antibiotics should be started before confirmatory testing is complete. The choice of antimicrobials should be based on the infant's status, exam, and other medical care. Coverage for staph species should be considered. If the infant has been hospitalized, is older than 7 days, and has been receiving support, the possibility of nosocomial infection should be considered and coverage should be modified to cover suspected sources of infection.

Independent of the timing of infection, when a causative agent is identified the antimicrobials used should be narrowed to be specific to that pathogen.

Treatment should include ongoing surveillance for improvement in clinical status, any abnormal labs, abnormal vital signs, and signs of bleeding.

Nursing-specific care and treatment includes:

■ Monitoring and support of airway, breathing, and circulation

■ Infant comfort and pain control during procedures

■ Administration of antimicrobials and screening for complications of infection

■ Family support (Family support during this time cannot be overemphasized. Not only do families have the stress of a sick newborn, but perhaps the guilt of an infection that was potentially transmitted by the mother.)

■ Breastfeeding support

PROGNOSIS

Prognosis depends on the pathogen that infected the neonate and the presence of meningitis. Term infants with rapid recognition and treatment of infection seldom have long-term consequences. The incidence of neurologic sequelae may be as high as 15% to 30% if the infant has meningitis. The incidence of long-term sequelae is higher in the preterm infant, especially if shock was present (Bodin, 2014).

PREVENTION

Infection prevention is an integral part of nursing care. Good hand hygiene and aseptic technique has been shown to prevent many infections.

OMPHALITIS

Omphalitis is an infection of the umbilical stump. It usually presents as a cellulitis around the cord, but may progress to necrotizing fasciitis and systemic disease. Omphalitis is rare in industrialized countries, but remains a significant cause of neonatal death in areas with unhygienic delivery practices. The majority of omphalitis cases are polymicrobial (Gallagher, 2014) and this should be considered when antibiotics are being chosen. Suggested antibiotics are an anti-staphylococcal penicillin or vancomycin and gentamicin. Many cases of omphalitis are culture positive for anaerobes; metronidazole or clindamycin can provide anaerobic coverage (Gallagher, 2014). Topical antimicrobials are also sometimes used, but their use is not well studied (Gallagher, 2014).

Local customs and care of the umbilical stump have been implicated in the incidence of omphalitis. Using clean equipment to cut the cord and assessment of local practices around care of the cord are of utmost importance. The American Academy of Pediatrics (Riley & Stark, 2012) and the WHO recommend dry cord care after delivery for the majority of infants. WHO recommends daily cleaning of the cord with chlorhexidine for the first week of life if the infant is born at home in an area with high neonatal mortality (WHO, 2013b).

FUNGAL INFECTIONS

The neonate is at risk for infections from fungal pathogens as well. Candida species are frequently found in humans and are the most frequently occurring. Topical infections with candida species such as thrush and monilial diaper rashes are not unusual in the newborn period and are easily treated with oral and topical medications.

Invasive fungal disease is unusual, except in the premature infant with a history of invasive procedures, indwelling lines, parenteral nutrition, and multiple courses of broad spectrum antibiotics. Prolonged antibiotic use may lead to fungal overgrowth in the gastrointestinal system and put the infant at risk for systemic disease. Fungal sepsis should be considered in any small, septic-appearing infant who is not responding to standard antimicrobial therapy. If an infant develops cultures positive for fungus, the infant will be screened to determine the extent of the disease and ultrasound may be used to look for vegetations in the eye, kidney, and heart. These infants can develop infections of the central nervous system with significant sequelae and even death.

Some neonatal units provide fungal prophylaxis with oral nystatin or IV fluconazole. Because of the risk of these agents and the risk of developing drug resistance, these programs are generally targeted at the smallest infants with the most risk factors (Weitkamp, Ozdas, LaFleur, & Potts, 2008).

Treatment of active systemic fungal infections generally uses the antifungal agent amphotericin B. Some other newer agents are available, but evidence to support its use in neonates is still limited. All of these drugs have significant potential nephrotoxic and bone marrow effects. Neonates need to be monitored carefully during the administration of antifungal agents.

CONGENITAL INFECTIONS

The micro-organisms responsible for congenital infections have been traditionally grouped together as the TORCH infections; however, as the number of infections has grown Maldonado et al. (2011) have recommended that the acronym be expanded to TORCHES CLAP.

TO Toxoplasma gondii

R   Rubella

C   Cytomegalovirus (CMV)

H   Herpes simplex virus (HSV)

E Enteroviruses

S Syphilis (*Treponema pallidum*)

C Chicken pox (varicella-zoster virus)

L Lyme disease (*Borrelia burgdoferi*)

A Acquired immunodeficiency syndrome (AIDS/human immunodeficiency virus [HIV])

P Parvovirus B9

The most effective treatment for most congenital infections is prevention. Good maternal prenatal care and immunizations can limit their prevalence. Outcomes can be highly variable and are dependent on the timing and severity of illness. A cursory review of a select group of these pathogens, their presentation, and their treatment can be found in Table 6.1. HIV will be addressed separately.

HUMAN IMMUNODEFICIENCY VIRUS

The incidence of HIV and AIDS varies by geography. The rate of maternal infant transmission of HIV is 25% to 30% if the mother did not receive antiretroviral therapy (ART). Treating an infected mother and her infant with ART has significantly lowered this rate of transmission. Depending on the timing and types of ART, this transmission rate may fall to 1.8% to 8.3% (McLean, 2014).

Many countries have recommendations for screening pregnant women, prophylaxis during pregnancy, and neonatal prophylaxis. In the United States, the National Institutes of Health (NIH) have guidelines that recommend universal screening of pregnant women, prophylaxis during pregnancy, and zidovudine prophylaxis in the newborn. This prophylaxis should start soon after birth. Zidovudine with or without nevirapine is recommended for varying lengths of time depending on the mother's current treatment and disease. Current guidelines can be downloaded from http://aidsinfo.nih.gov/guidelines. The WHO has also developed guidelines for ART prophylaxis. Their recommendations take into consideration the resources available. The WHO frequently review and revise these

TABLE 6.1 Short Review of Selected Congenital Infections

Condition	Transmission	Symptoms	Treatment/Nursing Considerations	Outcomes
Toxoplasmosis	Protozoa transmission to mother per uncooked meat or animal feces	May be asymptomatic or mild symptoms in mother. Infant presentation is highly variable: from normal appearing at birth to hydrocephalus, retinitis, intracranial calcifications, and hydrops. New lesions may develop for years.	Prevention and early recognition are best treatments. Treatment: pyrimethamine + sulfonamides daily for 2–6 months, then three times weekly for 1 year Leucovorin may be given concurrently or after this therapy. Nursing care: supportive	Dependent on the extent of disease and treatment Deafness, microcephaly, and low IQ

(continued)

TABLE 6.1 Short Review of Selected Congenital Infections (*continued*)

Condition	Transmission	Symptoms	Treatment/Nursing Considerations	Outcomes
Rubella	Virus German measles infection during pregnancy	Infection prior to 20 weeks gestation may cause neonatal birth defects: auditory, ophthalmic (cataracts), cardiac, neurologic, and growth restriction Treatment of active infection after birth is rare. New symptoms may appear for years.	Prevention and immunization prior to pregnancy are the most effective treatments. Nursing care: supportive	Dependent on the severity of birth defects Persistent shedding of virus may occur for the first year of life; pregnant women should avoid contact.
CMV	DNA virus	By adulthood, most people have been exposed to CMV and developed antibodies.	Evaluation: urine culture, IgG, and IgM titers.	Highly variable Generally, outcomes are worse if the primary infection occurred during pregnancy.

| | Methods of transmission: transplacental, contact with blood and body fluids, including breast milk | Symptoms in the mother are usually fatigue, fever, and liver complications. Neonatal symptoms: IUGR, microcephaly, deafness, blindness, cataracts, profound intellectual deficits, hepatosplenomegaly, and jaundice. Classic pattern of petechiae "blueberry muffin syndrome." | Treatment: supportive, immunoglobulin therapy, vaccines, and chemotherapy are all under development. Valacyclovir, ganciclovir, and valganciclovir have been used in the treatment of neonates (Hamilton et al., 2014) Chemotherapy may be toxic and there is limited data to demonstrate improvement in long-term outcomes. Nursing care: preventive and supportive | 26% of severely infected infants die, 90% of symptomatic infected infants will have sequelae. |

(continued)

TABLE 6.1 Short Review of Selected Congenital Infections (continued)

Condition	Transmission	Symptoms	Treatment/Nursing Considerations	Outcomes
Herpes	DNA virus may be dormant for extended periods Transmission: ascending infection from vaginal vault or transmission from infected fluids during delivery	Wide range of symptoms from asymptomatic to severe disseminated disease that presents with CNS problems, multisystem organ failure, and frequent death. Three categories: 1. Localized infections of skin, eyes, and mouth 2. Patients with encephalitis (may not have vesicles) 3. Disseminated disease (may not have vesicles)	Prevention is the best treatment strategy. Active HSV outbreak is a contraindication for vaginal delivery. It is not recommended that women with HSV have internal monitoring used. Acyclovir is the recommended mode of therapy; it is an inhibitor of viral replication. The recommended dosage is 30 mg/kg/day divided every 8 hours.	Outcome is dependent on category of disease and rapid detection and treatment. Infants who present with encephalitis have a rate of neurologic sequelae of approximately 50%.

Rate of transmission is much higher during primary infections than during recurrent outbreaks. Transmission has also been documented from lesions on the breast or oral lesions.	Multiple laboratory tests can now identify HSV.	Nursing care: supportive and prevention education	Infants who present with disseminated disease present with multisystem organ failure. The CNS in involved in 70%–90% of these infants.

(continued)

TABLE 6.1 Short Review of Selected Congenital Infections (*continued*)

Condition	Transmission	Symptoms	Treatment/Nursing Considerations	Outcomes
Syphilis	Spirochete; vertical transmission may occur at any time during pregnancy.	Maternal history, snuffles, hepatosplenomegaly, jaundice, low birth weight, osteochondritis, and peeling of the palms of the hands and the soles of the feet.	Prevention and prevention of incomplete maternal treatment Evaluation: includes maternal and infant serologic screening, CSF analysis, and bone x-rays. Treatment is with aqueous penicillin G for 10–14 days.	Infection can be treated, but outcome is dependent on organ damage during development.

CMV, cytomegalovirus; CNS, central nervous system; CSF, cerebrospinal fluid; HSV, herpes simplex virus; IUGR, intrauterine growth restricted.

Source: Unless otherwise noted, data was extracted from Bodin (2014).

guidelines. The current recommendations include the use of zidovudine prophylaxis and other medications for the infant. WHO guidelines can be downloaded from http://www.who.int/hiv/pub/en.

Breastfeeding is contraindicated in HIV women. The only exception to this is if the woman and her infant live in an area with no safe water supply. If the risk of death from formula made with unclean water is higher than the risk of HIV transmission, maternal daily prophylaxis with nevirapine may reduce transmission (McLean, 2014). Nursing considerations (McLean, 2014):

- Maternal education should include:
    - Importance of compliance with ART regimes
    - Breastfeeding not recommended
    - Mother not sharing food she has chewed with her infant
    - Importance of compliance with infant ART and follow-up
- Infants receiving ART should be assessed and monitored for anemia and neutropenia.
- Infants at risk for HIV/AIDS should be monitored for unexplained fever, recurrent infections, yeast infections, diarrhea, hepatosplenomegaly, lymphadenopathy, and failure to thrive.

EMERGING THREATS

Periodically, new pathogens present that may put the infant at risk. One recent example is the Zika virus. Information about these emerging infections and their management changes quickly. It is recommended that a clinician use established sources such as the WHO (http://www.who.int/mediacentre/factsheets/zika/en), the Centers for Disease Control (http://www.cdc.gov/zika), and a national health system to keep abreast of the most recent recommendations for emerging diseases.

CONCLUSION

The immature immune system of the neonate puts the infant at greater risk for acquiring almost every type of infection and offers a limited ability to respond to pathogens and localized infections.

The signs and symptoms of infection in the neonate are nonspecific. The nurse has a critical role in identifying early, subtle signs of infection; assessing for complications; safely administering antimicrobials; and providing the family information and support.

REFERENCES

Bodin, M. B. (2014). Immune system. In C. Kenner & J. W. Lott (Eds.), *Comprehensive neonatal nursing care* (5th ed., pp. 278–298). New York, NY: Springer Publishing Company.

Gallagher, P. G. (2014). *Omphalitis*. Retrieved from http://emedicine.medscape.com/article/975422-overview

Hamilton, S. T., van Zuylen, W., Shand, A., Scott, G. M., Naign, Z., Hall, B., ... Rawlinson, W. C. (2014). Prevention of congenital cytomegalovirus complications by maternal and neonatal treatments: A systematic review. *Reviews in Medical Virology, 24*, 420–433.

Healthy Newborn Network. (2015). *Newborn numbers*. Retrieved from http://www.healthynewbornnetwork.org/page/newborn-numbers

Liu, L., Oza, S., Hogan, D., Perin, J., Rudan, I., Lawn, J. E., ... Black, R. E. (2014). Global, regional, and national causes of child mortality in 2000-13, with projections to inform post-2015 priorities: An updated systematic analysis. *Lancet, 385*(9966), 430–440.

Lott, J. W., & Kilb, J. R. (1992). The selection of antibacterial agents for treatment of neonatal infection. *Neonatal Pharmacy Quarterly, 1*(1), 19–29.

Maldonado, Y. A., Nizet, V., Klein, J. O., Remington, J. S., & Wilson, C. B. (2011). Current concepts of infections of the fetus and newborn infant. In J. S. Remington, J. O. Klein, C. B. Wilson, C. Nizet, & Y. A. Maldonado (Eds.), *Infectious diseases of the fetus and newborn* (7th ed., pp. 23–67). Philadelphia, PA: Elsevier.

McLean, K. R. (2014). Emerging infections. In C. Kenner & J. W. Lott (Eds.), *Comprehensive neonatal nursing care* (5th ed., pp. 619–639). New York, NY: Springer Publishing Company.

Riley, L. E., & Stark, A. R. (Eds.). (2012). *Guidelines for perinatal care* (7th ed., p. 302). Elk Grove Village, IL and Washington, DC: American Academy of Pediatrics and American College of Obstetricians and Gynecologists.

Weitkamp, J. -H., Ozdas, A., LaFleur, B., & Potts, A. L. (2008). Fluconazole prophylaxis for prevention of invasive fungal infections in targeted highest risk preterm infants limits drug exposure. *Journal of Perinatology, 28*, 405–411.

World Health Organization. (2013a). Compilation of WHO recommendations on maternal, newborn, child and adolescent health. Retrieved from http://www.who.int/maternal_child_adolescent/documents/mnca-recommendations/en

World Health Organization. (2013b). *Pocket book of hospital care for children.* Retrieved from Apps.who.int/iris/bitstream/10665/81170/1/9789241548373_eng.pdf

ADDITIONAL CHAPTER RESOURCES

American Academy of Pediatrics Subcommittee on Hyperbilirubinemia, Maisels, M. J., Baltz, R. D., Bhutani, V. K., Newman, T. B., Palmer, H., ... Weinblatt, H. (2004). Clinical practice guideline: Management of hyperbilirubinemia in the newborn infant ≥ 35 weeks of gestation. *Pediatrics, 114,* 297–316.

Bhutani, V. K., & The Committee on Fetus and Newborn. (2011). Phototherapy to prevent severe neonatal hyperbilirubinemia in the newborn infant 35 or more weeks gestation. *Pediatrics, 128*(4), e1046–e1052.

Bhutani, V. K., Stark, A., Lazzeroni, L., Poland, R., Gourley, G. R., Kazmierczak, S., ... Initial Clinical Testing Evaluation and Risk Assessment for Universal Screening for Hyperbilirubinemia Study Group. (2013). Predischarge screening for severe neonatal hyperbilirubinemia identifies infants who need phototherapy. *Journal of Pediatrics, 162*(3), 477–482.

Brites, D., Fernandes, A., Gordo, A. S., Silva, R. F., & Brito, M. A. (2009). Biological risks for neurological abnormalities associated with hyperbilirubinemia. *Journal of Perinatology, 29*(Suppl. 1), S8–S13.

Chima, R. S., Johnson, L. H., & Bhutani, V. K. (2001). Evaluation of adverse effects due to exchange transfusion in term and near-term newborns. *Pediatric Research, 49,* 324A.

Clark, M. (2013). Clinical update: Understanding jaundice in the breastfed infant. *Community Practitioner, 86*(6), 41–45.

Hansen, T. (2011). Prevention of neurodevelopmental sequelae of jaundice in the newborn. *Developmental Medicine & Child Neurology, 53*(Suppl. 4), 24–28.

Kaplan, M., & Hammerman, C. (2009). The need for neonatal glucose-6-phosphate dehydrogenase screening: A global perspective. *Journal of Perinatology, 29*(Suppl. 1), S46–S52.

Lauer, B., & Spector, N. (2011). Hyperbilirubinemia in the newborn. *Pediatrics in Review, 32*(8), 341–349.

Maisels, M. J., Watchko, J. F., Bhutani, V. K., & Stevenson, D. K. (2012). An approach to the management of hyperbilirubinemia in the preterm infant less than 35 weeks of gestation. *Journal of Perinatology, 32*(9), 660–664.

National Association of Neonatal Nurses (NANN). (2010). *Position statement on prevention of bilirubin encephalopathy and kernicterus in newborns.* Glenview, IL: Author.

Newman, T. B. (2009). Universal bilirubin screening, guidelines, and evidence. *Pediatrics, 124*(4), 1199–1202.

Panel on Treatment of HIV-Infected Pregnant Women and Prevention of Perinatal Transmission. (2016). *Recommendations for use of antiretroviral drugs in pregnant HIV-1-infected women for maternal health and interventions to reduce perinatal HIV transmission in the United States.* Retrieved from http://aidsinfo.nih.gov/contentfiles/lvguidelines/PerinatalGL.pdf

Riskin, A., Tamir, A., Kugelman, A., Hemo, M., & Bader, D. (2008). Is visual assessment of jaundice reliable as a screening tool to detect significant neonatal hyperbilirubinemia? *Journal of Pediatrics, 152*(6), 782–787.

Schwoebel, A., & Gennaro, S. (2006). Neonatal hyperbilirubinemia. *Journal of Perinatal and Neonatal Nursing, 20*(1), 103–107.

Stark, A., & Lannon, C. M. (2009). Systems changes to prevent hyperbilirubinemia and promote breastfeeding: Pilot approaches. *Journal of Perinatology, 29*(Suppl. 1), S53–S57.

Stokowski, L. (2006). Fundamentals of phototherapy for neonatal jaundice. *Advances in Neonatal Care, 6*(6), 303–312.

Vandborg, P., Hansen, B., Greisen, G., & Ebbesen, F. (2012). Dose-response relationship of phototherapy for hyperbilirubinemia. *Pediatrics, 130*(2), e352–e357.

Vouloumanou, E. K., Plessa, E., Karageorgopoulos, D. E., Mantadakis, E., & Falagas, M. E. (2011). Serum procalcitonin as a diagnostic marker for neonatal sepsis: A systematic review and meta-analysis. *Intensive Care Medicine, 37*(5), 747–762.

Watchko, J., & Tiribelli, C. (2013). Bilirubin-induced neurologic damage-mechanism and management approaches. *New England Journal of Medicine, 369*(21), 2021–2030.

World Health Organization. (2010). *Antiretrovial drugs for treating pregnant women and preventing HIV infections in infants.* Retrieved from http://www.who.int/hiv/pub/mtct/PMTCTfactsheet/en

II

Special Care Considerations in Neonatal Nursing

Nutrition

Ruth Lucas and Carrie-Ellen Briere

OVERVIEW

IMPORTANCE OF BREAST MILK

Breast milk is universally recommended as the best nutrition for infants (American Academy of Pediatrics [AAP], 2012). Premature and ill newborns in the neonatal intensive care unit (NICU) are vulnerable to illness and breast milk provides both immunity to disease and better long-term health outcomes (AAP, 2012). An ideal goal is that all infants who receive NICU care should have an exclusive human breast milk diet (mother's own milk as the first choice, followed by donor human milk) (AAP, 2012). The Baby-Friendly Hospital Initiative Ten Steps to Successful Breastfeeding has recently been expanded to include guidance for NICUs and all providers should be aware of these recommendations.

PHYSIOLOGY OF LACTATION

During pregnancy, the breast begins remodeling to prepare for lactation. This preparation is referred to as secretory differentiation (previously known as lactogenesis I) (Anderson, Rudolph, McManaman, & Neville, 2007). Once the placenta has been delivered, the drop in progesterone leads to the next phase in lactation, known as secretory activation (previously known as lactogenesis II), which signals the production of milk (Anderson et al., 2007). Mothers who deliver prematurely have an interruption in normal breast development of pregnancy and may be at increased risk for challenges in milk production after birth. NICU providers must recognize the importance of breast milk and provide appropriate education and support for these high-risk mothers to initiate and maintain lactation.

SUPPORTING BREASTFEEDING IN THE NICU

Depending on the medical stability of the premature infant, most mothers in the NICU will have to initiate lactation by expression (by hand or pump) rather than by an infant feeding directly at their breast. Supporting lactation and breastfeeding in the NICU requires collaboration between NICU staff, maternal care staff, and the mother. Pumping education is often the first step to build and maintain a milk supply for mothers of infants who are not able to orally feed at birth.

Implement strategies to support breast milk production and breastfeeding:

■ Educate mothers on breast milk pumping and provide instruction on pumping technique (hand expression, manual, and/or electric pump).

■ Initiate pumping within 6 hours of birth.

■ Initiate skin-to-skin contact as soon as possible after birth and promote frequent sessions.

■ Pump at least 8 times every 24 hours.

■ Provide emotional support and acknowledge differences between breast pumping and direct breastfeeding an infant.

■ Initiate direct breastfeeding (feeding the infant directly at the breast) prior to introduction of bottles.

■ Support semi-demand breastfeeding (infant put to breast whenever signs of waking or hunger, and not fed according to a schedule).

Although breast milk provides the ideal nutrition for infants, it is recommended that fortification (especially of protein) is used in infants less than 1,500 g to support growth that is similar to intrauterine growth (AAP, 2012; Adamkin & Radmacher, 2014).

PEER SUPPORT

Peer support should be used both during hospitalization and once home. Benefits of support include:

■ Increased duration of breastfeeding and provision of breast milk.

■ Mothers perceive peer support as trustworthy and valuable because these peers understand the difficulties in breastfeeding a preterm infant.

BENEFITS OF DIRECT BREASTFEEDING

All breastfeeding infants should receive their first oral feeding at the breast, with support of continued direct breastfeeding during hospitalization. Feeding infants directly at the breast (direct breastfeeding) has additional benefits over feeding expressed breast milk in a bottle. Direct breastfeeding provides a more stable feeding environment with infants more likely to maintain appropriate oxygenation levels (Buckley & Charles, 2006). In addition, direct breastfeeding provides the freshest breast milk, skin-to-skin contact, and better infant oral development (Buckley & Charles, 2006). Direct breastfeeding can be initiated once an infant is stable (extubated and off continuous positive airway pressure), and should not be limited by an infant's gestational age.

TRANSITIONING TO DIRECT BREASTFEEDING AND DISCHARGE

If infants have not achieved exclusive direct breastfeeding before discharge, the following strategies should be used to support the transition after discharge:

■ Continued encouragement of skin-to-skin contact at home

■ Clear discharge plan for breastfeeding and supplementation guided by input from the mother and family

■ Education and participatory guidance on "triple feeding" during the transition (direct breastfeeding followed by pumping and bottle feeding); consider the recommendations of Meier, Patel, Wright, and Engstrom (2013)

■ Consistent breastfeeding follow-up and support at home

BREASTFEEDING AND DRUGS

Most drugs are approved for lactation and specific guidelines can be found in the book series *Medications and Mother's Milk*. However, there are certain drugs or medications that may be contraindicated for breastfeeding. The characteristics for a safe drug for lactation include a short half-life with no active metabolites, high protein binding, high molecular weight (large molecules), low pH, low oral bioavailability, having a milk-to-plasma (M/P) ratio more than 1, and relative infant dose (RID) that is less than 10% of the maternal dose. A greater number of maternal medication is present in colostrum than in mature milk because of the immature mammillary cells. However, the small volume of colostrum limits infants' risk (Casey, 2012).

Terms to understand about breastfeeding and drugs

■ M/P Ratio: The M/P ratio compares the peak concentration of the maternal drug in milk to the peak drug concentration in maternal plasma. A ratio of 1 indicates the drug is equally distributed. An M/P ratio less than 1 indicates a drug that is less distributed to the breast milk, while more than 1 demonstrates accumulation of the drug in breast milk.

■ RID: Drug doses are calculated on a per kilogram (kg) basis: a 500-mg drug dose given to a 50-kg woman results in a relative dose of 10 mg/kg. An infant weighing 5 kg given the same dose directly would be receiving 100 mg/kg. A theoretical guide for infant safety is if the infant's weight-adjusted dose is 10% of the maternal dose. Preterm infants may receive high doses of maternal drug due to their low body weight and immature liver function (see Table 7.1).

TABLE 7.1 Medication Pregnancy Fetal Risk and Lactation Infant Risk Categories

Lactation Risk Categories	Designation	Description	Examples
L1	Safest	■ No observed adverse effects ■ Controlled studies fail to demonstrate a risk ■ Possibility of harm is remote ■ Not orally bioavailable to the infant	Acetaminophen[a] Ampicillin[a] Amoxicillin[a] Cefazolin[a] Domperidone[e] Famotidine[a] Heparin[a] Insulin[a] Ibuprofen[a] Vitamins[a]
L2	Safe-limited studies	■ Safety studied with limited breastfeeders without adverse effects	Caffeine[f] Carbamazepine[g] Citalopram[g] Fluoxetine[g] Fluvoxamine[g] Gentamicin[a] Interferon[a] Meperidine[h] Metoclopramide[e] Nicotine[f] Propranolol[a] Sertraline[g] St. John's wort[d] Valproic acid[g]

(continued)

TABLE 7.1 Medication Pregnancy Fetal Risk and Lactation Infant Risk Categories (*continued*)

Lactation Risk Categories	Designation	Description	Examples
L3	Moderately safe	■ No controlled studies in breastfeeders ■ Possible risks should be given only if potential benefit justifies the potential risk to the infant	Alcohol[f] Amphetamines[b] Aspirin[h] Benzodiazepines[b] Buprenorphine[c] Chamomile[d] Diazepam[g] Codeine[h] Echinancea[d] Fenugreek[d,e] Ginkgo[d] Ginseng[d] Lamotrigine[g] Lithium[g] Lorazepam[b] Methadone[c] Metoprolol[a] Morphine[h] Naproxen[h] Oxycodone[h] Pseudoephedrine[f] Valerian[d]
L4	Possibly hazardous	■ Evidence of risk to infant or to breast-milk production ■ Benefits to mothers may be acceptable despite the risk to the infant	Black cohosh[d] D2 antagonist[i] Thioridazine[i] Thorazine[i] Radiophar-maceuticals[b]

(*continued*)

Lactation Risk Categories	Designation	Description	Examples
L5	Contra-indicated	■ Significant documented risk or high risk of causing significant damage to the infant ■ If another medication in the drug class will treat the mother effectively and allow the mother to breastfeed, a medication treatment plan needs to be discussed by the maternal and infant caregiver team	Blue cohosh[d] Cannabis[b] Chemotherapy[b] Cocaine[b] Doxepin[g] Heroin[b] Kava[d] Metham-phetamines[b] Methylenedioxy-methamphetamine (ecstasy)[b] Phencyclidine (PCP)[b] Yohimbe[d]

TABLE 7.1 Medication Pregnancy Fetal Risk and Lactation Infant Risk Categories (*continued*)

Notes: a, approved by AAP; b, not recommended by AAP; c, less infant withdrawal symptoms with Buprenorphine; d, not recommended by AAP due to lack of studies; e, galactagogues; f, council mothers to decrease drug intake; g, SSRIs; h, morphine preferred maternal narcotic; i, antipsychotics.

Source: D'Apolito (2013).

REFERENCES

Adamkin, D. H., & Radmacher, P. G. (2014). Fortification of human milk in very low birth weight infants (VLBW < 1500 g birth weight). *Clinical Perinatology*, *41*(2), 405–421. doi:10.1016/j.clp.2014.02.010

American Academy of Pediatrics. (2012). Breastfeeding and the use of human milk. *Pediatrics*, *129*(3), e827–e841.

Anderson, S. M., Rudolph, M. C., McManaman, J. L., & Neville, M. C. (2007). Key stages in mammary gland development. Secretory activation in the mammary gland: It's not just about milk protein synthesis! *Breast Cancer Research*, *9*(1), 204. doi:10.1186/bcr1653

Buckley, K. M., & Charles, G. E. (2006). Benefits and challenges of transitioning preterm infants to at-breast feedings. *International Breastfeeding Journal*, *1*, 13.

Casey, G. (2012). Breastfeeding and drugs. *Kai Tiaki Nursing New Zealand*, *18*(2), 20–24.

D'Apolito, D. (2013). Breastfeeding and substance abuse. *Clinical Obstetrics and Gynecology*, *56*(1), 202–211.

Meier, P., Patel, A. L., Wright, K., & Engstrom, J. L. (2013). Management of breastfeeding during and after the maternity hospitalization for late preterm infants. *Clinical Perinatology*, *40*(4), 689–705. doi:10.1016/j.clp.2013.07.014

ORAL FEEDINGS

Ksenia Zukowsky

OVERVIEW

Human breast milk is the recommended food of choice for all infants—term and preterm—rather than formula and other substances. Research has demonstrated that infants have better outcomes in the areas of development, immunology, infectious disease, and childhood obesity when fed human milk. Additionally, there are also better maternal outcomes noted for mothers who feed their infants human milk (AAP, 2005, 2012).

The enteral caloric recommendations for healthy newborn infants vary according to sources. Recommendations may range from 98 to 120 kcal/kg/day for adequate growth and development

(American Academy of Pediatrics Committee on Nutrition, 1985; Merves, 2012). Enteral caloric recommendations for premature infants are a little higher—110 to 135 kcal/kg/day for growth (Agostoni et al., 2010). These enteral nutrition recommendations are based on the goal of duplicating the rates of intrauterine accretion of the fetus (Pointdexter & Schanler, 2012). The goal of nutritional intake for this population is for the premature infant to grow in extrauterine life at the same rate and composition as the fetus of the same gestational age. This extrauterine goal poses a challenge to attain for the premature low-birth-weight infant.

PREMATURE NEONATES

Premature low-birth-weight neonates generally have one or more comorbidities to contend with that may compromise their growth. These may include one or more diseases such as bronchopulmonary dysplasia, severe intraventricular hemorrhage, necrotizing enterocolitis, or sepsis, which may contribute to additional demands for the premature infant's ability to grow (Pointdexter & Schanler, 2012). Preterm infants also have limited body stores, an increase in energy expenditure, and/or an immaturity and inability to tolerate enteral feedings. These issues all affect the preterm infant's ability to grow sufficiently over time. Therefore, parenteral nutrition is generally given immediately after birth to these infants and enteral feedings are introduced in small amounts over time (Pointdexter & Schanler, 2012).

Studies have demonstrated that small volumes of feedings over time, called trophic feedings, that are given early to preterm low-birth-weight infants yield better outcomes in advancement and tolerance of feedings. Importantly, using this modality and method of enteral feeding has demonstrated that these neonates may be on total parenteral nutrition for fewer total days (Pointdexter & Schanler, 2012; Slagle & Gross, 1988). The initiation of trophic feedings and titration of increasing enteral feedings decrease parenteral nutrition, usually over a period of several days to weeks. Human milk remains the preferred enteral feeding using these strategies. The initiation of trophic feedings may begin with 10 mL/kg/day and advance by 10 to

20 mL/kg/day until total enteral intake is equal to 150 mL/kg/day (Ehrenkranz, 2007).

The total caloric intake of enteral feedings for premature infants may range between 110 and 135 kcal/kg/day (Agostoni et al., 2010). These caloric requirements are derived from the preterm low-birth-weight infant's energy expenditure. Within the energy expenditure, the infant's resting metabolic rate is the largest component of the total estimated energy requirement. Other energy expenditures that contribute to energy requirements are movement, activity, thermoregulation, and growth. Compromising these entities is that the preterm infant has limited energy storage of fat and lean mass. The preterm also has energy losses that are due to incomplete absorption of nutrients and immature body organs (Pointdexter & Schanler, 2012). Enteral nutrition and preterm low-birth-weight infant feeding may be increased over time as the neonate tolerates. A mean weight gain for the preterm infant is approximately 15 g/kg/day. Regaining the neonate's birth weight by the seventh to fourteenth day of life is one goal that may utilize these approaches (Cloherty, Eichenwald, & Stark, 2012). As with all nutrition, the major components of enteral nutrition are protein, fat, and carbohydrates. The preterm low-birth-weight infant is at a disadvantage when trying to feed and absorb these nutrients.

PROTEIN

Gastric acid is required for protein breakdown. The preterm infant's gastric acid levels are lower than those of term infants (Anderson, 2014). Protein requirements for very low-birth-weight and premature infants are 4 g/kg/day. A recommended intake of enteral protein by fortified human milk and/or premature formula would need to supply 3.2 to 4.1 g protein/100 kcal. Fortified human milk and/or premature formula is derived to yield an increased protein accretion and improved weight gain without causing toxicity to the infant (AAP, 2012; Pointdexter & Schanler, 2012).

FAT

Human milk contains fat, a major energy source. Fat comprises nearly 50% of breast milk's calories, although the fat content varies from mother to mother. Fat may adhere to collection containers, feeding tubes, and/or syringes when administering and/or storing human milk. Because of this, human milk administration is performed judiciously. Times and dates are noted when it is being administered to premature low-birth-weight infants (Pointdexter & Schanler, 2012). Fats are broken down to triglycerides and fatty acids by enzymes located in the infant's lingual secretions, from the pancreas, and in the intestines (Anderson, 2014). A recommended intake of fat for enteral-fed premature low-birth-weight infants ranges between 4.8 and 6.6 g/kg/day. Medium-chain triglycerides are the major source of fat in formula (Agostoni et al., 2010; Pointdexter & Schanler, 2012). Fat makes up 40% to 50% of total caloric intake of either human milk or formula (Anderson, 2014).

CARBOHYDRATES

Lactose is the primary carbohydrate in human milk. Lactase (*beta-galactosidase*) is an intestinal enzyme that hydrolyzes lactose to glucose and galactose in the small intestine. The preterm infant, due to his or her immaturity, has a lower level of lactase yet will tolerate lactose in human milk well (Pointdexter & Schanler, 2012). Glucose polymers are found as the source of carbohydrate in premature formula. Glucose polymers have an advantage in that they increase caloric density without a rise in osmolality. Recommended carbohydrate intake for premature infants is 11.6 to 13.2 g/kg/day (Agostoni et al., 2010; Pointdexter & Schanler, 2012).

READINESS FOR ORAL FEEDING

The premature infant's coordination of sucking, swallowing, and breathing is a highly organized behavior (Medoff-Cooper, Verklan, & Carlson, 1993). This coordination occurs around 32 to 34 weeks gestational age (Delaney & Arvedson, 2008; Jones, 2012).

The coordination of swallowing and breathing matures around 37 weeks corrected gestational age (Amaizu, Shulman, Schanler, & Lau, 2008; Koenig, Davies, & Thach, 1990; Lau, Smith, & Schanler, 2003). It has been noted that in clinical practice oral feeding initiation may occur as early as 28 to 32 weeks (DeMauro, Patel, Medoff-Cooper, Posencheg, & Abbasi, 2011; Kirk, Alder, & King, 2007).

The preterm infant has immature organs that contribute to enteral feeding issues. There is a relaxation of the lower esophageal sphincter, which contributes to the reflux. A delay in gastric emptying and a decrease in intestinal motility also are noted. Intestinal motility usually starts to improve around 32 weeks gestation (Anderson, 2014). There is an incompetence of the ileocecal valve, which acts as a barrier between the small and large intestine. There is also an impaired retro sphincter reflux that can be noted in a delay in stool evacuation (Anderson, 2014).

CALCIUM AND PHOSPHOROUS

Calcium and phosphorus are essential for all neonates. The premature infant requires greater quantities of calcium and phosphorus than the term infant; these quantities are not available in human milk. Calcium and phosphorus are necessary for 99% and 85%, respectively, of bone mass. Human milk contains calcium and phosphorus that is ionized easily; thus, it is better absorbed than the calcium and phosphorous that is contained in formula (Pointdexter & Schanler, 2012).

Although the calcium and phosphorous in human milk are better absorbed by neonates, in the preterm infant the amount of calcium and phosphorus in human milk is not adequate enough to attain the intrauterine accretion growth rates. This is exhibited in low serum and urine phosphorous concentrations, elevated serum alkaline phosphatases, and elevated urine calcium concentrations (Pointdexter & Schanler, 2012).

Human milk supplementation of calcium and phosphorus improves retention of these minerals in the preterm infant. Preterm formulas are fortified with greater amounts of calcium and phosphorous than term infant formulas (Pointdexter & Schanler, 2012).

PARENTERAL NUTRITION

The largest component of the total estimated energy requirement is that needed for the resting metabolic rate. When nourished parenterally, the premature infant has less fecal energy loss, generally fewer episodes of cold stress, and somewhat lesser activity so that the actual energy needs for growth are lowered to 80 to 100 kcal/kg/day for the first week of life (Schanler, 2015).

Parenteral nutrition initiated early in this population minimizes weight loss, improves growth and neurodevelopmental outcome, and appears to reduce the risk of mortality and morbidity. There is literature to support better neurodevelopmental outcomes with initiation of higher protein intake (Christmann et al., 2013; Ehrenkranz et al., 2011; Moyses, Johnson, Leaf, & Cornelius, 2013).

PROTEIN

Recommendations are that 1.5 g/kg/day of protein be started within the first 24 hours after birth and then increased to 3.5 to 4 g/kg/day by 0.5 to 1 g/kg/day increments. There are not significant increases in blood urea nitrogen (BUN) and/or acidosis with this higher protein initiation (Burattini et al., 2013; Clark, Chace, & Spitzer, 2007; Klein, 2002; Porcelli & Sisk, 2002; Schanler, 2015; Schanler, Shulman, & Prestridge, 1994; Tan & Cooke, 2008). Essential and nonessential amino acids are necessary to attain a positive nitrogen balance leading to attainment of growth (Malloy, Rassin, & Richardson, 1984).

Studies have shown that administering protein of ≥ 4 g/kg/day was well tolerated and yielded an association of lower rates of bronchopulmonary dysplasia when compared with lower protein (Malloy et al., 1984). Currently, recommendations are to start protein/amino acids administration immediately after birth with an infusion rate of 3.5 g/kg/day. There is an improved nitrogen balance and stable serum BUN or glucose concentrations with these higher doses (te Braake, van den Akker, Wattimena, Huijmans, & van Goudoever, 2005; Thureen, Melara, Fennessey, & Hay, 2003). Infants who receive protein on the first day of life have a positive nitrogen balance with no side effects from the amino acids (Ibrahim, Jeroudi, Baier, Dhanireddy, & Krouskop, 2004; Poindexter & Ehrenkranz, 2015).

As for toxicity, there are no differences between 3 g/kg/day compared with 1 g/kg/day in serum BUN (Paisley, 2000). Estimated parenteral protein requirements for premature infants who are low birth weight are 3 to 3.5 g/kg/day. Estimates for term infants are 2.5 to 3 g/kg/day (Poindexter & Denne, 2012).

TrophAmine is a brand of amino acid solution that yields normal amino acid plasma concentrations (Thureen et al., 2003). TrophAmine and Premasol supply amino acids L-tyrosine and N-acetyl-L-Tyrosine. Aminosyn-PF and Primene do not supply substanial tyrosine. Cysteine is not in most parenteral amino acid solutions. The ideal intravenous amino acid is not known for parental nutrition (Poindexter & Ehrenkranz, 2015).

GLUCOSE

As with enteral nutrition, carbohydrates and fat primarily provide the calories for energy. The percentages of nonprotein calories are carbohydrates 40% and lipids 45% (Schanler, 2015). Others have noted the fat to glucose ratio can mimic human milk 60:40 (Poindexter & Ehrenkranz, 2015). Glucose is the source of carbohydrate used in parenteral nutrition. Initially, exogenous glucose is often needed until the infant can begin to mobilize glycogen stores and produce glucose.

Term infants, due to their utilization and glucose production, need 3 to 5 mg/kg/minute. Preterm infants' demands are greater: 8 to 9 mg/kg/minute. Preterm infants may start at a glucose infusion rate of 6 mg/kg/day and increase as high as 10 to 12 mg/kg/minute as long as hyperglycemia does not occur. Glucose infusion rates of 5 to 8 mg/kg/minute may be needed. The primary source of energy for the neonatal brain is glucose (Poindexter & Ehrenkranz, 2015). Very-low-birth-weight infants who weigh 1,000 g or more will usually tolerate 10% glucose–dextrose solution. Infants that weigh less than 1,000 g may require 5% glucose–dextrose solution (Poindexter & Ehrenkranz, 2015).

FAT

Fat emulsions are important to prevent essential fatty acid deficiency and serve as a nonprotein energy source. These emulsions are from soybean oil, olive oil, medium chain triglycerides, and fish oil. The fish oil emulsions contain very long chain omega-3 fatty acids, docosahexaenoic acid, and eicosapentaenoic acid (Mayer & Schafer, 2006; Poindexter & Ehrenkranz, 2015). Lipids can be given 3 mg/kg/day. Plasma lipid clearance improves when intravenous lipids are given continuously over 24 hours (Poindexter & Ehrenkranz, 2015).

REFERENCES

Agostoni, C., Buonocore, G., Carnielli, V. P., De Curtis, M., Darmaun, D., Decsi, T., ... ESPGHAN Committee on Nutrition. (2010). Enteral nutrient supply for preterm infants: Commentary from the European Society for Paediatric Gastroenterology, Hepatology, and Nutrition (ESPGHAN) committee on nutrition. *Journal of Pediatric Gastroenterology Nutrition, 50*(1), 85–91.

Amaizu, N., Shulman, R. J., Schanler, R. J., & Lau, C. (2008). Maturation of oral feeding skills in preterm infants. *Acta Pediatric, 97*(1), 61–67.

American Academy of Pediatrics. (2005). Breastfeeding and the use of human milk, policy statement. *Pediatrics, 115*(2), 496–506.

American Academy of Pediatrics. (2012). Breastfeeding and the use of human milk section on breastfeeding. *Pediatrics, 129*(3), e837–e841.

American Academy of Pediatrics Committee on Nutrition. (1985). Nutritional needs of low-birth-weight infants. *Pediatrics, 75*(5), 976–986.

Anderson, D. (2014). Nutrition management of the preterm infant. In C. Kenner & J. W. Lott (Eds.), *Comprehensive neonatal nursing: An interdisciplinary approach* (5th ed.). New York, NY: Springer Publishing Company.

Burattini, I., Bellagamba, M. P., Spagnoli, C., D'Ascenzo, R., Mazzoni, N., Peretti, A., ... Marche Neonatal Network. (2013). Targeting 2.5 versus 4 g/kg/day of amino acids for extremely low birth weight infants: A randomized clinical trial. *Journal of Pediatrics, 163*(5), 1278–1282.

Clark, R. H., Chace, D. H., & Spitzer, A. R. (2007). Pediatrix amino acid study group. Effects of two different doses of amino acid supplementation on growth and blood amino acid levels in premature neonates admitted to the neonatal intensive care unit: A randomized, controlled trial. *Pediatrics, 120*(6), 1286–1296.

Cloherty, J. P., Eichenwald, E. C., & Stark, A. R. (Eds.). (2012). *Manual of neonatal care* (7th ed.). Philadelphia, PA: Wolters Kluwer/Lippincott Williams & Wilkins.

Christmann, V., Visser, R., Engelkes, M., de Grauw, A. M., van Goudoever, J. B., & van Heijst, A. F. J. (2013). The enigma to achieve normal postnatal growth in preterm infants–using parenteral or enteral nutrition? *Acta Paediatric, 102*(5), 471–479.

Delaney, A. L., & Arvedson, J. C. (2008). Development of swallowing and feeding: Prenatal through first year of life. *Developmental Disability Research Review, 14*(2), 105–117.

DeMauro, S. B., Patel, P. R., Medoff-Cooper, B., Posencheg, M., & Abbasi, S. (2011). Postdischarge feeding patterns in early- and late-preterm infants. *Clinic in Pediatrics, 50*(10), 957–962.

Ehrenkranz, R. A. (2007). Early, aggressive nutritional management for very low birth weight infants: What is the evidence? *Seminar Perinatology, 31*(2), 48–55.

Ehrenkranz, R. A., Das, A., Wrage, L. A., Poindexter, B. B., Higgins, R. D., Stoll, B. J., & Oh, W. (2011). Early nutrition mediates the influence of severity of illness on extremely LBW infants. *Pediatric Research, 69,* 522–529.

Ibrahim, H. M., Jeroudi, M. A., Baier, R. J., Dhanireddy, R., & Krouskop, R. W. (2004). Aggressive early total parenteral nutrition in low birth weight infant. *Journal of Perinatology, 24*(8), 482–486.

Jones, L. R. (2012). Oral feeding readiness in the neonatal intensive care unit. *Neonatal Network, 31*(3), 148–155.

Kirk, A. T., Alder, S. C., & King, J. D. (2007). Cue-based oral feeding clinical pathway results in earlier attainment of full oral feeding in premature infants. *Journal of Perinatology, 27*(9), 572–578.

Klein, C. J. (2002). Nutrient requirements for preterm infant formulas. *Journal Nutrition, 132*(6), 1295S–1577S.

Koenig, J. S., Davies, A. M., & Thach, B. T. (1990). Coordination of breathing, sucking, and swallowing during bottle feedings in human infants. *Journal of Applied Physiology, 69*(5), 1623–1629.

Lau, C., Smith, E. O., & Schanler, R. J. (2003). Coordination of suck-swallow and swallow respiration in preterm infants. *Acta Pediatric, 92*(6), 721–727.

Malloy, M. H., Rassin, D. K., & Richardson, C. J. (1984). Total parenteral nutrition in sick preterm infants: Effects of cysteine supplementation with nitrogen intakes of 240 and 400 mg/kg/day. *Journal of Pediatric Gastroenterology & Nutrition*, 3(2), 239–244.

Mayer, K., & Schafer, M. B. (2006). Fish oil and the critically ill: From experiment to clinical data. *Current Opinion Clinical Nutrition Metabolic Care*, 9(2), 140–148.

Medoff-Cooper, B., Verklan T., & Carlson, S. (1993). The development of sucking patterns and physiologic correlates in very-low-birth-weight infants. *Nursing Research*, 42(2), 100–105.

Merves, M. H. (2012). Newborn assessment. In M. Tschudy & M. Jones (Eds.), *Harriet lane* (19th ed.). Philadelphia, PA: Elseiver.

Moyses, H. E., Johnson, M. J., Leaf, A. A., & Cornelius, V. R. (2013). Early parenteral nutrition and growth outcomes in preterm infants: A systematic review and meta-analysis. *American Journal Clinical Nutrition*, 97(4), 816–826.

Paisley, J. E. (2000). Safety and efficacy or low versus high parental amino acids in extremely low birth weight neonates immediately after birth. *Pediatric Research*, 47(4), 293A.

Poindexter, B. B., & Denne, S. C. (2012). Parenteral nutrition. In C. S. Gleason & S. Devaskar (Eds.), *Avery's diseases of the newborn* (9th ed., pp. 963–972). Philadelphia, PA: Elsevier Health Science.

Poindexter, B., & Ehrenkranz, R. (2015). Nutrient requirements and provision of nutrition supporting the preterm infant. In R. J. Martin, A. A. Fanaroff, & M. C. Walsh (Eds.), *Fanaroff and Martin's neonatal-perinatal medicine: Diseases of the fetus and infant* (10th ed.). Philadelphia, PA: Saunders/Elsevier.

Pointdexter, B. B., & Schanler, R. J. (2012). Enteral nutrition for the high risk neonate. In C. S. Gleason & S. Devaskar (Eds.), *Avery's diseases of the newborn* (9th ed., pp. 952–962). Philadelphia, PA: Elsevier Health Science.

Porcelli, P. J., & Sisk, P. M. (2002). Increased parenteral amino acid administration to extremely low-birth-weight infants during early postnatal life. *Journal of Pediatric Gastroenterology Nutrition*, 34(2), 174–179.

Schanler, R. J. (2015). *Parenteral nutrition in premature infants*. Retrieved from http://www.uptodate.com/contents/parenteral-nutrition-in-premature-infants?source=search_result&search=Parenteral+Nutrition+in+premature&selectedTitle=1~150

Schanler, R. J., Shulman, R. J., & Prestridge, L. L. (1994). Parenteral nutrient needs of very low birth weight infants. *Journal of Pediatrics*, 125(6), 961–968.

Slagle, T. A., & Gross, S. J. (1988). Effect of early low-volume enteral substrate on subsequent feeding tolerance in very low birth weight infants. *Journal of Pediatrics, 113*(3), 526–531.

Tan, M. J., & Cooke, R. W. (2008). Improving head growth in very preterm infants—A randomised controlled trial I: Neonatal outcomes. *Archives Disease Child Fetal & Neonatal Education, 93*, F337–F341.

te Braake, F. W., van den Akker, C. H., Wattimena, D. J., Huijmans, J. G., & van Goudoever, J. B. (2005). Amino acid administration to premature infants directly after birth. *Journal of Pediatrics, 147*(4), 457–461.

Thureen, P. J., Melara, D., Fennessey, P. V., & Hay, W. W., Jr. (2003). Effect of low versus high intravenous amino acid intake on very low birth weight infants in the early neonatal period. *Pediatric Research, 53*(2), 24–32.

Surgical Care for the Neonate

Michele DeGrazia

OVERVIEW

This section provides guidance on general considerations of the surgical newborn, inclusive of commonly observed (noncardiac) conditions and interventions.

GENERAL CONSIDERATIONS IN THE MANAGEMENT OF THE SURGICAL NEONATE: CONSENT, FAMILY-CENTERED CARE, FLUID AND ELECTROLYTE AND PAIN MANAGEMENT

Denise Casey and Donna Armstrong

OVERVIEW

The care of the surgical neonate requires considerable skill and expertise. To care for a surgical neonate, nurses must possess the skills to provide routine well newborn care, deliver care to those with isolated surgical conditions, as well as those with multiple, complex, medical, and surgical diagnoses (Kelly, Liddell, & Davis, 2008). Nurses must advocate, monitor, and identify concerns related to the surgical neonate, and provide holistic, family-centered care to the family. This section will touch briefly on the topics of consent, family-centered care, fluid and nutrition management, and pain management.

CONSENT

Informed consent is the initial process of educating the patient or surrogate person who is responsible for the care of the patient.

■ In the case of a neonate, the responsible person is usually the parent(s), but sometimes it is another family member or surrogate. For simplicity, we will use parent(s) throughout this section, knowing that in some situations a family member or surrogate may be substituted (Sudia-Robinson, 2015).

Education of the parent should include specific information about the surgical procedure that is to be performed. This education should be delivered in the form of a discussion where families feel comfortable asking questions to enhance their understanding. This will ensure parents remain engaged and involved in the decision-making process. During informed consent, the provider must use clear language and minimize the use of medical terminology that can be misinterpreted or misunderstood by the parent(s).

Prior to the consent process, consider the following:

■ Primary language of the person receiving the information

■ Is an interpreter needed?

■ Education level of the individual

■ Language used to explain the procedure should be done at the individual's educational level.

Obtaining surgical procedure informed consent includes:

■ Indications for the procedure

■ Potential benefits, risks, side effects

■ Likelihood of achieving the goals of the procedure

■ Reasonable alternatives to the procedure (if any)

■ Risks and benefits associated with not receiving the procedure (if any)

■ What is involved in the procedure?

Obtaining anesthesia informed consent includes:

■ Obtaining a separate consent for anesthesia.

■ Discussing the indication, type of anesthesia, and method of administration; in addition, consent for anesthesia should include potential benefits, risks, side effects, and reasonable alternatives to the procedure (if any).

Nursing responsibilities during informed consent:

■ Understand institutional policies and procedures for obtaining informed consent

■ Identify and document the name of the person responsible for giving informed consent and his or her contact information in the chart

■ Confirm that the person giving consent fully understands what he or she is consenting to

   ■ If the information is not understood, it is the responsibility of the nurse to notify the provider that more education regarding the procedure is needed.

FAMILY-CENTERED CARE

When a newborn infant is admitted to a neonatal intensive care unit (NICU) and needs to undergo surgery, it can be very scary and overwhelming to parents. Family-centered care focuses not only on the patient but the entire family. The family takes an active role in participating, decision making, and advocating, which has been shown to improve safety as well as outcomes (Gephart & McGrath, 2012; McGrath, 2014).

ENCOURAGING A FAMILY-CENTERED CARE ENVIRONMENT

■ Orient the patient and family to the hospital and NICU surroundings

   ■ Waiting room

   ■ Self-care facilities (bathrooms, parents rooms, laundry)

   ■ Dining options, lactation services, rooms, and supplies

■ Orient them to available support services

   ▩ Social worker

   ▩ Lactation

   ▩ Chaplain

   ▩ Center for families

■ Develop and maintain open and honest communication

   ▩ Assist the family with establishing realistic expectations and goals about their infant's hospitalization as well as surgery. You may want to ask them, "What is your understanding of the surgical procedure and what will it achieve?"

   ▩ Describe the operating room (OR) procedures and postoperative course (cardiorespiratory needs, pain control, goals/expectations, expected time frame for the procedure) (Curley, Meyer, Scoppettuolo, McGann, Trainor, Rachwal, & Hickey, 2012, pp. 1133-1139).

   ▩ Empower parents to be involved as advocates for their infant.

      • Involve the parents in decision making for their newborn

      • Encourage the parents' presence on rounds

         ◦ Rounding with the patient care team

      • Encourage the parents' presence during procedures

         ◦ Have a dedicated team member (family facilitator) available to explain what is taking place as it is happening.

         ◦ If parents are unable to stay or if they choose not to be present then provide regular updates during the procedure.

■ Hold routine family meetings

   ▩ Give scheduled updates

   ▩ Include patient's current status, plan, or goals for the day, week, or month

■ Use a team approach in meetings; include (if applicable):

   ▩ Surgeon

   ▩ Neonatologist

- Nurse practitioner
- Fellow or resident physicians
- Nurse
- Social worker
- Appropriate consulting team representatives

■ Allow time for questions

- Describe what is known and not known
- Encourage family members to voice concerns they have regarding their newborn

■ Involvement and learning new skills

- On admission and throughout the hospitalization, assess the parents' readiness to learn new skills
- Identify how the parents learn best
  - Written information
  - Demonstration
  - Hands on
  - Reinforcement of new skills
- Anticipate which skills parent(s) will need when caring for their newborn following surgery
  - Teach parent(s) in the care of their newborn and, when possible, have them participate in their infant's care (taking temperature, changing diaper, bathing/dressing, and feeding) (Sprull, 2015)

FLUID AND ELECTROLYTE MANAGEMENT

Approximately 75% of the total body weight of the term infant consists of water and approximately 80% to 85% of the preterm infant's total body weight is water (O'Brien & Walker, 2014). The more premature the infant is, the greater the percentage of total body weight is water. Within the first week of life, the infant experiences a postnatal diuresis. During this diuresis, the term infant will typically lose 5% to 10% of his or her birth weight while the preterm infant will lose 10% to 20% (Lorenz, 1997). This diuresis consists of water and electrolyte losses, mainly sodium, potassium, and glucose (Snyder, 2015).

Demands on the infant transitioning to extrauterine life will affect fluid hemostasis and necessitate close monitoring of his or her fluid status. The need for surgery within this time frame will further complicate fluid and electrolyte management. Fluid homeostasis status is necessary to maintain good perfusion, prevent cellular damage, and avoid acidosis. Nurses must be vigilant with close monitoring of their patients' fluid balance in order to maintain homeostasis (Koletzko et al., 2005).

PERIOPERATIVE MAINTENANCE OF FLUID HOMEOSTASIS

- Strictly monitor total fluid intake and output
- Consider the gestational age of the infant when determining his or her fluid needs (Davies et al., 2008)
  - Premature infants experience increased insensible water losses (IWLs).
- Assess risks for IWL
  - Decreased gestational age
  - Environmental losses
  - Body temperatures
  - Skin breakdown or open wounds
  - Congenital defects (tracheoesophageal fistula/esophageal atresia [TEF/EA], abdominal wall defects, bowel perforation)
  - Open warmer (choose isolette or similar containment to decrease IWL)
  - Phototherapy
  - Ventilator
    - Humidity (decreases IWL)

■ Maintain detailed calculation of all fluid losses
- Urine
- Stool (diarrhea/ostomy)
- Nasogastric/orogastric (NG/OG) drainage
- Cerebrospinal fluid (CSF) (ventricular drainage)
- Blood

POSTOPERATIVE ASSESSMENT OF FLUID AND ELECTROLYTE STATUS

Vigilant monitoring of fluid status should be done for every postoperative patient, inclusive of the following assessments:

■ Physical exam

■ Vital signs

■ Acid–base balance

■ Respiratory
   ■ Inadequate oxygenation and ventilation can lead to a respiratory acidosis; monitor for:
   - Abdominal distention
   - Ascites
   - Fluid overload

■ Cardiac
   ■ Poor tissue perfusion may cause acidosis; monitor for:
   - Low cardiac output
   - Sepsis

■ Renal
   ■ Impaired renal function may lead to metabolic acidosis; monitor for:
   - Decreased output
   - Acute tubular necrosis (ATN)
   - Premature kidney

■ Weight

 ■ Assess fluid gains/losses

 ■ Obtain daily weights for all stable postoperative patients (consider twice daily weights for infant with excessive fluid changes, especially premature infants)

■ Skin/mucosa

 ■ Evaluate for dry mucous membranes, altered turgor, sunken fontanelle, and edema

■ Cardiovascular

 ■ Assess for tachycardia from too little extracellular fluid (hypovolemia) and/or anemia

 ■ Check for delayed capillary refill from low cardiac output

  • Monitor for hypotension (later sign)

  • Use inotropes to support blood pressure with excessive losses

■ Blood loss

 ■ Estimate blood loss during procedure to assess for anemia

  • Was it replaced in the OR?

  • Does the patient require further blood products?

  • Bleeding—is the patient continuing to bleed?

  • Monitor hematocrit and bleeding studies; transfuse as needed

   ◦ Packed red blood cells (PRBCs)

   ◦ Platelets

   ◦ Fresh frozen plasma (FFP)

   ◦ Cryoprecipitate

■ Intake and output

 ■ Perform close monitoring of maintenance fluid and total output

 ■ Conduct close monitoring of tube output from surgically placed drain(s)

  • Consider replacement of surgical drain/tube output if excessive (> 2 mL/kg/hr)

- Replacement fluids are given in addition to maintenance fluids
  - Gastric losses: NG tube output, vomiting, gastrointestinal (GI) bleed
  - Drains: chest tube, Jackson–Pratt
  - Urine losses
  - Stool output: dumping syndrome, diarrhea
  - Insensible losses: open wounds, exposed abdominal organs
- Replacement fluid chosen is based on the type of fluid losses. Fluid is typically replaced milliliter for milliliter or a fraction of the total volume lost over a certain time period (4 or 8 hours).
- Fluids typically used:
  - Normal saline (NS)
  - One half NS
  - Lactated Ringer's (caution must be taken because it does contain electrolytes, but does not contain glucose)
    - Typically fluid with potassium is not used due to the potential for hyperkalemia.

■ Nutritional requirements
  ■ If the enteral feedings are delayed (for > 48–72 hours), initiate parenteral nutrition and lipids as soon as possible (Koletzdo et al., 2008)
  ■ Determine feeding advancement plan if feeding via the enteral route

■ Lab evaluation
  ■ Serum electrolytes
  ■ Urine output
  ■ Urine electrolytes
  ■ Blood urea/serum creatinine

- Arterial blood gas (ABG) (low pH and bicarbonate may indicate poor perfusion)
- Develop routine schedule for laboratory studies (i.e., every 4, 8, or 24 hours)
- Notify prescriber of abnormal values (see Table 8.1 for normal values and causes of electrolyte imbalances) so that a treatment plan can be implemented
  - Consider obtaining repeat sample if aberrant values do not fit with the patient's clinical status

TABLE 8.1 Electrolyte Abnormalities

Sodium	Normal Range	Hyponatremia	Hypernatremia
	135–145	< 135 Fluid losses Inadequate intake Third spacing	> 145 Excessive fluid intake Sepsis Paralysis
Potassium	**Normal Range**	**Hypokalemia**	**Hyperkalemia**
	3.5–5.5 mEq/mL	Fluid losses nasogastric losses Inadequate supplementation	Acidosis Excessive intake Renal failure
Glucose	**Normal Range**	**Hypoglycemia**	**Hyperglycemia**
	60–100 mg/dL	Inadequate intake Low glycogen stores (premature and intrauterine growth restricted [IUGR] infants) Diabetic mother (excessive production of insulin)	Extreme prematurity IUGR Stress Sepsis Steroids Excessive intake

■ Blood sampling of electrolytes and glucose

  ■ If laboratory values are abnormal, take the following into consideration:

    • A slow return of blood can yield false labs due to hemolysis or breakdown of red blood cells and release of electrolytes into serum.

    • Dextrose in the tubing of the line may cause a false elevation in blood glucose level.

DOCUMENTATION

■ Vital signs

■ Accurate intake and output

■ Tissue perfusion

■ Laboratory values and management of aberrant values

■ Symptoms of electrolyte drop and abnormality

PAIN MANAGEMENT

Neonatal pain management has evolved tremendously over the past two decades. Pain assessment is now considered the fifth vital sign for all patients, including premature infants and neonates. Pain management for all infants requires a multimodal approach. The combination of nonpharmacologic and pharmacologic measures should be utilized to optimize the benefits to the patient while decreasing the total amount of opioids the patient will receive.

NONPHARMACOLOGIC MEASURES

■ Minimize exposure to painful or stressful procedures

■ Provide opportunities for nonnutritive sucking

■ Offer oral sucrose (24% solution)

■ Swaddle infant when condition permits

■ Arrange for kangaroo mother care (KMC) sessions with parents

PHARMACOLOGIC MEASURES

- Nonnarcotic analgesics: acetaminophen, administered alone or as adjunct treatment
- Opioids: morphine or fentanyl
- Sedatives: midazolam is a useful adjunct treatment; however, always address pain first

GOAL OF POSTOPERATIVE PAIN MANAGEMENT AND ASSESSMENT

The goal of postoperative pain management is to utilize the lowest amount of analgesia necessary to provide adequate pain relief while also minimizing the side effects of the agents (Walker, 2014). Pain management is a collaborative process that involves the nurse, anesthesiologist, surgeon, neonatologist, and the parents. Management of postoperative pain should begin preoperatively with a thoughtful discussion from all services and with the development of a pain management plan. When developing the pain management plan, consider the type of procedure, airway management, desired sedation, pain estimate, and previous opioid or benzodiazepine exposure. Establishment of the pain plan preoperatively allows for seamless pain management as soon as the patient returns from surgery.

PAIN ASSESSMENT SCALES

There are several reliable and valid pain assessment scales for the neonatal population (McNair et al., 2004; Suraseranivongse et al., 2006). The nurse should use the appropriate scale based on the age of the infant and the hospital's standard:

- PIPP—Premature infant pain profile (Stevens, Johnston, Petryshen, & Taddio, 1996)
- CRIES—Crying, requires increased oxygen administration, increased vital signs, expression, and sleeplessness (Krechel & Bildner, 1995)
- FLACC—Face, legs, activity, cry, and consolability (Merkel, Voepel-Lewis, Shayevitz, & Malviya, 1997)

POSTOPERATIVE PAIN PROTOCOLS

Standardized postoperative pain protocols should be established at institutions caring for the surgical infant. These protocols should include select opioids for minor surgical procedures or interventions as well as those for moderate to major surgical procedures. Minor surgical procedures may be treated with nonpharmacologic measures (i.e., sucrose, swaddling) to intermittent opioids (i.e., fentanyl or morphine). Major surgical procedures may be treated with intermittent or continuous opioids for 24 to 48 hours (i.e., morphine or fentanyl infusion) postoperatively. Minor and major surgical procedures should be defined in order to standardize treatment for surgical procedures.

It is recommended that routine postoperative pain assessment occur with relative frequency; at a minimum every 1 to 4 hours.

If pharmacologic agents are used, reassessment should be completed within a short time of administration to ensure adequate pain relief is achieved (within 1 hour).

Epidurals are defined as regional anesthesia that numbs or blocks pain sensation/feeling in a certain part of the body. Epidurals are managed by the anesthesia or pain team in the institution.

■ Common epidural anesthetics include:

■ Chloroprocaine

■ Rarely used epidural anesthetics for patients who are younger than 1 month:

■ Bupivicaine (rarely used in patients under a month of age)

■ Ropivacaine (rarely used in patients under a month of age)

■ The addition of small amounts of fentanyl or clonidine has proven effective in enhancing the anesthetic effects in the epidural agents; however, use with caution due to their potential toxic effects (Krane, 2005).

POSTOPERATIVE NURSING ASSESSMENT

■ Close monitoring of vital signs: respiratory depression can be a common side effect (Table 8.2)

■ Monitor for toxicity

TABLE 8.2 Medications Commonly Used in the Postoperative Phase

Medication		Dosing (Lexicomp Online, 2015)		Side Effects	Special Considerations
Classification	Name	Bolus	Continuous		
Sedative	Midazolam	0.05–0.2 mg/kg	0.03–0.06 mg/kg/hr	Hypotension Respiratory insufficiency Bradycardia Tolerance and dependency	Due to reduced clearance of the metabolites and seizurelike myoclonus reported, avoid using in premature infants (< 35 weeks) Reversal agent: Flumazenil
Analgesics	Morphine	0.05–0.2 mg/kg/ dose every 4 hours	0.01–0.02 mg/kg/hr	Urinary retention Seizures Tolerance and dependency	Reversal agent: Naloxone

Fentanyl	0.5–4 mcg/kg/dose every 2–4 hours	0.5–5 mcg/kg/hr	Chest wall rigidity (rapid administration)	Give IV slow push Reversal agent: Naloxone
Acetaminophen	*Oral:* 10–15 mg/kg/dose every 4–6 hours *Rectal:* 10–20 mg/kg/dose every 4–6 hours			Adjunct for low to moderate pain to decrease total amount of overall opioids
Sucrose	1–10 dips on pacifier or 2 mL	N/A		Use for heel sticks, with starting IVs
Local Anesthetic	LMX4 (lidocaine topical)	Apply 1 × 1 in. to intact skin 30 minutes prior to venipuncture/injection		Cover with bio-occlusive dressing. Analgesia lasts 1 hr. Do not exceed 2 g/24 hr.

Source: Welcome to Lexicomp Online (2015).

- Close monitoring of insertion site
- Monitor for drainage: Leaking from the epidural catheter is common with epidurals
- Monitor comfort level of patient

REFERENCES

Curley, M. A. Q., Meyer, E. C., Scoppettuolo, L. A., McGann, E. A., Trainor, B. P., Rachwal, C. M., & Hickey, P. A. (2012). Parent presence during invasive procedures and resuscitation. *American Journal of Respiratory and Critical Care Medicine, 186* (11), 1133–1139. doi: 10.1164/rccm.201205-0915OC

Davies, P., Hall, T., Ali, T., & Lakhoo, K. (2008). Intravenous postoperative fluid prescriptions for children: A survey of practice. *BMC Surgery, 8*, 10.

Gephart, S., & McGrath, J. (2012). Family-centered care of the surgical neonate. *Newborn Infant Nurse Review, 12*(1), 5–7.

Kelly, A., Liddell, M., & Davis, C. (2008). The nursing care of the surgical neonate. *Seminars in Pediatric Surgery, 17*(4), 290–296.

Koletzko, B., Goulet, O., Hunt, J., Krohn, K., Shamir, R., Parenteral Nutrition Guidelines Working Group, ... European Society of Paediatric Research (ESPR). (2005). Guidelines on paediatric parenteral nutrition of the European Society of Paediatric Gastroenterology, Hepatology and Nutrition (ESPGHAN) and the European Society for Clinical Nutrition and Metabolism (ESPEN), supported by the European Society of Paediatric Research (ESPR). *Journal of Pediatric Gastroenterology and Nutrition, 41*(Suppl. 2), S1–87. PubMed PMID: 16254497.

Krane, E. (2005). *Pediatric pain management in children.* Retrieved from http://pedsanesthesia.stanford.edu/downloads/guideline-pain.pdf

Krechel, S. W., & Bildner, J. (1995). CRIES: A new neonatal postoperative pain measurement score. Initial testing of validity and reliability. *Paediatric Anaesthesia, 5*(1), 53–61.

Lorenz, J. (1997). Assessing fluid and electrolytes status in the newborn. *Clinical Chemistry, 43*(1), 205–210.

McGrath, J. M. (2014). Family: Essential Partner in Care. In C. Kenner & J. W. Lott (Ed.), *Comprehensive neonatal nursing care* (5th ed.). New York, NY: Springer Publishing Company.

McNair, C., Ballantyne, M., Dionne, K., Stephens, D., & Stevens, B. (2004). Postoperative pain assessment in the neonatal intensive care unit. *Archives of Disease in Childhood—Fetal and Neonatal Edition, 89*(6), F537.

Merkel, S. I., Voepel-Lewis, T., Shayevitz, J. R., & Malviya S. (1997). The FLACC: A behavioral scale for scoring postoperative pain in young children. *Pediatric Nursing, 23*(3), 293–297.

O'Brien, F., & Walker, I. A. (2014). Fluid hemostasis in the neonate. *Pediatric Anesthesia, 24*, 49–59.

Snyder, C. (2015). *Fluid management for the pediatric surgical patient.* Retrieved from http://emedicine.medscape.com/article/936511-overview

Sprull, C. T. (2015). Developmental support. In M. T. Verklan & M. Walden (Eds.), *Core curriculum for neonatal intensive care nursing* (5th ed.). St. Louis, MO: Elsevier Saunders.

Stevens, B., Johnston, C., Petryshen, P., & Taddio, A. (1996). Premature infant pain profile: Development and initial validation. *Clinical Journal of Pain, 12*(1), 13–22.

Sudia-Robinson, T. (2015). Ethical issues. In M. T. Verklan & M. Walden (Eds.), *Core curriculum for neonatal intensive care nursing* (5th ed.). St. Louis, MO: Elsevier Saunders.

Suraseranivongse, S., Kaosaard, R., Pornsiriprasert, S., Karnchana, Y., Kaopinpruck, J., & Sangjeen, K. (2006). A comparison of postoperative pain scales in neonates. *British Journal of Anaesthesia, 97*(4), 540–544.

Walker, S. (2014). Neonatal pain. *Paediatric Anaesthesia, 24*(1), 39–48.

Welcome to Lexicomp Online. (n.d.). *Lexicomp Online Login.* N.p., n.d. Web. 09 February 2015.

SURGICAL DRAINS, TUBES, LINES, AND AIRWAY

Caitlin Bradley and Melissa Roberts

ABDOMINAL DRAINS

DEFINITION

Abdominal drains are soft, flexible drains inserted into the peritoneal space for evacuation of pneumoperitoneum, excess fluids, and/or infectious material identified on radiographic study(s).

CLINICAL INDICATION(S)

Designed to drain the peritoneal cavity of free air, excess fluids, and infectious material, abdominal drains can be used for very premature infants that are too unstable for transport to the OR or infants with significant ascites or abscesses.

Very preterm infants with spontaneous intestinal perforation (SIP) may benefit from drain placement; drain placement may help avoid an operative procedure. For necrotizing enterocolitis (NEC), infants may have drains placed until they are stable enough to tolerate a laparoscopic procedure (Chiu et al., 2006; Premkumar, 2012; Rao, Basani, Simmer, Samnakay, & Deshpande, 2011).

PREOPERATIVE ASSESSMENT AND NURSING CARE

■ Perform abdominal radiograph and/or ultrasound (US) prior to drain placement
■ Make infants nothing per os (NPO or by mouth) for 4 to 6 hours
■ Place peripheral IV line
■ Begin maintenance IV fluids
■ Obtain informed consent

Placement

■ Abdominal drains are placed by surgeons or interventional radiologists (IRs).
  ■ They can be placed at the bedside, which is an advantage for an unstable infant.

POSTOPERATIVE ASSESSMENT AND NURSING CARE

■ Allow drainage from abdominal drains to flow into the gauze or a diaper
■ Describe and measure drainage for accurate intake and output
■ Keep NPO in the immediate postoperative period; extent depends upon the condition being treated

- Feed infants being treated for abscesses or ascites if clinically stable
- Administer antibiotic treatment for coverage of known or suspected intra-abdominal processes and skin flora
- Provide parenteral nutrition for infants that will be NPO for greater than 5 to 7 days

DOCUMENTATION

- Location of the drains
- Appearance of the drain site
- Presence and integrity of sutures
- Drainage appearance

CENTRAL VENOUS LINES

DEFINITION

Central venous catheters (CVCs) are IV catheters placed in large veins, such as the internal and external jugular, saphenous, femoral, and subclavian. CVCs should be considered in the following patient scenarios: long-term IV access (> 1–2 weeks), poor vascular access, ongoing hemodynamic monitoring, and failed placement of peripheral-inserted central catheter (PICC) (Hansen, Greene, & Puder, 2009; Heffner & Androes, 2014a).

CLINICAL INDICATION(S)

- Clinical indications for CVCs include administration of medications, fluids, parenteral nutrition, central venous pressure (CVP) monitoring, and blood sampling.
- A vascular access decision-making algorithm can be an objective aid when determining the most appropriate CVC.

■ Consider the patient's condition, duration of therapy, specific procedure requirements, and history of vascular access problems when choosing the appropriate CVC device.

PREOPERATIVE ASSESSMENT AND NURSING CARE

■ Confirm parent or guardian has given consent

■ Obtain surgical and anesthesia team consents if CVC placement is going to occur in OR

■ Secure peripheral IV access for infusion of maintenance fluids and medications

■ Assess complete blood count (CBC) and coagulation tests for risk of bleeding and presence of anemia

■ Evaluate the patient for signs of infection; blood cultures should be negative for at least 48 hours if the infant is being treated for an infection to decrease the risk of seeding the new CVC with infectious material or infectious debris

■ Place infant on NPO status 4 to 6 hours prior to CVC placement

SURGICAL PROCEDURE

■ Common CVCs used in the NICU are femoral lines or those placed in the neck or upper chest.

■ When deciding on a single, double, or triple lumen CVC, consider the size of the vessel and the patient's needs (infusions, medications, etc.).

■ Past studies (Centers for Disease Control and Prevention and Healthcare Infection Control Practices Advisory Committee, 2011; Palefski & Stoddard, 2001) have shown an increased risk of infection with CVCs placed in the femoral area; current evidence refutes this finding, demonstrating no increased risk for femoral placement (Marik, Flemmer, & Harrison, 2012).

■ CVCs may be nontunneled or tunneled (Hansen et al., 2009; Heffner & Andres, 2014a):

■ Nontunneled CVCs are placed percutaneously and often sutured into place. Nontunneled CVCs are meant for short-term access (typically < 2 weeks). These types of catheters tend to be less flexible and lack the decreased thrombogenicity that tunneled CVCs offer.

■ Tunneled CVCs follow a subcutaneous tunnel between the catheterized veins to the exit site located on the skin. They are frequently placed in the upper chest or neck. These lines are typically used for longer term access, as they are more pliable, are at decreased risk for infection, and have less thrombogenicity and have a cuff that is placed under the infant's skin. Over time the original external sutures remain, but with time the cuff becomes secured in the infant's subcutaneous tissue and the line's stability will be enhanced.

POSTOPERATIVE ASSESSMENT AND NURSING CARE

Confirmation of placement

■ Confirm placement of the CVC with a chest radiograph

■ Ideal positioning (Hansen et al., 2009; Heffner & Androes, 2014b)

■ An upper body placed CVC is considered central if the tip resides at the superior vena cava (SVC) and the right atrium junction.

■ A lower body placed CVC is considered central if it resides within the inferior vena cava (IVC).

■ Caution should be exercised when CVCs terminate in the right atrium, as significant complications may arise.

■ Confirm proper placement of tip with a prescriber prior to use

Dressing

■ Maintain sterile occlusive dressings on CVCs at all times

■ Maintain visibility of the insertion site so it can be continually assessed for swelling, drainage, leakage, and erythema

■ Assess the site for pain with hourly (or more frequent) site checks

■ Change the dressing weekly, or more frequently if it becomes nonocclusive or soiled

Blood sampling

■ Follow individual, institutional evidence-based policies for accessing the CVC

■ General procedures for accessing the CVC include:

  ■ Pause infusions for 1 minute prior to obtaining a blood sample to ensure accuracy of the specimen, if the line has a continuous infusion

  ■ Perform hand hygiene and don clean gloves

  ■ Clean the hub with an approved antiseptic agent such as alcohol or chlorhexidine pads, scrubbing the hub for 15 (for alcohol) or 30 seconds (for chlorhexidine), and allow to dry

  ■ Flush the CVC with 1 to 3 mL NS (volume dependent upon the size of the catheter and fluid goals for the patient) in a pulsating manner

  ■ Withdraw 1 to 3 mL of blood (referred to as waste)

  ■ Depending on the catheter size and hospital policy, you may or may not return this waste

    • If returning the waste, ensure the sterility of the syringe during the blood draw and throughout the procedure.

  ■ Slowly withdraw your laboratory sample, removing the minimum amount of blood needed for the desired laboratory study(s)

    • Return waste (when applicable) after cleaning the hub (as mentioned earlier) and allowing it to dry

    • Return the waste to the infant slowly

  ■ Clean the hub again, allowing it to dry

  ■ Flush the tubing with NS in a pulsating manner

  ■ Reconnect to IV tubing and resume infusions, if applicable

COMPLICATIONS

CVC line days, sedation/paralysis, and exposure to multiple surgical procedures all increase the incidence of CVC complications (Bairdain et al., 2014).

Infection

- Maintain vigilant monitoring for infection, a major risk of CVC placement
  - Cellulitis: Continually assess the insertion site for signs of localized infection including erythema, swelling, and drainage.
  - Central line associated bloodstream infection (CLABSI): Continually assess the patient for signs of systemic infection that include escalation in respiratory support, pallor, increase in apnea/bradycardia/desaturations, fever, feeding intolerance, and change in vital signs.
- If local/skin infection (cellulitis) or CLABSI is suspected:
  - Obtain a CBC and blood culture
  - Determine the infection source by obtaining both peripheral and CVC line cultures
  - Administer prescribed broad-spectrum antibiotics after cultures are drawn for symptomatic infants
    - Narrow or revise antibiotic coverage when cultures yield an organism
    - Discontinue antibiotics if infection is ruled out
- Minimize infection risk by securing the CVC and IV tubing toward the head of the patient and never secure the CVC tubing in or around the diaper area (Hansen et al., 2009; Heffner & Androes, 2014a).

Malposition

- Accidental entrance or migration into an anatomical area not intended for the CVC
- Diagnose with chest radiograph, echocardiogram, and US

■ Removal of the line may be needed along with treatment for related complications

■ Treatment of related complications depend on the clinical scenario and infant's condition

■ Malposition can lead to pneumothorax, hemothorax, and/or cardiac tamponade depending on location of migrated catheter

■ Assess for symptoms of malposition including pain when infusing, tachypnea, bradycardia, respiratory distress, hypoxia, ventilation/perfusion (VQ) mismatch, and hypotension

Hemothorax

■ Caused by atrial trauma during insertion causing blood to collect in the pleural space

■ Assess for respiratory distress symptoms

Cardiac tamponade

■ This refers to blood or fluid that accumulates around the pericardium. This collection prevents effective contraction of the ventricles. This leads to lack of proper oxygen delivery to tissues.

■ Signs include those findings of tachypnea, bradycardia, respiratory distress, hypoxia, VQ mismatch, and hypotension, along with venous engorgement of the face and neck, paradoxical pulse, and cardiac arrest.

Arrhythmia

■ Abnormal heart rhythm

■ Caused by malposition, typically in the atria

■ Reposition the CVC and obtain x-ray confirmation

■ Perform hemodynamic monitoring until the arrhythmia subsides and the line is repositioned or removed

Venous thrombosis

- Results from a fibrin clot formation surrounding the tip of the CVC
- Removal of the line and anticoagulation may be necessary depending on the size of the clot and risk of dislodgement

SVC syndrome

- Results from obstruction to venous drainage from the SVC, due to thrombosis or a CVC that fills the vessel
- Treat by raising the head of the bed, monitoring respiratory status, and considering/alleviating the cause

Catheter occlusion

- Blockage of fluids from infusing and inability to withdraw blood from the CVC
- Ensure that the entire length of the CVC tubing is not kinked or clamped
- Restore patency of the occluded CVC lumen; utilizing a sterile technique, remove the injection cap and try gently flushing the line with a small amount of NS
- Consult the prescriber if patency cannot be restored with these measures
  - Prescribe tissue plasminogen activator (TPA), if indicated, to dislodge the occlusion
  - Instill this solution using sterile technique using only enough to fill the volume of the catheter, as more would lead to undesired systemic effects
  - Leave the solution to dwell in the catheter for the prescribed time (usually 30–60 minutes)
  - Aspirate the solution following the desired dwell time
  - Check for patency by attempting to flush the line (Hansen et al., 2009; Heffner & Androes, 2014b)

DOCUMENTATION

- Size of the catheter and priming volume (this should be recorded in the operative note)
- Hourly site assessments for erythema, drainage, and swelling
- Dressing integrity (should be occlusive, clean, dry, and intact)
- Length of external visible catheter to recognize migration of the catheter during routine daily assessments

CHEST TUBES

DEFINITION

Chest tubes can be made of silicone or polyvinyl chloride (PVC); they come in varying sizes, including the small bore pigtail catheter type. Chest tubes are used during surgical procedures to treat isolated pneumothoraces and to drain the chest of fluids such as chylous fluid, blood, esophageal leakage, and many more conditions.

- The benefits to pigtail catheters include reduced pain; however, their small bore makes drainage of viscous or proteinaceous fluids difficult.

CLINICAL INDICATION(S)

There are many clinical indications for chest tube placement, including drainage of both air and fluids from the pleural and extrapleural cavities. Chest tubes are often placed during operative procedures involving the chest and esophagus including patent ductus arteriosus (PDA) ligation, EA, TEF, congenital diaphragmatic hernia (CDH), chylothorax, and pneumothoraces that occur as a result of the operative procedure.

The size and type of the chest tube are dependent on the patient size, goals of treatment, and anticipated drainage. For example, a 12 French catheter may be placed for a full-term patient with a chylothorax. While a smaller chest tube, such as 8 French, can be used for a preterm infant following PDA ligation (Hansen & Lillehei, 2009).

PREOPERATIVE ASSESSMENT AND NURSING CARE

- Conduct a complete respiratory assessment
- Develop a plan for pain management
- Perform other preoperative assessments and nursing care relevant to the infant's clinical condition and diagnosis
- Select the chest drainage system to be used postoperatively

SURGICAL PROCEDURE

- Chest tubes are placed by trained providers under sterile conditions.
- Drainage of air
  - The smallest possible chest tube size should be used; 8 French is used for extremely low-birth-weight infants, and 10 or 12 French for near-term or term infants.
  - The infant should be given narcotic for pain control during placement.
  - A lidocaine injection may also be given for local analgesia.
  - The infant should be positioned with the side of placement up and the head of the bed elevated to 30° to 45°. This facilitates evacuation of air.
  - To avoid injury to the nipple, muscle, and major blood vessels, the chest tube is placed at the anterior axillary line, fourth intercostal space.
    - The entire area should be cleaned by the provider according to institutional policies and procedures.
    - The intended positioning of the chest tube is anterior to facilitate air drainage.
  - There will potentially be an audible rush of air when evacuated. The chest tube must be immediately connected to the drainage system (see text that follows for the postoperative placement instructions) (Gomella, Cunningham, & Eyal, 2013; Hansen & Lillehei, 2009).

■ Drainage of fluid

■ The smallest possible chest tube should be placed, with consideration to the type of fluid to be evacuated.

- In general, drainage of blood requires a larger bore chest tube (12 French) due to the risk of clotting and subsequent need for replacement. However, a chylothorax may be drained using a 10 French or pigtail catheter.

■ Narcotics should be given, prior to placement, for pain control.

■ To avoid injury to the nipple, muscle, and major blood vessels, the chest tube is placed at the anterior axillary line, fourth intercostal space.

- The entire area should be cleaned by the provider according to the institution's policies and procedures.

- US may be used for placement guidance.

- The intended positioning of the chest tube is posterior to facilitate fluid drainage (Gomella et al., 2013; Hansen & Lillehei, 2009).

■ The chest tube is connected to the drainage system.

■ Chest tubes are sutured in place for stabilization.

■ This is followed by placement of an occlusive dressing.

■ The use of a petroleum gauze dressing forms a secure seal around the tube insertion site.

■ The site is then covered with dry gauze before placement of the final transparent dressing over the entire site.

POSTOPERATIVE ASSESSMENT AND NURSING CARE

■ Secure (immediately following placement) the chest tube with tape, just outside of the dressing, for stabilization using a chevron style method.

■ Use a small piece of tape (about 2 in. long) wrapped around the tubing to form a tab or anchor.

- Utilize a pin to attach the anchor to the patient's bedding to prevent accidental dislodgement.
- Ensure connection of the chest tube to the drainage system.
  - Move, in order, from the patient to the drainage system
    - Inspect the chest tube at the site: ensure the holes for drainage are not protruding from the incision
      - For the functional drainage of air or fluid, the holes must remain inside the chest cavity.
    - Inspect the dressing; petroleum gauze should encircle the chest tube at the incision site, and the dressing should be occlusive
    - Ensure the chest tube is connected securely to the drainage system
      - A Christmas tree–style adaptor is sometimes needed to form a secure attachment between the chest tube and tubing from the drainage apparatus.
      - Each connection down to the drainage system must be methodically inspected.
    - Evaluate for any escape of air, fluid, or other drainage at all connections
    - Consult with the provider to determine the level of suction; generally, it is set between 15 and 20 cm H_2O, negative pressure (Hansen & Lillehei, 2009)
      - For postoperative CDH repairs on extracorporeal membrane oxygenation (ECMO), 5 or 10 cm H_2O of negative pressure may be used to avoid damage and/or hemorrhage while the infant is being anticoagulated and for reestablishment of the thoracic cavity.
- Provide adequate pain management
  - For silicone or PVC catheters
    - Continuous narcotic drips (morphine or fentanyl) should be administered.

- If properly managed, low doses can be effective.
- Bolus doses of narcotics should be administered when moving the patient.

■ For pigtail catheters

- Each patient's pain should be evaluated and addressed on an individual basis.
- Continuous drips may be used, but they may not be needed for the entire length of time the pigtail is indwelling.

■ Assist the provider with removal

- Removal should be considered when there is no further air or fluid evacuated for approximately 24 hours (Gomella et al., 2013; Hansen & Lillehei, 2009).
  - An exception is with EA repairs: Chest tubes will remain in place and may be put to water seal until a contrast study evaluates the site of anastomosis for leakage.
  - During the esophagram study, contrast is injected into the upper esophagus.
  - If there is a leakage at the anastomosis, the contrast will be visualized moving into the chest cavity.
  - If the anastomosis leaks, the chest tube remains in place until the study is repeated (typically 1–2 weeks).
  - If the contrast does not leak, the chest tube can be removed.
- A trained provider removes the chest tube.
- When no air or fluid is drained, the chest tube will remain in place, but the suction is turned to 0 cm H_2O; this is called *placing the chest tube to water seal.*
- If the patient demonstrates respiratory distress or other symptoms of reaccumulation of air or fluid, a chest radiograph should be obtained and the negative pressure suction may be resumed.

■ Obtain a chest radiograph prior to removal of the chest tube to ensure there has been no reaccumulation of air or fluid

▨ Administer narcotics prior to chest tube removal to ensure proper pain control

▨ Remove upon inspiration when the patient is on continuous positive airway pressure (CPAP) or intubated, and remove upon expiration when the patient is not intubated or on CPAP (Gomella et al., 2013)

▨ Place a petroleum gauze dressing over the incision site immediately after removal, followed by a gauze sponge and transparent occlusive dressing

  • This dressing is left in place for at least 24 hours, as instructed by the provider.

DOCUMENTATION

■ Respiratory assessment

■ Chest tube site and dressing integrity

■ Goals of the chest tube and progress toward removal

■ Specific characteristics

  ▨ Type and amount of drainage

  ▨ Amount of suction

■ Patient tolerance to the chest tube

■ Pain medication requirements and response

■ Untoward respiratory symptoms prior to and following removal

GASTROSTOMY TUBES

DEFINITION

Surgically placed gastrostomy tubes (G-tubes) are used for a variety of purposes, but generally are meant to provide enteral nutrition, fluids and/or medications, and gastric decompression for infants with a variety of clinical conditions (i.e., risk of aspiration including vocal cord paralysis, discoordination in suck, swallow, and breathe, and muscle weakness; airway or GI anomalies [microgastria];

oral aversion; neurologic or metabolic conditions; congenital heart disease; congenital syndromes esophageal atresia and TEF, and prolonged ileus [Duro, Bousvaros, & Puder, 2009]).

CLINICAL INDICATION(S)

■ Inability to orally consume sufficient calories for growth and hydration

■ Inability to safely feed or take medications orally

PREOPERATIVE ASSESSMENT AND NURSING CARE

Obtain history

■ Obtain a complete history of the presenting problem from the parent or surrogates

  ■ Document a history of vomiting/reflux

■ Assess growth (anthropometric measurements including weight, head circumference, and length)

  ■ In general, infants should be more than 2 kg before having their G-tube placed. This will decrease the potential for surgical complications.

■ Evaluate ability to orally feed at bedside and via swallow study

  ■ There are two types of swallow studies: conventional and modified barium swallow (MBS). Both are fluoroscopic evaluations of the infant's swallow, as well as presence or absence of aspiration.

  ■ The conventional swallow study provides additional information about the esophageal and gastric anatomy and should be chosen when there is concern for TEF and/or esophageal atresia, or an obstruction (Duro et al., 2009).

■ Obtain a chest radiograph if there is a new suspected case of aspiration, or in the event of chronic aspiration

■ Assess the adequacy of home resources and supports

Perform examination

■ Evaluate the gag reflex in neurologically compromised and hypotonic infants

■ Assess signs and symptoms consistent with lung or heart disease

■ Appraise primitive reflexes prior to any oral feeding, including rooting and sucking

■ Monitor coordination of suck, swallow, and breathe during feedings. Speech therapists or occupational therapists can be of great assistance in evaluating an infant's feeding skills

Secure laboratory evaluation

■ Obtain nutrition labs: CBC with differential, electrolytes, calcium, phosphorous, albumin/total protein, and liver function tests (LFTs) and assess for abnormalities

  ▪ Laboratory studies will be normal, or consistent with a specific disorder.

  ▪ Genetic and neurologic studies are sent when there is a suspicion for a specific disorder.

Preoperative readiness

■ Choose the correct feeding tube in consultation with neonatology, nursing, surgery, gastroenterology, radiology, and speech therapy as applicable

■ Maintain NPO for 4 to 6 hours prior to placement of the G-tube

■ Place a peripheral IV if infant does not have central line access

■ Infuse maintenance IV fluids

■ Obtain signed informed consents

SURGICAL PROCEDURE

There are several techniques used in placing a G-tube. Techniques include percutaneous endoscopic gastrostomy (PEG) placement, Stamm (open) gastrostomy, laparoscopic gastrostomy, or Seldinger technique (placed by IR). The Seldinger and PEG procedures are the least invasive, the laparoscopic slightly more invasive, and the Stamm is the most invasive G-tube placement method (Baker, Emil, & Baird, 2013; Duro et al., 2009).

■ G-tubes are placed by surgeons, gastroenterologists, and/or IRs that have training in surgical feeding tube placement.

■ G-tubes will consistently have two ports: one for feeding and the other to inflate and deflate the balloon.

  ▦ Depending on the brand and type of the G-tube, there may also be a port for medication administration.

POSTOPERATIVE ASSESSMENT AND NURSING CARE

Management of the G-tube

■ Place the G-tube to drain while any postoperative ileus resolves

  ▦ Minimal drainage may be expected and is typically serosanguinous or clear.

  ▦ Some bilious drainage may be observed if there is a temporary ileus.

■ If there is no drainage after 4 to 6 hours, clamp or disconnect from drainage for several hours, prior to enteral feeding

■ Irrigate the G-tube with NS or sterile water to ensure patency (if unable to withdraw irrigant, notify a nurse practitioner [NP] or MD)

■ Achieve pain control through the use of opioids in conjunction with acetaminophen

■ Prophylactic antibiotics may be prescribed and given for 24 hours

■ Ensure securement of the G-tube

  ▦ There are two types of G-tube location of the securement; these depend on the desired anatomic placement.

    • External securement on the abdomen with medical tape is done for at least 6 weeks to avoid tract enlargement and dislodgement (from movement of the tube).

      • This facilitates normal healing of the G-tube tract.

- If a flange or disk is present, external securement is achieved by stabilizing the dressing onto the abdomen.
  - Internal securement such as a balloon or bolster is used for internal stabilization on some G-tubes.
- Place a hydrocolloid wound dressing between skin and tape, taking care to avoid excessive traction if there is skin breakdown or irritation
  - Excessive traction can affect the healing site and may cause leakage around the G-tube.
- Check balloon inflation weekly, on a consistent day of the week
  - Balloons may have different volumes; during each check, aspirate the fluid from the balloon and ensure it is the correct amount.
  - The operative note is a good source for accurate information related to volume in the balloon.
  - If there is a discrepancy in volume, there may be a mechanical issue with the tube and the surgeon should be notified.
- Assess for gastric content or feeding residuals by gently aspirating stomach contents via the G-tube
- Maintain patency by flushing the G-tube with warm water (sterile water is used with immune-compromised infants)
- Flush the G-tube before and after feeding/medication administration
  - Flush twice daily to maintain patency if the G-tube port is not being used
- Vent the G-tube to decrease the risk for reflux, aspiration, and to alleviate gastric distention when infants are on noninvasive ventilation

Feedings

- Administer bolus or continuous feedings via G-tubes after a period of observation following surgery and approved by the surgeon
  - If the infant has tolerated bolus feedings, they should be resumed after G-tube placement.

Dressings, bathing, and skin care

■ Change dressings once or twice per day

■ Inspect the peristomal site, noting the site's integrity, erythema, and drainage

■ Cleanse skin with saline or water

  ■ If there is crust at the site, use one-fourth strength hydrogen peroxide (mixed with sterile water or saline), then rinse with saline.

■ Dry the skin before reapplying the dressing

■ Apply a split 2- × 2-inch gauze around the insertion site

  ■ Small amounts of drainage are appropriate.

  ■ Consider using an absorbent dressing to wick moisture away from the skin.

  ■ Drainage and skin irritation may indicate leakage of gastric contents onto skin.

  ■ Reassess tube stabilization and the balloon inflation if leakage occurs.

  ■ Leakage could be due to inadequate balloon volume; check balloon volume and add appropriate fluid if needed and consider replacing the tube if balloon leakage is noted.

■ Resume tub baths for stable infants on postoperative day (POD) 7 if the site is healing well

■ Notify providers of complications

  ■ The majority of complications occur during the first year following placement (McSweeney, Jiang, Deutsch, Atmadja, & Lightdale, 2013). Notify the surgeon if the complication is significant.

Dislodgement

■ Never try to reinsert the G-tube that dislodges

  ■ If the person trying to reinsert the tube is not properly trained, the tract could be disrupted.

■ Cover the G-tube site with gauze and seek the attention of a trained provider to reinsert

　■ Less than 12 weeks post-op: Only a surgeon can replace the G-tube

　■ Greater than 12 weeks post-op: MD, NP, or RN with specialty training may perform replacement

Occlusion

■ Milk or flush tubing with 5 to 10 mL warm water or NS tubing if occlusion in the tubing is noted

■ Establish patency by contacting a prescriber to order an enzymatic solution to manage an obstruction not relieved with an NS or water flush

■ Replace the tube if patency is not achieved, via flush or the administration of an enzymatic solution

■ Consider causes (incompatibility, flushing frequency, thick formula) of occlusion when patency is reestablished

　■ Prevent future occlusion through anticipatory guidance

Skin breakdown

■ Check for leakage at the site

　■ Application of a colloidal oatmeal soak or domeboroaluminum acetate solution can decrease moisture at the site

■ Infection (cellulitis) is treated with antibiotics including Augmentin, cephalexin, or clindamycin

■ Treat cellulitis targeting for specific organisms (i.e., bactroban ointment may be used for *Staphylococcus*)

Worsening reflux

■ Worsening of reflux may result from G-tube placement.

■ Minimize reflux by lengthening the feeding time if reflux worsens following G-tube placement.

▨ Conversion to a postpyloric feeding tube can be considered if reflux is severe and noninvasive methods do not alleviate the symptoms.

Bleeding

▨ Assess for granulation tissue and skin integrity

  ▨ Ensure there isn't excessive traction on the tube

  ▨ Manage granulomas as described here

Granulation

▨ Movement of the G-tube can lead to development of granulation tissue.

  ▨ Cauterization of the granuloma is performed daily with silver nitrate sticks until granuloma is flat.

   • Apply a barrier to protect surrounding skin with petrolatum ointment when treating with silver nitrate

   • Cauterized granuloma tissue will turn gray or black during treatment

  ▨ Triamcinolone cream 0.5% applied three times daily for 7 to 10 days has been shown to decrease the granuloma size.

Other rare complications

▨ Early onset, but less prevalent complications include: colonic perforation, duodenal hematoma, and necrotizing fasciitis (Duro et al., 2009)

  ▨ This would manifest as abdominal distention, tenderness, discoloration of the abdomen, and other signs consistent with sepsis.

  ▨ Surgery should be notified if these are suspected.

▨ Late onset, less prevalent complications include gastrocolic fistula (Duro et al., 2009)

  ▨ Presenting symptoms include abdominal pain, diarrhea, vomiting.

  ▨ Surgery should be notified if this is suspected.

DOCUMENTATION

- Include G-tube type, length, and diameter
- Type of securement(s)
- Dressing applied
- Amount of fluid to fill the balloon
- Date balloon is due for a check
- Peristomal and stomal appearance
- Presence of leakage
- Presence of granuloma including size and location in clock hours and treatment

GASTRO-JEJUNAL TUBES

DEFINITION

Surgically placed gastro-jejunal (G-J) tubes are used for a variety of purposes, but generally are meant to provide enteral nutrition, fluids and/or medications, and gastric decompression for infants with certain clinical indications (i.e., due to risk of aspiration including vocal cord paralysis, discoordination of suck, swallow, and breathe, and muscle weakness; and airway or GI anomalies [microgastria], oral aversion, neurologic or metabolic conditions, congenital heart disease, congenital syndromes EA and TEF, and prolonged ileus) in infants with an inability to tolerate gastric feeding (Duro et al., 2009).

CLINICAL INDICATION(S)

Postpyloric feedings are indicated for infants with the following situations:

- Unable to tolerate NG or OG feedings
- High risk of aspiration
- Delayed gastric emptying

- Dysmotility with risk of reflux and aspiration
- Anatomic abnormalities, such as microgastria

PREOPERATIVE ASSESSMENT AND NURSING CARE

Many preoperative evaluations take place to determine the necessity and appropriateness of a G-J tube. Consultation with neonatology, nursing, surgery, gastroenterology, radiology, and speech therapy is needed. Discussion with family or guardians throughout the process must take place, as well as evaluation of home resources.

Prior to placement, infants should be NPO for 4 to 6 hours, peripheral IV should be placed, maintenance fluids should be infusing, and consents should be signed.

Evaluation frequently includes similar components such as G-tube placement. The preoperative assessment and care presented here are specific for management of G-J tubes.

History

- Growth and ability to orally feed and tolerate gastric feedings
    - Anthropometric measurements (weight, head circumference, and length)
- In general, infants should be more than 2 kg before having their surgical feeding tube placement.
    - This will decrease the potential for surgical complications.
- Obtain a chest radiograph if there are new suspected aspiration events or in the event of chronic aspiration
- Evaluate for a history of vomiting/reflux

Examination

- Evaluation of a gag reflex is critical in neurologically compromised and hypotonic infants
    - Infants with a lack of a gag reflex are at extremely high risk for aspiration and are extremely limited or have no ability to coordinate suck/swallow/breathe.

- Assess for the presence of signs consistent with lung or heart disease, especially if exacerbated by reflux and aspiration
- Evaluate for uncoordinated feeding ability and risk for reflux/aspiration using a swallow study
- Measure stomach clearance with a gastric emptying study when concerned for delayed emptying
- Perform an evaluation of an infant's feeding skills using experts from speech or occupational therapy

Laboratory evaluation

- Obtain ordered labs for genetic and neurologic studies (specific to suspected disorder) and nutritional labs: CBC with differential, electrolytes, calcium, phosphorous, albumin/total protein, and LFTs
  - Laboratory studies will be normal, but in the event of a specific disorder they can yield etiology of the infant's oral feeding ability or inability

SURGICAL PROCEDURE

- G-J tube placement is done after the G-tube is placed.
- The J-tube is advanced through the G-tube, under fluoroscopy, and into the jejunum.
  - Placement is confirmed with contrast in the OR or IR.

POSTOPERATIVE ASSESSMENT AND NURSING CARE

Management of the G-J tube

Surgically placed G-J tubes have a G, J, and balloon port.

- Leave the gastric portion to gravity and clamp the jejunal portion for 6 to 8 hours in the immediate postoperative period.
  - This is done to avoid vomiting and aspiration due to temporary ileus.
- Monitor for drainage from the G-tube port.
  - Minimal drainage is expected.

▨ Drainage is typically serosanguinous or clear.

▨ Some bilious drainage may be observed if there is a temporary ileus or due to consistent stenting of the pylorus.

■ Irrigate the G-tube port with NS (sterile water should be used with immunocompromised patients) to ensure patency.

▨ If unable to withdraw irrigantion solution, notify the NP, MD, or surgeon.

■ Clamp the G-tube port when there is no drainage, or not a large amount of drainage, as there may be normal gastric secretions. Enteral feeds can begin if the infant can tolerate clamping the G-tube port and there is no vomiting of gastric secretions.

■ Manage postoperative pain control. Opioids are used in conjunction with acetaminophen.

■ Administer prescribed antibiotics prophylactically for 24 hours or longer if there is a concern for infection.

■ Communicate the type of G-J tube to all care providers; not all G-J tubes will have internal securement.

■ Internal securement may be accomplished with a balloon or bolster.

■ Apply external securement on the abdomen for at least 6 weeks to avoid tract enlargement and dislodgement.

▨ This facilitates healing of the tract.

▨ It is similar to G-tube securement.

▨ If an external flange or disk is present, stabilize the dressing onto the abdomen with tape.

■ Place a hydrocolloid wound dressing between the skin and tape if there is skin breakdown or irritation, taking care to avoid excessive traction.

▨ Excessive traction can interfere with healing and may cause leakage.

■ Check the balloon volume weekly, on a consistent day.

▨ Each balloon may have different volumes, so ensure correct volume for the balloon is used.

■ The operative note is a good source for accurate information related to volume in the balloon.

■ During each check, aspirate the fluid from the balloon and ensure it is the correct amount and report discrepancies to the surgeon.

• Discrepancies can occur from mechanical issues.

■ Vent the G port to decrease the risk of reflux and aspiration, and alleviate gastric distention when infants are on noninvasive ventilation.

■ Flush the G and J ports before and after feeding/medication administration

■ Warm water is used for flushing the ports.

■ Sterile water flushes are used for immunocompromised patients.

■ Flushing of unused ports

■ Flush the G port twice daily if not being used.

■ Flush the J port every 4 hours if not being used.

Feeding

■ Administer jejunum feeds continuously

■ Never give feeds by bolus to jejunum due to discomfort and a risk of intestinal perforation.

Dressing, bathing, and skin care

■ Change dressings once or twice per day

■ Inspect the peristomal site: note integrity, erythema, and drainage

■ Small amounts of drainage are appropriate.

■ Drainage and skin irritation indicate leakage of gastric contents onto skin.

• Reassess for adequate tube stabilization and balloon inflation

■ Cleanse skin with saline or water

■ If there is crust at the site, use one-fourth strength hydrogen peroxide.

■ Rinse with saline or water.

■ Dry skin prior to reapplying dressing

  ▨ Use a split 2- × 2-inch gauze placed around the insertion site if there is drainage. If there is significant drainage, use an absorbent dressing to wick moisture away from the skin.

■ If the site is healing well and the infant is stable, tub baths can be resumed on POD 7.

Dislodgement

■ Never try to reinsert the G-J tube that dislodges

  ▨ If the person trying to reinsert the tube is not properly trained, the tract could be disrupted.

■ Cover the G-tube site with gauze and seek the attention of a trained provider to reinsert

  ▨ Less than 12 weeks post-op

    • Temporary replacement can only be performed by a surgeon.

    • Replacement is completed in interventional radiology under fluoroscopy for position confirmation.

  ▨ Greater than 12 weeks post-op

    • A trained MD, NP, or RN may place a temporary G-tube to maintain patency of the tract.

      ◦ Placement confirmation should be completed prior to use for medications or feedings.

    • The G-J is replaced in IR under fluoroscopy to confirm placement.

Occlusion

■ Milk or flush tubing with 5 to 10 mL warm water or NS tubing if occlusion in the tubing is noted

■ Establish patency by contacting a prescriber to order an enzymatic solution to manage an obstruction that is not relieved with an NS or water flush

■ Replace the tube if patency is not achieved, via flush or the administration of an enzymatic solution

■ Consider causes (incompatibility, flushing frequency, thick formula) of occlusion when patency is reestablished

　■ Prevent future occlusion through anticipatory guidance

Skin breakdown

■ Check for leakage at the site

　■ Application of a colloidal oatmeal soak or domeboro-aluminum acetate solution can decrease moisture at the site

■ Infection (cellulitis) is treated with antibiotics including Augmentin, cephalexin, or clindamycin

■ Treat cellulitis targeting for specific organisms (i.e., bactroban ointment may be used for *Staphylococcus*)

Bleeding

■ Assess for granulation tissue and skin integrity

　■ Ensure there is not excessive traction on the tube

　■ Manage granulomas as described in the following

Granulation

■ Movement of the G-tube can lead to development of granulation tissue.

　■ Cauterization of the granuloma is performed daily with silver nitrate sticks until the granuloma is flat.

　　• Apply a barrier to protect surrounding skin with petrolatum ointment when treating with silver nitrate.

　　• Cauterized granuloma tissue will turn gray or black during treatment.

　■ Triamcinolone cream 0.5% applied three times daily for 7 to 10 days has been shown to decrease the granuloma size.

Residual checks

■ Do not perform residual checks via J-tube port.

    ■ The narrow lumen of the J portion precludes residual check as suction cannot be applied to the J port.

■ Residual checks can be performed on the G-tube portion.

Complications

The majority of complications occur during the first year postplacement (McSweeney et al., 2013).

■ Notify the prescriber if a complication is suspected.

■ Notify the surgeon if the complication is significant.

Other rare complications

■ Early-onset rare complications that can occur (in the first 2 weeks) include colonic perforation, duodenal hematoma, and necrotizing fasciitis (Duro et al., 2009).

    ■ Surgery should be notified if these are suspected.

■ A late-onset complication, gastrocolic fistula, is a significant complication.

    ■ Surgery should be notified if this is suspected.

DOCUMENTATION

■ Include tube type, length, and diameter

■ Type of securement(s)

■ Dressing applied

■ Amount of fluid to fill the balloon

■ Date the balloon check is due

■ Peristomal and stomal appearance

■ Presence of leakage

■ Presence of granuloma including size and location in clock hours and treatment

TRACHEOSTOMY

DEFINITION

Tracheostomy is a procedure that exposes, incises, and cannulates the trachea to create a surgical airway. The size and type of tracheostomy depend on the infant's anatomy and size.

CLINICAL INDICATION(S)

■ Conditions that may require treatment with tracheostomy include airway obstruction, chronic lung disease, vocal cord paralysis, chronic aspiration, congenital airway anomalies, laryngomalacia, tracheomalacia, respiratory failure, congenital central hypoventilation syndrome, and neuromuscular weakness.

■ Tracheostomies can reduce the risk of subglottic and tracheal stenosis in infants requiring long-term intubation and mechanical ventilation, as well as decrease complications related to long-term intubation.

■ The tracheostomy tube may be attached to a ventilator or a system for humidification.

■ It may be used for airway suctioning and also administration of aerosolized medications (Lowinger & Ohlms, 2009; Overman et al., 2013).

PREOPERATIVE ASSESSMENT AND NURSING CARE

■ Maintain NPO for 4 to 6 hours prior to the procedure, if on non-fortified breast milk feedings

■ Up to 8 hours may be needed if fortified feedings are being administered

■ Confirm surgical and anesthesia team consents are obtained

■ Secure peripheral IV access for infusion of maintenance fluids and medications

General assessment

■ Assess respiratory status, tolerance to ventilator support and weaning, and blood gas measurement for all patients undergoing a tracheostomy

■ Communicate symptom management and respiratory status to the entire care team

■ Evaluate for appropriate somatic weight gain that is critical for infants requiring a tracheostomy

■ Suspend enteral feedings and support with parenteral nutrition or dextrose/electrolyte-containing IV fluids

Testing

■ Diagnose suspected airway anomalies with flexible and direct laryngoscopy

■ Perform diagnostic tests including airway imaging, such as dynamic airway CT

■ Assess for genetic anomalies or syndromes, neuromuscular problems, and difficulties swallowing (Lowinger & Ohlms, 2009)

Medications

■ Manage respiratory status with systemic medications including diuretics, methylxanthines, and steroids

■ Use inhaled medications as adjunct respiratory management therapy including bronchodilators and steroids

Reduce infection risk

■ Minimize risk for aspiration and pneumonia through the use of ventilator-associated pneumonia (VAP) bundles

▪ Respiratory bundles include elevation of the head of the bed, frequent mouth care, and in-line tracheal suctioning.

SURGICAL PROCEDURE

■ The infant's airway is secured prior to the operative procedure, typically with an endotracheal tube (ETT).

■ The infant is then positioned with a shoulder roll and head ring to expose the neck. The neck is incised and subcutaneous fat is removed.

■ Incisions to the second and third tracheal rings are made.

■ The tracheostomy tube, with predetermined diameter and length, is placed by the surgeon (or most qualified provider if placed emergently).

■ Bilateral air entry is confirmed at the end of the procedure (Lowinger & Ohlms, 2009).

POSTOPERATIVE ASSESSMENT AND NURSING CARE

Immediate postoperative period

■ Obtain chest radiograph to ensure proper placement, as well as lung expansion postoperatively

■ Minimize infant movement through PODs 5 to 7 to allow for the stoma and tract to heal

   ▪ Movement of the head and neck during the first 5 to 7 days will increase stoma size, resulting in tissue damage, leakage of air, and bleeding.

   ▪ Excessive movement will encourage the formation of granulomas, which can bleed and cause leakage around the stoma.

   ▪ Limit manipulation of the tracheostomy to the otolaryngology (ORL) service until the initial tracheostomy change on POD 5 to 7.

■ Document the tracheostomy inner diameter and length

■ Ensure "stay sutures" remain fixed to the chest and secured with a transparent dressing

   ▪ These are intact and secured in the immediate postoperative period.

■ Keep a spare tracheostomy tube of the same size (length and diameter) and another that is one size smaller, scissors, oxygen, suction and suction catheters, and a syringe for cuffed tubes at the bedside

Sedation

■ Control pain, decrease agitation, and limit movement using a combination of opioids with benzodiazepines

■ Maintain moderate sedation until the initial tracheostomy change on POD 5 to 7

Mechanical ventilation

■ Support of breathing postoperatively while patient is sedated and treated for pain

■ Wean from mechanical ventilation if able to, depending upon the infant's diagnosis and degree of lung disease

■ Humidify air entering the trachea, even after infant is weaned from mechanical ventilation, since it now bypasses the nares

Suctioning

■ Clear the airway with routine care and as needed to ensure patency.

■ Scant bloody secretions may be noted in the immediate postoperative period.

■ Minimize infection by suctioning with an in-line catheter or open suction using sterile technique (sterile gloves and sterile catheter).

■ Minimize airway trauma and irritation by advancing the suction catheter to the appropriate depth (to the end of the tracheostomy tube, and not beyond) as determined by ORL and respiratory therapy.

Nutrition

■ Maintain NPO on parenteral nutrition or dextrose/electrolyte-containing IV fluids until bowel activity (bowel sounds and passage of gas) resumes.

■ Restart or begin enteral feedings and advance as tolerated once bowel activity returns.

■ Until safety with oral feeding is established, feedings should be administered through a feeding tube placed via the NG/OG routes or surgically.

   ▪ Surgically placed feeding tubes may be placed at the same time as the tracheostomy if the infant is not expected to PO feed.

■ A feeding team evaluation and MBS should be done to evaluate the safety of oral feedings for infants with a tracheostomy with a perceived ability to orally feed.

Routine tracheostomy site care (started after initial tracheostomy change)

■ Gather supplies, perform hand hygiene, and put on gloves before loosening tracheostomy ties and cleaning the site

■ Have medical ORL provider present for tracheostomy changes if required by institutional policy

■ Clean secretions or drainage from the stoma site using cotton-tip applicators dampened with sterile water, sterile NS, and/or hydrogen peroxide/water solution (50/50 solution; optional)

■ Allow the site to air dry briefly

■ Observe site for redness or cellulitis

■ Apply prescribed treatments (such as mupirocin) in a thin layer followed by the dressing

   ▪ Apply a split-gauze dressing to the stoma if there is scant drainage and the site is intact

   ▪ Use a moisture wicking dressing if there is significant drainage and breakdown of the site

Change tracheostomy ties

■ Have two health care providers present for the procedure

   ▪ One provider is responsible for securing the tracheostomy flanges while the second provider manages the tracheostomy ties.

- Cut the new tracheostomy ties so the Velcro straps do not overlap
- Taper the edges to 45° to make threading through the flanges easier
- Loosen the old ties and cleanse skin underneath
- Allow the skin to dry
- Apply prescribed medication (i.e., mupirocin to treat cellulitis or antifungal cream to treat a yeastlike rash)
- Thread the ends of the new tracheostomy ties, one at a time
- The free ends of the tracheostomy ties should be brought to the back of the neck
- Fasten Velcro ends of each tracheostomy tie, one at a time
- Ensure correct tightness, check to see if one small finger fits between the neck and ties
- Readjust if too loose or too tight

Complications

Initial:

- Hemorrhage manifests as bleeding at the site, blood during suctioning, and respiratory distress.
- Pneumothorax and pneumomediastinum manifest as respiratory, and potentially cardiovascular, instability and distress.
- Loss of airway/dislodgement: If the tracheostomy becomes dislodged, the infant will manifest respiratory distress that is not relieved by bag-mask ventilation.
- Infection (local cellulitis) manifests as erythema and drainage around the site.

Later:

- Granulation tissue, suprastomal collapse, subglottic stenosis, erosion, and tracheocutaneous fistula are long-term complications that will manifest as difficulty weaning from the ventilator and the need for increased ventilator support.

- Speech delay is a long-term complication that must be assessed using speech therapy. Ideally, speech therapy should begin as early as possible to avoid this delay.

When matched for gestational age, infants with tracheostomies have a higher mortality rate and complications increase those risks of mortality. Discussion with family around these risks is necessary prior to tracheostomy placement.

DOCUMENTATION

- Tracheostomy type, size, and presence or absence of a cuff
- Inflation or deflation of cuff
  - Quantity of fluid with cuff inflation (to assess for leakage)
- Date of tracheostomy change
- Respiratory examination and toleration of weaning
- Stoma site assessment and drainage
- Presence, appearance, and quantity of secretions
- Parental response
- Parental education

REFERENCES

Bairdain, S., Kelly, D., Tan, C., Dodson, B., Zurakowski, D., Jennings, R., & Trenor, C. (2014). High incidence of catheter-associated venous thromboembolic events in patients with long gap esophageal atresia treated with the Foker process. *Journal of Pediatric Surgery, 49*(2), 370–373.

Baker, L., Emil, S., & Baird, R. (2013). A comparison of techniques for laparoscopic gastrostomy placement in children. *Journal of Surgical Research, 184*(1), 392–396.

Centers for Disease Control and Prevention (CDC) and Healthcare Infection Control Practices Advisory Committee. (2011). *Guidelines for the prevention of intravascular-catheter related infections.* Retrieved from http://www.cdc.gov/hicpac/BSI/04-bsi-background-info-2011.html

Chiu, B., Pillai, S., Almond, S., Madonna, M. B., Reynolds, M., Luck, S., & Arensman, R. (2006). To drain or not to drain: A single institution's experience with neonatal intestinal perforation. *Journal of Perinatal Medicine, 34*, 338–341.

Duro, D., Bousvaros, A., & Puder, M. (2009). Feeding tubes. In A. Hansen & M. Puder (Eds.), *Manual of neonatal surgical intensive care* (2nd ed., pp. 323–336). Shelton, CT: People's Medical Publishing House.

Gomella, T., Cunningham, M., & Eyal, F. (2013). *Chest tube placement. Neonatology: Management, procedures, on-call problems, diseases, and drugs* (7th ed.). New York, NY: McGraw Hill Education.

Hansen, A., Greene, A., & Puder, M. (2009). Vascular access. In A. Hansen & M. Puder (Eds.), *Manual of neonatal surgical intensive care* (2nd ed., pp. 42–52). Shelton, CT: People's Medical Publishing House.

Hansen, A., & Lillehei, C. (2009). Respiratory disorders. In A. Hansen & M. Puder (Eds.), *Manual of neonatal surgical intensive care* (pp. 159–223). Shelton, CT: People's Medical Publishing House.

Heffner, A., & Androes, M. (2014a). Overview of central venous access. In T. W. Post (Ed.), *Up-to-date*. Waltham, MA: UpToDate, Inc.

Heffner, A., & Androes, M. (2014b). Placement of femoral venous catheters. In T. W. Post (Ed.), *Up-to-date*. Waltham, MA: UpToDate.

Lowinger, D., & Ohlms, L. (2009). Otolaryngology, head and neck surgery. In A. Hansen & M. Puder (Eds.), *Manual of neonatal surgical intensive care* (2nd ed., pp. 71–118). Sheldon, CT: People's Medical Publishing House.

Marik, P., Flemmer, M., & Harrison, W. (2012). Risk of catheter-related blood stream infection with femoral venous catheters as compared to subclavian and internal jugular venous catheters: A systematic review of the literature and meta-analysis. *Critical Care Medicine, 40*(8), 2479–2485.

McSweeney, M., Jiang, H., Deutsch, A., Atmadja, M., & Lightdale, J. (2013). Long-term outcomes of infants and children undergoing percutaneous endoscopy sastrostomy tube placement. *Journal of Pediatric Gastrostomy and Nutrition, 57*(5), 663–667.

Overman, A., Liu, M., Kurachek, S., Shreve, M., Maynard, R., Mammel, M., & Moore, B. (2013). Tracheostomy for infants requiring prolonged mechanical ventilation: 10 years' experience. *Pediatrics, 131*(5), 1–6.

Palefski, S., & Stoddard, G. (2001). The infusion nurse and patient complication rates of peripheral-short catheters. A prospective evaluation. *Journal of Intravenous Nursing, 24*, 113–123.

Premkumar, M. (2012). Necrotizing enterocolitis. In J. Cloherty, E. Eichenwald, & A. Hansen (Eds.), *Manual of neonatal care* (7th ed., pp. 340–349). New York, NY: Lippincott Williams and Wilkins.

Rao, S. C., Basani, L., Simmer, K., Samnakay, N., & Deshpande, G. (2011). Peritoneal drainage versus laparotomy as initial surgical treatment for perforated necrotizing enterocolitis or SIP in preterm low birth weight infants. *Cochrane Database Systemic Reviews*, *15*(6). doi:10.1002/14651858.CD006182.pub2

SURGICAL DISORDERS OF THE BRAIN AND SPINAL CANAL

Eileen C. Dewitt and Noel Dwyer

HYDROCEPHALUS

DEFINITION

Hydrocephalus is a disorder in which an excessive amount of CSF accumulates within the cerebral ventricles and/or subarachnoid spaces, which are dilated (Carey, Tullous, & Walker, 1994). In infants and children, hydrocephalus is almost always associated with increased intracranial pressure (ICP). In most cases, this is caused by excess CSF accumulation in the cerebral ventricles due to disturbances of CSF circulation. This is known as obstructive or noncommunicating hydrocephalus. Hydrocephalus results from an imbalance between the intracranial CSF inflow and outflow. It is caused by obstruction of CSF circulation, by inadequate absorption of CSF, or, rarely, by overproduction of CSF (Beni-Adrani, Biani, Ben-Sirah, & Constantini, 2006). Regardless of the etiology, excessive volume of CSF causes increased ventricular pressure and leads to ventricular dilatation.

PRESENTATION

Hydrocephalus can be congenital or acquired. Congenital forms can result from central nervous system malformations such as neural tube defects, infection, intraventricular hemorrhage, genetic defects, trauma, and teratogens (Jeng, Gupta, Wrensch, Zhao, & Wu, 2011).

Acquired forms include infections, tumors, and posthemorrhagic hydrocephalus. Regardless of etiology, the signs and symptoms of hydrocephalus can be nonspecific and result from increased ICP and dilatation of the ventricles. Pain results from distortion of the meninges and blood vessels, and can be intermittent or persistent (Kirkpatrick, Engelman, & Minns, 1989). Affected patients often have changes in behavior such as irritability. As hydrocephalus worsens, midbrain and brainstem dysfunction can result in lethargy. Increased ICP in the posterior fossa often leads to nausea, vomiting, and decreased appetite.

DIAGNOSIS

Physical exam findings are due to the effects of increased ICP.

- Distortion of the brainstem can result in vital sign changes such as bradycardia, hypertension, and altered respiratory rate.
- Excessive head growth may be noted on serial measurements of head circumference.
  - Effects of hydrocephalus on the head are most common in infants while the cranial sutures are still open.
    - The anterior fontanelle may become full or distended.
    - The sutures become more widely split due to an enlarging head circumference.
    - The scalp veins may appear dilated and prominent.
    - Pressure on the midbrain may result in impairment of upward gaze, known as sun-setting sign because of the appearance of the sclera visible above the iris.
    - Stretching of the fibers from the motor cortex around the dilated ventricles may result in spasticity of the extremities, especially the legs (Kirkpatrick, Engelman, & Minns, 1989).
- Along with physical exam, the diagnosis of hydrocephalus is confirmed with neuroimaging.
  - Ultrasonography is the preferred technique in the newborn because it is portable and avoids ionizing radiation.

▓ Serial US tests should be performed because signs of evolving hydrocephalus such as rapid head growth, full anterior fontanelle, and separated cranial sutures do not appear for days to weeks after ventricular dilatation has commenced.

■ In older infants with suspected hydrocephalus, MRI is generally the modality of choice; it provides superior visualization of pathologic processes in the CSF pathway, including CSF flow dynamics.

■ MRI helps to distinguish obstructive or noncommunicating hydrocephalus from absorptive or communicating hydrocephalus.

▓ This distinction informs treatment decisions about shunting versus third ventriculostomy.

PREOPERATIVE ASSESSMENT AND NURSING CARE

■ Conduct a thorough physical exam to assess for signs of hydrocephalus and increasing ICP

■ Obtain a daily occipital frontal circumference (OFC) measurement just above the infant's ear

■ Conduct weekly growth assessment of the head (Verklan, 2015)

■ Assist with serial cranial US of the head

■ Facilitate neurosurgical consultation

■ Support the infant by decreasing noxious stimuli

■ Position head to avoid pressure points

■ Provide family support/education

■ Obtain preoperative lab work, CBC, coagulation studies, type, and screen

SURGICAL PROCEDURE

■ Lumbar puncture (LP) is an invasive but nonsurgical therapeutic approach to decreasing CSF in the early stages of communicating hydrocephalus (Horinek, Cihar, & Tichy, 2003).

■ The nurse has a key role in positioning the patient and monitoring oxygen saturations, heart rate, respiratory rate, and color.

■ The nurse notes opening and closing pressures and monitors the puncture site for CSF leakage.

■ If the LP proves to be inefficient, an external ventricular drain (EVD) is the next invasive step in the management of hydrocephalus.

■ The catheter is inserted into the dilated anterior horn of the right lateral ventricle.

■ The proximal end of the catheter is subcutaneously tunneled to a site on the scalp and connected to a drainage system (Horinek et al., 2003).

■ The amount of CSF drained can be adjusted by elevating or lowering the level of the drip chamber.

■ A subcutaneous reservoir is another frequently used option in the management of hydrocephalus.

■ Reservoirs can be tapped up to two to three times per day.

■ A drawback with the reservoir is that the removal of CSF is intermittent.

■ The fluid buildup and resulting rise in ICP between taps could be problematic to the infant.

■ Endoscopic third ventriculostomy (ETV) is a procedure in which a perforation is made to connect the third ventricle to the subarachnoid space (Chumas, Tyagi, & Livingston, 2001).

■ This has been useful in the treatment of obstructive hydrocephalus and as an alternative to shunt placement.

■ When successful, it provides a treatment that is relatively low cost, durable, and involves no surgically placed hardware.

■ Ventriculoperitoneal shunt placement is a permanent solution to managing excess CSF.

■ A mechanical shunt system is placed in order to prevent the excessive accumulation of CSF.

■ A catheter is placed into one of the lateral ventricles.

■ The catheter is connected to a one-way valve system that opens when the pressure in the ventricle exceeds a certain value.

■ The distal end of the system is connected to a catheter that is placed in the peritoneal cavity where the fluid is absorbed.

POSTOPERATIVE ASSESSMENT AND NURSING CARE

■ Monitor vital signs and respiratory status

■ Observe fontanelle and head circumference; changes can be critical and need to be reported immediately

■ Observe and document neurologic vital signs

■ Observe and document physical exam

■ Reestablish feedings once return of bowel function occurs postanesthesia

Care specific to EVD

■ Maintain clean, dry, and intact scalp dressing

■ Level the system and clamp the system with each patient repositioning

■ Watch for changes in CSF flow, volume, and patency of the system (minimum every hour)

Care specific to shunt

■ Monitor for shunt malfunction

■ Shunt malfunction from mechanical failure such as obstruction of the catheter may result in over- or underdrainage:

■ Overdrainage will result in a sunken anterior fontanelle.

■ Underdrainage will result in symptoms associated with elevated ICP.

■ Perform close assessment for symptoms of infection such as fever, erythema at insertion site, lethargy, and poor feeding

■ Symptoms of infection should prompt an immediate sepsis evaluation.

- ▨ Shunt infection is a common complication, occurring in 5% to 15% of procedures (Simon et al., 2009).
- ■ Careful positioning is crucial in order to prevent skin breakdown.
  - ▨ Gel pillows may diminish skin breakdown and provide a source of comfort.
- ■ Provide postoperative pain management guided by unit-based scoring systems or tools to assess comfort

DOCUMENTATION

- ■ Head circumference
- ■ Neurologic assessment including description of fontanelles and suture position
- ■ Respiratory assessment
- ■ Feeding irregularities including vomiting
- ■ Assessment of skin at defect site and wound healing
- ■ Pain assessment and management postoperatively

MYELOMENINGOCELE

DEFINITION

Myelomeningocele (a congenital neural tube defect) is the saclike protrusion of the spinal meninges through an opening in the spinal column. This defect is also known as spinal dysmorphism or spina bifida aperta. The majority of myelomeningoceles occur in the lumbar region (Mclone & Bowman, 2014). Findings associated with this defect can include frontal bone scalloping, cerebellum abnormalities, Chiari II malformation, hydrocephaly, microcephaly, and encephalocele. A majority of patients with myelomeningocele have hydrocephalus. Hydrocephalus results from an obstruction of the fourth ventricular outflow, or the flow of CSF through the posterior fossa, called Chiari II malformation.

PRESENTATION

Standard of care is to screen for an elevation in the maternal serum alpha-fetoprotein (AFP) at 16 weeks gestation. Elevated AFP is an indication for further diagnostic testing via US to evaluate for a neural tube defect. In utero surgery may be an option although it is associated with increased risk of premature birth (Ditzenberger & Blackburn, 2014). A scheduled cesarean section is the preferred delivery method to reduce the risk of rupturing the meningeal sac.

DIAGNOSIS

- Confirmation of the neural tube defect is made during the physical exam at birth.
- A head US is usually indicated to diagnose Chiari II malformation (a smaller than normal space between the bones at the lower base of the skull, leading to downward protrusion of the cerebellum and brainstem into the foramen magnum and into the upper spinal canal) (Soul & Madsen, 2009).
- A thorough neurologic exam will show variations in motor control and reflexes from hip to foot, depending upon the level of the lesion.
- Assess for associated anomalies including clubfeet, cleft lip and palate, imperforate anus, and cryptorchidism.

PREOPERATIVE ASSESSMENT AND NURSING CARE

- Monitor for hydrocephalus (and resulting ICP) by assessing head circumference, fontanelles, and sutures
- Position the infant prone with the lesion covered with wet sterile dressings (to protect the lesion as well as minimize insensible fluid losses)

- Place a roll between the legs at hip level to maintain abduction of the legs
- Reposition frequently to help prevent skin breakdown and contractures
- Protect the defect from contamination with stool and urine
- Administer prophylactic IV antibiotics as prescribed
- Clean intermittent catheterization (CIC) should be practiced until renal and urologic functions are understood
- Use nonlatex gloves and equipment to prevent development of latex allergy
- Obtain a head US soon after birth to assess for obstructed CSF flow and hydrocephalus
- Monitor for seizures
- Perform regular neurologic exams to assess upper and lower extremity motor and sensory function, as well as anal wink

SURGICAL PROCEDURE

Repair of the lesion within 24 to 48 hours is optimal. The abnormal end of the spinal cord, called the placode, is dissected from any possible adhesions; surrounding skin that is too thin to use in the repair is removed. The placode is formed into a more normal shape and sutured. The area around the placode and within the spinal canal is assessed for tethers. The dural edge is separated from the lumbar fascia, rolled around the dura, and closed watertight. Subcutaneous and cutaneous layers are closed with the goal of having a well-vascularized and watertight closure (Soul & Madsen, 2009). A ventriculoperitoneal shunt may be placed at the time of first surgery but is often postponed pending further monitoring for hydrocephalus.

POSTOPERATIVE ASSESSMENT AND NURSING CARE

- Keep in prone or side-lying position with occlusive dressing in place until wound is healed

- Monitor head circumference daily
- Assess for ICP including irritability, bulging fontanelles, vomiting, feeding difficulties, stridor, and apnea
- Monitor urologic function and renal status closely
  - Consider a renal US, voiding cystourethrogram (VCUG), urinalysis, and serum creatinine
- Perform CIC every 4 hours to assess for postvoid residuals
  - CIC may be continued long term, depending on urologic function.
- Reestablish feedings once return of bowel function occurs postanesthesia
- Provide postoperative pain management guided by unit-based scoring systems or tools to assess comfort

DOCUMENTATION

- Head circumference
- Neurologic assessment including description of fontanelles and suture position
- Respiratory assessment
- Feeding irregularities including vomiting
- Assessment of skin at defect site and wound healing
- Urine output via catheterization and diaper voids
- Pain assessment and management postoperatively

TETHERED CORD

DEFINITION

A tethered cord is characterized by a prolonged conus (or lower end of the spinal cord) and abnormal filum; fixation of the caudal end of the cord is by fibrous bands (Volpe, 2008).

PRESENTATION

In the newborn period, the physical characteristics (of an occult dysraphic state) such as abnormal collections of hair, subcutaneous mass, superficial cutaneous abnormalities, or cutaneous dimples or tracts raise suspicion of a disorder of caudal neural tube formation including tethered cord (Volpe, 2008).

DIAGNOSIS

Noninvasive evaluation by US is preferred over plain radiograph given the poor ossification of the posterior spinal elements. Visualization of the spinal cord, subarachnoid space, conus medullaris, and filum terminale, along with real-time observation of the mobility of the cord, have allowed identification of a variety of occult dysraphic states. If US is normal and no neurologic signs exist, further radiologic study is not necessary in the neonatal period and clinical follow-up is appropriate. If an abnormality is present, proceed to MRI for better sagittal and coronal topography of the intravertebral and extravertebral components.

PREOPERATIVE ASSESSMENT AND NURSING CARE

- Observe and document the neurologic exam to include overall muscle tone as well as lower limb movement and reflexes
- Observe and document the physical exam

SURGICAL PROCEDURE

Surgical release of the tethered cord combined with removal of any cysts can prevent deterioration or reverse deficits. Surgery is performed primarily to prevent development of neurologic deficits. Neurologic deficits may present suddenly from vascular insufficiency produced by tension on the tethered cord.

POSTOPERATIVE ASSESSMENT AND NURSING CARE

- Assess the surgical site for signs of infection and drainage
- Evaluate bladder function in the newborn

■ Assess neurologic function

■ Follow the movement of the lower extremities and muscle tone closely

■ Carefully position the infant to include side-to-side and prone positioning in the immediate postoperative period

■ Reestablish oral feedings once return of bowel function occurs postanesthesia

■ Provide postoperative pain management guided by unit-based scoring systems or tools to assess comfort

DOCUMENTATION

■ Evaluation of surgical site

■ Neurologic evaluation

■ Urine output

■ Pain assessment and management postoperatively

REFERENCES

Beni-Adrani, L., Biani, N., Ben-Sirah, L., & Constantini, S. (2006). The occurrence of obstructive v. absorptive hydrocephalus in newborns and infants: Relevance to treatment choices. *Childs Nervous System, 22*(12), 1543–1563.

Carey, C. M., Tullous, M. W., & Walker, M. L. (1994). Hydrocephalus: Etiology, pathologic effects, diagnosis, and natural history. In W. R. Cheek (Ed.), *Pediatric neurosurgery* (3rd ed.). Philadelphia, PA: WB Saunders.

Chumas, P., Tyagi, A., & Livingston, J. (2001). Hydrocephalus, what's new. *Archives of Disease in Childhood, Fetal Neonatal Edition, 85*(3), F149.

Ditzenberger, G. R., & Blackburn, S. T. (2014). Neurologic system. In C. Kenner & J. W. Lott (Eds.), *Comprehensive neonatal nursing care* (5th ed., pp. 392–437). New York, NY: Springer Publishing Company.

Horinek, D., Cihar, M., & Tichy, M. (2003). Current methods in the treatment of posthemorhagic hydrocephalus in infants. *Therapy, 104*(11), 347–351.

Jeng, S., Gupta, N., Wrensch, M., Zhao, S., & Wu, T. W. (2011). Prevalence of congenital hydrocephalus in California, 1991–2000. *Pediatric Neurology, 45*(2), 67–71.

Kirkpatrick, M., Engelman, H., & Minns, R. A. (1989). Symptoms and signs of progressive hydrocephalus. *Archives of Disease in Childhood*, 64(1), 124–128.

Mclone, D. G., & Bowman, R. (2014). *Overview of the management of myelomeningocele (spina bifida)*. Waltham, MA: Up to Date—Wolters-Kluwer Health.

Simon, T. D., Hall, M., Riva-Cambrin, J., Albert, J. E., Jeffries, LaFleur, B., Dean, J. M., Kestle, J. R. W., & Hydrocephalus Clinical Research Network. (2009). Infection rates following initial cerebrospinal fluid shunt placement across pediatric hospitals in the United States. *Journal of Neurosurgical Pediatrics*, 4(2), 156–165. doi: 10.3171/2009.3.PEDS08215

Soul, J., & Madsen, J. R. (2009). Neurological disorders, part 1 neonatal hydrocephalus. In A. R. Hansen & M. Puder (Eds.), *Manual of neonatal surgical intensive care* (2nd ed., Chap. 9, pp. 444–458). Shelton, CT: BC Decker.

Verklan, M. T. (2015). Neurological disorders. In M. T. Verklan & M. Walden (Eds.), *Core curriculum for neonatal intensive care nursing* (5th ed., pp. 734–766). St. Louis, MO: Elsevier Saunders.

Volpe, J. (2008). *Neurology of the newborn* (5th ed., pp. 21–22). Philadelphia, PA: Elsevier Saunders.

SURGICAL DISORDERS OF THE BRONCHOPULMONARY TREE AND DIAPHRAGM

Maura Heckmann and Mary-Jeanne Manning

BRONCHOPULMONARY SEQUESTRATION

DEFINITION

Bronchopulmonary sequestration (BPS) is composed of extraneous and nonfunctioning lung tissue that has separated itself from the normal pulmonary structure. It is a congenital thoracic malformation that develops as a cystic or solid mass that does not communicate with the tracheobronchial tree and has an anomalous systemic blood supply. Its blood supply is from systemic circulation rather than the pulmonary circulation. Multiple feeding vessels may be present in 15% to 20% of cases. The two forms of pulmonary sequestration are intrapulmonary lung sequestration (ILS), which is surrounded by normal lung tissue, and extrapulmonary lung sequestration (ELS), an accessory lung that is enclosed in its own pleural sac, most commonly on the left side. Hybrid lesions exist that contain features of both ILS and ELS.

Pulmonary sequestration represents approximately 6% of all congenital pulmonary malformations. Intrapulmonary sequestrations are the most common form, and 60% of these are found in the posterior basal segment of the left lower lobe. Overall, 98% occur in the lower lobes. Bilateral involvement is uncommon. Other congenital anomalies may be seen in about 10% of the cases (DeParedes, Pierce, Johnson, & Waldhausen, 1970; Flye, Conley, & Silver, 1976).

PRESENTATION

■ BPS usually presents as a lung infection on physical examination and chest imaging. Intralobar sequestration generally presents later in childhood with recurrent cough or pneumonia, and occurs equally between the sexes. Extralobar sequestration presents more typically in males, often in infancy, with respiratory distress and chronic cough.

DIAGNOSIS

■ Chest radiography, CT scan of the thorax, and MRI permit increased definition of a particular lesion and serve as the primary tools for diagnosing BPS.

PREOPERATIVE ASSESSMENT AND NURSING CARE

■ Provide supportive care, ranging from oxygen supplementation to mechanical ventilation

■ Administer prescribed antibiotics in children with lesions complicated by pneumonia

SURGICAL PROCEDURE

■ Treatment of BPS depends on defect location and neonatal status.

■ Even asymptomatic patients may benefit from repair to prevent chronic cough and pneumonia.

■ Surgical resection is the treatment of choice for patients who present with infection or symptoms resulting from compression of normal lung tissue.

■ Surgical management BPS involves lobectomy or segmentectomy.

■ Extrapulmonary lesions can usually be excised without loss of normal lung tissue.

■ Intrapulmonary lesions often require lobectomy because the margins of the sequestration may not be clearly defined.

■ Complete thoracoscopic resection of pulmonary lobes in infants and children has been described with low mortality and morbidity (Albanese & Rothenberg, 2007).

POSTOPERATIVE ASSESSMENT AND NURSING CARE

■ See "Postoperative Assessment and Nursing Care" for Congenital Pulmonary Airway Malformation (CPAM).

CDH IN THE NEONATE

DEFINITION

CDH is a developmental defect of the diaphragm in which the abdominal viscera herniate into the chest through an abnormal opening in the diaphragm. The presence of the abdominal organs in the thoracic cavity leads to pulmonary hypoplasia and pulmonary hypertension.

■ It is one of the most common major congenital anomalies.

■ The incidence is reported as 1 in 3,000 live births worldwide (Wynn et al., 2013).

■ Infants with CDH can have lung hypoplasia and increased pulmonary vascular resistance (Curley & Harmon, 2001).

PRESENTATION

Respiratory distress or failure is seen within the first hours to days of life. The degree of respiratory compromise is related to the severity of the defect and often with the side of the defect (right side, less common often thought to be worse) (Wynn et al., 2013). A large defect allows for more organs to enter the chest including the bowel, stomach, and liver. Pulmonary hypoplasia and pulmonary hypertension are more severe in cases where more organs herniate into the chest during fetal development.

DIAGNOSIS

■ It is often found on prenatal US.

■ A chest radiograph postnatally to evaluate respiratory distress demonstrates the CDH.

■ Physical exam reveals signs of respiratory distress, barrel-shaped chest, scaphoid-appearing abdomen, and the absence of breath sounds on the ipsilateral side. Left-sided defects may lead to displacement of the heart and heart sounds; the point of maximal intensity (PMI) is shifted to the right (Curley & Harmon, 2001).

PREOPERATIVE ASSESSMENT AND NURSING CARE

■ The goal is to avoid conditions that increase pulmonary vascular resistance, including hypoxemia, acidosis, hypothermia, and hypoglycemia, as well as environmental stressors, noise, excessive light, and invasive procedures (Curley & Harmon, 2001).

■ Depending on the severity of the defect and the resulting pulmonary hypoplasia and pulmonary hypertension, patients may require support such as intubation, gentle ventilation, permissive hypercapnia, high-frequency oscillatory ventilation, and/or ECMO.

■ Major goals are maintaining permissive hypercapnia to avoid barotrauma and decrease pulmonary hypertension, as well as attaining cardiovascular stability (Wilson, Lund, Lillehei, & Vacanti, 1997).

Nursing assessment includes:

- Monitor preductal and postductal oxygen saturation, frequent blood gases to monitor for acidosis, and hypoxia and hypercarbia to evaluate respiratory function
  - Provide sedation, and possibly paralyze the infant if severe pulmonary hypertension is noted
- Obtain four extremity blood pressures and EKG to r/o cardiac anomalies
- Monitor perfusion
  - Inotropic support to maintain adequate peripheral perfusion
- Maintain umbilical venous catheter/umbilical arterial catheter (UVC/UAC) or other central lines
- Assess pupillary response, fontanelle size/tension, seizure activity, and signs of intraventricular/intraparenchymal bleeding
- Maintain a quiet environment and cluster cares
- Assess hematologic status
  - Report and respond to signs of bleeding (due to anticoagulation if on ECMO)
- Measure accurate intake and output
- Monitor electrolytes and diuretic treatment closely
- Obtain chest x-ray (CXR), ABG, electrolytes, CBC, lactic acid
- Treat with narcotics and sedatives to achieve desired pain control and activity level
- Administer parenteral nutrition

SURGICAL PROCEDURE

If the patient remains unstable despite maximal ventilatory measures, the use of ECMO may be necessary (Curley & Harmon, 2001). Repair is delayed until the patient's cardiovascular status is stabilized. A primary closure is performed for small defects and a patch closure is performed for larger or more complicated defects.

POSTOPERATIVE ASSESSMENT AND NURSING CARE

- Monitor preductal and postductal oxygen saturation, frequent blood gases to monitor for acidosis, and hypoxia and hypercarbia to evaluate respiratory function
- Monitor perfusion
    - Inotropic support to maintain adequate peripheral perfusion
- Assess pupillary response, fontanelle size/tension, seizure activity, and signs of intraventricular/intraparenchymal bleeding
- Maintain a quiet environment and cluster care
- Measure accurate intake and output
- Monitor electrolytes and diuretic treatment closely
- Obtain CXR, ABG, electrolytes, CBC, lactic acid
- Surgical wound assessment and care
- Chest tube maintenance (see section on "Tubes")
- Assess comfort
- Treat with narcotics and sedatives to achieve desired pain control and activity level
- Parenteral nutrition is administered until enteral feedings can be reestablished

DOCUMENTATION

- Vital signs
- Preductal and postductal oxygen saturations
- Perfusion
- Accurate intake and output
- Patient response to care and treatments
- Daily weights
- Wound assessment and management, including signs of infection

CONGENITAL PULMONARY AIRWAY MALFORMATION

DEFINITION

The most common malformations of the respiratory tract are CPAM, previously known as congenital cystic adenomatoid malformation (CCAM). In CPAM, usually an entire lobe of lung is replaced by a nonworking cystic piece of abnormal lung tissue. This abnormal tissue will never function as normal lung tissue.

There are currently five main types, which differ based on the embryologic level of origin and histologic features. 0 = tracheobronchial, 1 = bronchial/bronchiolar, 2 = bronchiolar, 3 = bronchiolar/alveolar, 4 and 5 = distal acinar. Although the pathogenesis of these lesions is poorly understood, they may have a common origin (Langston, 2003). Theories of their pathogenesis include abnormal proliferation of tissues, airway obstruction, and dysplasia and metaplasia of normal tissues. In most cases, it seems that the insult occurs during the pseudoglandular phase of lung development, between 7 and 17 weeks of gestation (Stocker, 2009). The reported incidence of CPAM ranges from 1 in 11,000 to 1 in 35,000 live births (Laberge et al., 2001).

PRESENTATION

Infants present prenatally via US and in the neonatal period. Research has demonstrated that a significant proportion of prenatal lesions decrease in size and may regress spontaneously; therefore, antenatal treatment is not usually required (Laberge et al., 2001).

Prenatal

Large lesions may be associated with the development of *hydrops fetalis* (a poor prognostic sign). Hydrops is thought to arise from compression of the IVC, which compromises venous return and leads to a decrease in cardiac output and the development of effusions. Fetal demise may result; therefore, premature delivery is attempted in order to save the fetus (Davenport et al., 2004).

Neonatal/Childhood

■ At least half of the patients diagnosed with CPAM antenatally are asymptomatic at birth.

■ Respiratory distress

■ This is the presenting symptom in most newborns with a diagnosis of symptomatic CPAM. It may range in severity from grunting, tachypnea, and a mild oxygen requirement to respiratory failure requiring aggressive ventilator support or ECMO.

■ Pulmonary hypoplasia may arise as a consequence of a large CPAM.

■ Mediastinal shift may compromise cardiac and respiratory function.

■ Spontaneous pneumothoraces may occur and air trapping within the cyst leads to compression of functional pulmonary tissue.

■ Recurrent infections develop when the CPAM has not been resected due to bronchial compression, air trapping, and inability to clear secretions.

■ Hemoptysis has occasionally been described as a manifestation of CPAM in the older child.

■ Dyspnea and chest pain may be a feature of pneumothorax, which has been described as a presenting feature of CPAM.

■ Cough, fever, and failure to thrive have all been reported in association with the presentation of CPAM (Parikh & Samuel, 2005).

DIAGNOSIS

■ Chest radiography typically identifies CPAM of sufficient size to cause clinical problems. The usual appearance is a mass containing air-filled cysts.

■ CT scan of the thorax provides a rapid means of defining the extent of CPAM in all age groups.

■ The typical appearance is of multilocular cystic lesions with thin walls surrounded by normal lung parenchyma. The presence of superimposed infection with the lesion may complicate the appearance.

■ MRI permits increased definition of a particular lesion.

■ Other imaging studies

■ Perform renal and cerebral ultrasonography in all newborns with CPAM in order to exclude coexisting renal and CNS anomalies.

■ Perform echocardiography in all newborns with CCAM to rule out any coexisting cardiac lesions. Furthermore, in infants with respiratory distress, echocardiography may provide evidence of persistent pulmonary hypertension (e.g., right-to-left shunting, increased pulmonary artery pressures).

PREOPERATIVE ASSESSMENT AND NURSING CARE

■ Provide supportive care, ranging from oxygen supplementation to mechanical ventilation.

■ Administer prescribed antibiotics in children with CPAM complicated by pneumonia.

SURGICAL PROCEDURE

■ Fetal surgery considered in patients with large CPAMs, and in cases complicated by hydrops with a prognosis, is poor (Adzick, Harrison, Crombleholme, Flake, & Howell, 1998).

■ Resection of CCAM in all children is recommended to remove the risk of complications, such as recurrent infection and pneumothorax. Additionally, the malignant potential of CCAM in later life has long been recognized (Adzick, 2003).

■ Children with asymptomatic CCAM that was diagnosed antenatally can be followed without surgical intervention as some lesions may decrease in size or resolve without intervention. If surgery is recommended, most suggest it be completed before the child is aged 12 months to enhance theoretical compensatory lung growth. Studies have not confirmed this hypothetical difference in lung function by age at the time of surgical resection (Kotecha et al., 2012).

■ Minimally invasive surgery is quickly becoming the standard of care. These procedures include intervening via thoracocentesis, thoracoamniotic shunt, laser ablation, or injection of a sclerosing agent into the feeding artery. Experience with these therapies is limited.

   ■ All removed tissue should be examined histologically as there can be discordance in radiologic and histologic diagnosis.

POSTOPERATIVE ASSESSMENT AND NURSING CARE

Postoperative care depends on the surgical technique utilized.

Thoracoscopic repair

Thoracoscopic repair generally requires a short hospital stay of 2 to 3 days.

■ Assess chest tube for evacuation of air and fluid as the lung heals.

■ Maintain clean, dry, and intact dressings over the chest incision(s) and the chest tube sites; these may be removed after 48 hours.

■ Resume the infant's normal diet once he or she has recovered from anesthesia.

■ Bathing the infant can be done beginning on POD 5.

   ■ Gently clean the incision and its closures with soap and water, then pat dry.

■ If tape strips are used over the incision, they will fall off on their own.

■ Administer acetaminophen (Tylenol) or ibuprofen (Advil) for pain.

Thoracotomy

Generally, a longer hospital stay (> 3 days) should be anticipated for a thoracotomy.

■ Monitor the surgical wound for drainage and wound infection

■ Monitor for signs and symptoms of systemic infection

■ Change the primary dressing according to the surgeon's instructions

■ Pain management is imperative postoperatively because it is essential for patients to take adequate breaths and move. They will be unable to do so if they have severe pain. There are various ways by which pain is managed, including:

■ Paravertebral

■ Methods conducted preoperatively or intraoperatively

■ Epidural catheters

■ IV nurse-controlled analgesia by IV drip

■ Oral analgesics (upon withdrawal of continuous pain control) for duration of time until they are pain free, including acetaminophen, NSAIDS, and narcotic agents

■ Monitor postoperative fluid balance closely

■ Maintain stable hemodynamics

■ Do not overhydrate the patient unless hemodynamics necessitate

■ Encourage oral feeding as soon as possible

■ Monitor chest tube for drainage and air leak

■ Prevent postoperative respiratory insufficiency by maintaining a clear airway, frequent repositioning of the infant, gentle chest physiotherapy, and the prevention of edema

REFERENCES

Adzick, N. S. (2003). Management of fetal lung lesions. *Clinics in Perinatology, 30*(3), 481–492.

Adzick, N. S., Harrison, M. R., Crombleholme, T. M., Flake, A. W., & Howell, L. J. (1998). Fetal lung lesions: Management and outcome. *American Journal of Obstetrics and Gynecology, 179*(4), 884–889.

Albanese, C. T., & Rothenberg, S. S. (2007). Experience with 144 consecutive pediatric thoracoscopic lobectomies. *Journal of Laparoendoscopic Advanced Surgical Techniques A, 17*(3), 339–341.

Curley, M. A. Q., & Harmon, P. A. (Eds.). (2001). Pulmonary critical care problems. In *Critical care nursing of infants and children* (Chap. 19, pp. 681–682). Philadelphia, PA: WB Saunders.

Davenport, M., Warne, S. A., Cacciaguerra, S., Patel, S., Greenough, A., & Nicolaides, K. (2004). Current outcome of antenally diagnosed cystic lung disease. *Journal of Pediatric Surgery, 39*(4), 549–556.

DeParedes, C. G., Pierce, W. S., Johnson, D. G., & Waldhausen, J. A. (1970). Pulmonary sequestration in infants and children: A 20-year experience and review of the literature. *Journal of Pediatric Surgery, 5*(2), 136–147.

Flye, M. W., Conley, M., & Silver, D. (1976). Spectrum of pulmonary sequestration. *Annals of Thoracic Surgery, 22*(5), 478–482. [Medline].

Kotecha, S., Barbato, A., Bush, A., Claus, F., Davenport, M., Delacourt, C., ... Midulla, F. (2012). Antenatal and postnatal management of congenital cystic adenomatoid malformation. *Paediatric Respiratory Reviews, 13*(3), 162–171.

Laberge, J. M., Flageole, H., Pugash, D., Khalife, S., Blair, G., Filiatrault, D., ... Wilson, R. D. (2001). Outcome of the prenatally diagnosed congenital cystic adenomatoid lung malformation: A Canadian experience. *Fetal Diagnostic Therapy, 16*(3), 178–186.

Langston, C. (2003). New concepts in the pathology of congenital lung malformations. *Seminars in Pediatric Surgery, 12*(1), 17–37.

Parikh, D., & Samuel, M. (2005). Congenital cystic lung lesions: Is surgical resection essential? *Pediatric Pulmonology, 40*(6), 533–537.

Stocker, J. T. (2009). Cystic lung disease in infants and children. *Fetal Pediatric Pathology, 28*(4), 155–184.

Wilson, J. M., Lund, D. P., Lillehei, C. W., & Vacanti, J. P. (1997). Congenital diaphragmatic hernia—A tale of two cities: The Boston experience. *Journal of Pediatric Surgery, 32*(3), 401–405.

Wynn, J., Krishnan, U., Aspelund, G., Zhang, Y., Duong, J., Stolar, C. J., ... Arkovitz, M. S. (2013). Outcomes of congenital diaphragmatic hernia in the modern era. *Journal of Pediatrics, 163*(1), 114–119.

SURGICAL DISORDERS OF THE TRACHEA AND ESOPHAGUS

Patricia Fleck and Monica A. Carleton

ESOPHAGEAL ATRESIA

DEFINITION

EA is the interruption in the continuity of the esophagus (El-Gohary, Gittes, & Tovar, 2010).

PRESENTATION

Prenatal diagnosis of EA is suspected when an US reveals a small or absent stomach bubble and polyhydramnios. When a small or absent stomach bubble coincides with polyhydramnios, the positive predictive value for having EA is 56% (Spitz, 2007). Preterm delivery occurs in 30% to 40% of cases, with an average gestational age of 36 weeks in the setting of polyhydramnios (Brantberg, Blaas, Haugen, & Eik-Nes, 2007).

DIAGNOSIS

■ The infant with EA may be well appearing at delivery or exhibit symptoms including:

  ▪ Excessive salivation

  ▪ Inability to swallow secretions

  ▪ Inability to pass an NG catheter

■ EA should be suspected when you are unable to pass an NG tube.

 ▨ The tube may pass 8 to 10 cm before meeting resistance.

 ▨ A chest radiograph will show the NG tube coiled in a dilated proximal esophageal pouch.

 ▨ The x-ray may demonstrate the presence of air in the intestine that differentiates isolated EA from EA with tracheoesophageal fistula (EA/TEF) and may reveal additional anomalies (Hansen & Lillehei, 2009).

PREOPERATIVE ASSESSMENT AND NURSING CARE

■ Place a double lumen (one lumen to apply suction for drainage removal and another to serve as an air vent) Replogle (1963) suction catheter in the upper esophageal pouch

 ▨ A physician or trained advanced practice nurse places the Replogle catheter.

 ▨ The catheter should be advanced to a predetermined length or until it meets resistance, and then pulled back 1 cm and secured with tape or occlusive dressing.

 ▨ Make a notation of the exit marking for the tube in the medical record.

 ▨ Connect the Replogle to continuous low wall suction (20–40 mmHg) to minimize the symptoms caused by excessive secretions.

■ Keep the catheter patent by irrigating the drainage removal port with 1 to 2 mL of air every 2 to 4 hours and as needed as secretions may be tenacious

■ Raise the head of the bed 30° to prevent aspiration of oral secretions and facilitate evacuation through the Replogle

■ Keep the infant NPO and administer IV fluids; consider parenteral nutrition until enteral nutrition through a gastrostomy tube can be initiated

 ▨ Parenteral nutrition is essential for good nutrition until surgical placement of a gastrostomy tube can be performed.

■ Monitor blood gases, electrolytes, CBCs; obtain blood type and cross match in preparation for surgery

■ Encourage oral stimulation and nonnutritive sucking to promote successful oral feedings postoperatively (Gupta & Sharma, 2008)

■ Encourage parental participation in care to facilitate maternal-infant attachment

SURGICAL PROCEDURE

■ End-to-end anastomosis or a primary repair is performed if the gap is less than three vertebral bodies.

■ If the gap is greater than three vertebral bodies, a delayed primary repair is the preferred method for surgical repair.

  ■ If the gap is greater than three vertebral bodies, consider transfer to a center with expertise in a growth induction procedure to induce natural growth of the esophagus (Foker, Kendall, Catton, & Khan, 2005; Zani et al., 2014).

■ In rare cases, if a delayed primary repair fails, a jejunal or colonic interposition in combination with a cervical esophagostomy or spit fistula may be performed (Spitz, 2007).

POSTOPERATIVE ASSESSMENT AND NURSING CARE

■ Maintain the neck in a flexed position to minimize tension on the anastomosis site

  ■ Use caution; do not apply tension on the anastomosis site; tension increases the risk of a leak or stricture

■ Consider paralysis to achieve the desired position and to facilitate healing

■ Adequate pain management is needed during paralysis based on sympathetic responses such as elevated heart rate and blood pressure; see Goal of Postoperative Pain Management and Assessment section

■ Conduct respiratory assessments frequently while infant is sedated and paralyzed

- Keep intubated until extubation readiness is established
- Vigilance toward mouth care, positioning, and closed suctioning should be considered to reduce the risk of VAP
- Continue to clear airway as needed
- Monitor thoracostomy tube drainage and consider removal when drainage is minimal and radiograph reveals no evidence of air leak or anastomosis leak
  - Excessive frothy output may indicate a leak at the anastomosis site.
- Provide gastric decompression via surgically placed NG tube
  - Avoid manipulation of tube and risk of injury to the anastomosis site.
- Perform a dye contrast study at 1 to 2 weeks or as prescribed postoperatively to ensure continuity of the esophagus prior to initiating oral feedings
- Establish oral feedings based on oral feeding cues, gestational age, and maturity (Montrowl, 2014)

DOCUMENTATION

- Vital signs
- Ventilation requirements and blood gas measurements
- Chest tube output
- NG tube placement
- Intake and output, including NG tube output
- Serum electrolytes, CBCs, and other laboratory values
- Sedation, state, and pain scores

EA WITH TRACHEOESOPHAGEAL FISTULA

DEFINITION

EA/TEF occurs from an abnormal septation between the trachea and esophagus. EA with distal TEF is the most common type. EA with proximal TEF and EA with proximal and distal TEF are the least common forms (Box 8.1).

Box 8.1. EA/TEF Variants and Incidence

- Esophageal atresia (EA) with distal tracheoesophageal fistula (TEF) (86%)
- Isolated EA without TEF (7%)
- H-type TEF without EA (4%)
- EA with proximal TEF (3%)
- EA with proximal and distal TEF (< 1%)

Adapted from Hansen and Lillehei (2009).

PRESENTATION

- Findings of an absent stomach bubble and maternal polyhydramnios during prenatal US may indicate EA/TEF.

- Delivery at a high-risk center should be arranged if EA/TEF is suspected.

- The infant may present with respiratory distress due to aspiration of secretions or reflux of stomach contents through a distal TEF.

- If a distal fistula is present, crying or bag-mask ventilation may force air into the stomach, causing progressive abdominal distention and decreased lung excursion (Gupta & Sharma, 2008).

- The inability to pass an NG tube beyond 8 to 10 cm may be an indication of EA/TEF.

DIAGNOSIS

- If EA is present, the radiograph will demonstrate the NG tube coiled in a dilated proximal esophageal pouch.

- If TEF is present, air will be noted in the intestine.

- An echocardiogram can be done to evaluate for congenital heart defects that are present in up to 50% of infants, and to determine the arch position for surgical approach.

■ Fluoroscopy, bronchoscopy, and endoscopy may be necessary to completely evaluate the defect.

　■ Evaluate vocal cord mobility prior to operative repair as injury to the recurrent laryngeal nerve may cause vocal cord paralysis, complicating the postoperative course (Mortellaro, Pettiford, St. Peter, Fraser, & Wei, 2011).

■ Approximately 10% of infants will have a sequence of anomalies known as VACTERL or VATER.

　■ These anomalies include: **V**ertebral, **A**nal atresia, **C**ongenital heart defects, **T**EF, **R**enal anomalies, and **L**imb deformities sequence.

■ Another EA/TEF-associated sequence of anomalies is called CHARGE.

　■ These anomalies include **C**oloboma, **H**eart defect, **A**tresia choanae, **R**etarded growth, **G**enital hypoplasia, and **E**ar anomalies (Hansen & Lillehei, 2009; Montrowl, 2014) (see Table 8.3).

PREOPERATIVE ASSESSMENT AND NURSING CARE

■ Clear secretions and provide supplemental oxygen as needed

■ Minimize gastric distention by limiting crying and positive pressure ventilation

■ Intubate and ventilate if clinically indicated to minimize gastric distention and the need for emergent gastrostomy for decompression (Hansen & Lillehei, 2009)

■ Assess abdomen frequently for distention that may compromise the infant's respiratory effort

　■ Excessive abdominal distention can lead to gastric perforation, diminished cardiac output, and death.

■ Manage secretions through placement of a Replogle® suction catheter in the upper esophageal pouch connected to continuous low wall suction

TABLE 8.3 EA/TEF, Evaluation of Associated Anomalies

	Evaluation	Key Elements
VACTERL		
Vertebral anomalies	Radiographs, US	Butterfly or hemi-vertebrae
Anus to anal atresia	Physical examination	Anal position, vaginal fistula, imperforate anus
Congenital heart defects	Echocardiogram	Situs, arch position, ASD, VSD, AV canal, TOF, pulmonary vein stenosis
TEF	Bronchoscopy	Proximal or distal fistula, tracheomalacia
EA	Radiograph, contrast study	Distance between proximal and distal segments determines gap
Renal anomalies	Abdominal US	Laterality, collecting system abnormalities, horseshoe kidney, hydronephrosis
Limb deformities	Physical examination, radiographs	Absent radius
CHARGE		
Coloboma	Ophthalmologic examination	Keyhole pupils
Choanal atresia	Physical examination, CT scan	Blockage of posterior nasal passages
Retarded growth	Physical measurements	Small for gestational age in parameters of weight, head circumference, and length

(continued)

TABLE 8.3 EA/TEF, Evaluation of Associated Anomalies (*continued*)

	Evaluation	Key Elements
Genital anomalies	Physical examination	Hydrospadias, microphallus, labial hypoplasia, rectovaginal fistula
Ear abnormalities	Physical examination	Microtia, auricular appendages, sinus

ASD, atrial septal defect; AV canal, atrioventricular canal; EA, esophageal atresia; TEF, tracheoesophageal fistula; TOF, Tetralogy of Fallot; US, ultrasound; VSD, ventricular septal defect.

- Keep the suction catheter patent by irrigating with 1 to 2 mL of air every 2 to 4 hours and as needed as secretions may be thick and cause plugging
- Prevent reflux of gastric secretions by raising the head of the bed 30°, especially in the setting of a distal TEF
- Position infants without a distal TEF prone or side lying to promote gravity drainage of secretions
- Keep the infant NPO and administer IV fluids; consider parenteral nutrition
  - This is essential for good nutrition until surgical placement of a gastrostomy tube can be performed.
- Encourage oral stimulation and nonnutritive sucking to promote successful oral feedings postoperatively
- Monitor blood gases, electrolytes, CBCs; obtain blood type and cross match in preparation for surgery
- Monitor vital signs
- Encourage parental participation in care to facilitate maternal-infant attachment

SURGICAL PROCEDURE

■ End-to-end anastomosis or primary repair is performed if the gap is less than three vertebral bodies.

■ If the gap is greater than three vertebral bodies, consider transfer to a center with expertise in a growth induction procedure to induce natural growth of the esophagus (Foker et al., 2005; Zani et al., 2014).

■ In rare cases, a jejunal or colonic interposition in combination with a cervical esophagostomy or spit fistula may be performed (Spitz, 2007).

POSTOPERATIVE ASSESSMENT AND NURSING CARE

■ Maintain the neck in a flexed position to minimize tension on the anastomosis site

■ Use caution; do not apply tension on the anastomosis site; tension increases the risk of a leak or stricture

■ Consider paralysis to achieve the desired position and to facilitate healing

■ Adequate pain management is needed during paralysis based on sympathetic responses such as elevated heart rate and blood pressure. See Goal of Postoperative Pain Management and Assessment section.

■ Conduct respiratory assessments frequently while infant is sedated and paralyzed

■ Keep intubated until extubation readiness is established.

■ Vigilance to mouth care, positioning, and closed suctioning should be considered to reduce the risk of VAP

■ Continue to clear the airway as needed

■ Use caution; do not apply tension on the anastomosis site

■ Tension increases the risk of a leak or stricture.

■ Monitor thoracostomy tube drainage and consider removal when drainage is minimal and radiograph reveals no evidence of air leak or anastomosis leak

■ Clear frothy (spit-like) drainage in the thoracostomy tube may be a sign of an anastomotic leak.

■ Provide gastric decompression via surgically placed NG tube

■ Avoid manipulation of the NG tube and risk of injury to the anastomosis site

■ Perform a dye contrast study at 1 to 2 weeks postoperatively to ensure continuity of the esophagus prior to initiating oral feedings

■ Establish oral feedings based on oral feeding cues, gestational age, and maturity

DOCUMENTATION

■ Vital signs
■ Ventilation requirements and blood gas measurements
■ Chest tube output
■ NG tube placement and output
■ Intake and output
■ Serum electrolytes and CBCs
■ Sedation, state, and pain scores

TRACHEOESOPHAGEAL FISTULA (ISOLATED)

DEFINITION

An isolated TEF forms from one or more abnormal connection(s) between the esophagus and the trachea in either the proximal and/or the distal segments. TEF frequently occurs with another birth defect known at EA (see TEF/EA). TEF without atresia occurs in approximately 4% of patients (Hansen & Lillehei, 2009).

PRESENTATION

- Infants with TEF may not have symptoms at birth.
- Presenting symptoms for infants with isolated TEF include:
  - Mild coughing or respiratory symptoms
  - Difficulty while eating
  - Frequent respiratory tract infections (Spitz, 2007)

DIAGNOSIS

- It may take several weeks to diagnose TEF.
- Bronchoscopy and, if necessary, contrast studies and endoscopy may be needed to determine the presence of an isolated TEF.
  - Use contrast material judiciously as the material can enter the lungs and cause injury (Hansen & Lillehei, 2009).

PREOPERATIVE ASSESSMENT AND NURSING CARE

- Position the infant to prevent aspiration of oral or gastric secretions
  - For infants with a distal TEF, raise the head of the bed 30° to prevent entry of secretions into the airway.
  - For infants with a proximal TEF, position flat and prone or side lying to promote gravity drainage of secretions
- Keep the infant NPO and administer IV fluids; consider parenteral nutrition
  - This is essential for good nutrition until surgical placement of a gastrostomy tube can be performed.
- Encourage oral stimulation and sucking skills to promote successful oral feedings postoperatively
- Implement jejunal tube feeds if needed to provide desired nutrition to prevent reflux and aspiration of stomach contents
- Monitor blood gases, electrolytes, CBCs; obtain blood type and cross match in preparation for surgery

SURGICAL PROCEDURE

■ TEFs do not close spontaneously; surgical repair is planned when the patient is stable.

■ Repair is performed via a thoracotomy, usually on the infant's right side (Spitz, 2007).

POSTOPERATIVE ASSESSMENT AND NURSING CARE

■ Keep the head of the bed elevated

■ Continue to provide airway clearance using sterile technique

■ Use great care suctioning; use precise suction catheter measurements to avoid contact with the surgical TEF repair site

■ Keep the infant intubated until readiness for extubation is established

■ Vigilance to mouth care, positioning, and closed suctioning should be considered to reduce the risk of VAP

■ Monitor thoracostomy tube drainage and consider removal when drainage is minimal and radiograph reveals no evidence of air leak

■ Continue gastric decompression via surgically placed NG tube

    ▪ Avoid manipulation of tube to avoid risk of injury to the surgical site

■ Optimize parenteral nutrition until enteral feeds are established

    ▪ Good nutrition is essential for growth and healing.

■ Feed using a surgically placed NG or jejunostomy feeding tube until the infant can receive oral feedings (Montrowl, 2014)

DOCUMENTATION

■ Vital signs

■ Ventilation requirements and blood gas measurements

■ Chest tube output

    ▪ Excessive frothy output may indicate a leak at the anastomosis site

- NG, gastrostomy, and/or jejunostomy tube placement
- Intake and output (include output from draining tubes)
- Serum electrolytes and CBCs
- Sedation, state, and pain scores

REFERENCES

Brantberg, A., Blaas, H.-G. K., Haugen, S. E., & Eik-Nes, S. H. (2007). Esophageal obstruction-prenatal detection rate and outcome. *Ultrasound Obstetrics and Gynecology, 30*, 180–187. doi:10.1002/uog.4056

El-Gohary, Y., Gittes, G. K., & Tovar, J. A. (2010). Congenital anomalies of the esophagus. *Seminars in Pediatric Surgery, 19*, 186–193.

Foker, J., Kendall, T. C., Catton, K., & Khan, K. M. (2005). A flexible approach to achieve a true primary repair for all infants with esophageal atresia. *Seminars in Pediatric Surgery, 14*, 5–8. doi:10.1053/j.sempedsurg.2004.10.021

Gupta, D. K., & Sharma, S. (2008). Esophageal atresia: The total care in a high-risk population. *Seminars in Pediatric Surgery, 17*, 236–243.

Hansen, A., & Lillehei, C. (2009). Respiratory disorders. Part 1: Esophageal atresia and tracheoesophageal fistula. In A. Hansen & M. Puder (Eds.), *Manual of neonatal surgical intensive care*. Hamilton, ON: BC Decker.

Montrowl, S. J. (2014). Gastrointestinal system. In C. Kenner & W. L. Lott (Eds.), *Comprehensive neonatal care* (5th ed., pp. 198–228). New York, NY: Springer Publishing Company.

Mortellaro, V. E., Pettiford, J. N., St. Peter, S. D., Fraser, J. D., & Wei, J. (2011). Incidence, diagnosis, and outcomes of vocal fold immobility after esophageal atresia (EA) and/or tracheoesophageal fistula (TEF) repair. *European Journal of Pediatric Surgery, 21*, 386–388. doi:10.1055/s-0031-1291269

Replogle, R. (1963). Esophageal atresia: Plastic sumo catheter for drainage of the proximal pouch. *Surgery, 54*, 296–297

Spitz, L. (2007). Oesophageal atresia. *Orphanet Journal of Rare Diseases, 2*(24). doi:10.1186/1750-1172-2-24

Zani, A., Eaton, S., Hoellwarth, M., Puir, P., Fasching, G., Bagolan, P., ... Pierro, A. (2014). International survey on the management of esophageal atresia. *European Journal of Pediatric Surgery, 24*(1), 3–8.

GASTROINTESTINAL SURGICAL CONDITIONS IN THE NEONATE

Julie Briere and Michelle LaBrecque

GI SURGERY GENERAL CONSIDERATIONS

Any segment of the GI tract may have an obstruction in the neonate, either due to a structural anomaly or a functional etiology (Table 8.4).

General symptoms that raise concern for a bowel obstruction in the neonate include:

- History of polyhydramnios

- Abdominal distension

- Emesis, often bilious

- Failure to pass meconium within 24 to 48 hours after birth

Advances in neonatology, neonatal surgery, and anesthesia have led to increased survival and overall decreased morbidity in neonates with GI issues. Prompt assessment, stabilization, and surgical intervention are essential in the management of a

TABLE 8.4 Common Types of Bowel Obstructions in Neonates	
Structural Anomalies: Anatomical Condition Affecting Bowel Continuity	**Functional Conditions: Mechanical Condition Either Due to Altered Peristalsis or a Blockage**
Esophageal atresia	Hirschsprung disease
Duodenal atresia	Meconium ileus
Malrotation/midgut volvulus	Meconium plug syndrome
Ileal/jejunal atresia	Necrotizing enterocolitis
Imperforate anus	

neonate with suspected bowel obstruction (Montrowl, 2014). Initial stabilization of a neonate with a suspected bowel obstruction includes:

■ Cessation of enteral feeds

■ Gastric decompression with a sump tube and replacement of excess gastric losses

■ IV hydration

■ Correction of fluid, acid–base, and electrolyte derangements

■ Antibiotic therapy (in most situations)

■ Fluid resuscitation (if fluid shifts occur from the vascular space into the bowel lumen, resulting in shock)

These therapies occur concurrently with surgical consultation and evaluation for a bowel obstruction with the following.

Radiologic studies

■ Abdominal x-ray (anteroposterior and left lateral decubitus or cross-table lateral views)

■ Upper GI contrast series

■ Contrast enemas

■ Ultrasonography (less often) based on presenting symptoms and patient history

Laboratory studies

■ CBC and differential, electrolytes, blood gas, blood culture, coagulation panel, and blood type and cross match (if surgery is anticipated)

Genetic evaluation

■ Consult the genetic service for evaluation of associated congenital anomalies or syndromes (as is often the case), following stabilization of the infant

DOCUMENTATION

- Bowel perfusion and color preoperatively (for gastroschisis and omphalocele)
- Strict input and output measurement, including gastric drainage
- Vital signs and abdominal girth
- Physical assessment with specific attention to abdominal assessment and bowel function
- Pain assessment and interventions
- Medication administration
- Document stoma appearance and drainage (if applicable)
- Peritoneal drain site appearance and drainage (if applicable)

DUODENAL ATRESIA

DEFINITION

Duodenal atresia is a congenital structural obstruction of the small intestine, typically distal to the ampulla of Vater. One of the more common areas of a bowel atresia, this condition is thought to result from a failure of recanalization of the bowel lumen during the first trimester when the midgut begins to form. The obstruction can be partial, such as a membranous web, or complete. Duodenal atresia has a reported incidence of 1 in 7,000 live births and is often, 50% to 70% occurrence, associated with other anomalies such as trisomy 21, congenital heart defects, and VACTERL (Choudhry, Rahman, Boyd, & Lakhoo, 2009; Cragan, Martin, Moore, & Khoury, 1993).

PRESENTATION

Newborns with duodenal atresia almost always have a maternal history of polyhydramnios. Shortly after birth, the infant presents with evidence of feeding intolerance, gastric distension, and emesis, which may be bilious depending on the location of the atresia. The majority of neonates with duodenal atresia will have the obstruction distal to the ampulla of Vater where the biliary ducts drain into the bowel, thus resulting in bilious emesis.

DIAGNOSIS

Duodenal atresia is diagnosed by history, clinical presentation, and abdominal x-ray (anteroposterior and left lateral decubitus). Duodenal atresia is typically seen on x-ray as a "double bubble" pattern: dilated air-filled stomach and proximal duodenum.

PREOPERATIVE ASSESSMENT AND NURSING CARE

- Discontinue enteral feedings
- Provide gastric decompression to decrease gastric distension and risk of aspiration of bilious emesis
- Establish IV access
- Collect laboratory studies including a CBC, chemistries, coagulation studies, and blood type and cross match (in anticipation of surgery and subsequent blood loss)
- Initiate IV hydration and correct any fluid and electrolyte abnormalities due to gastric losses
- Perform a cardiac evaluation, including a chest radiograph, electrocardiogram, and echocardiogram (due to the high incidence of associated cardiac anomalies)
- Administer perioperative antibiotics
- Obtain genetic service consultation to evaluate for trisomy 21 and other associated genetic abnormalities (This is not urgent and may be delayed until postoperatively, including obtaining genetic studies.)

SURGICAL PROCEDURE

- Goal of surgical repair is to restore duodenal continuity.
- Most often this surgery is a laparotomy, although some centers are now performing this as a laparoscopic procedure in larger, more stable neonates (Kay, Yoder, & Rothenberg, 2009).
- The affected segment of duodenum is resected and an end-to-end anastomosis, a duodenoduodenostomy, is completed.

POSTOPERATIVE ASSESSMENT AND NURSING CARE

- Continue gastric decompression until return of bowel function, which may occur over several days

- Monitor for excessive amounts of gastric drainage and the need for fluid replacement if excessive

- Continue maintenance IV fluids with electrolytes and begin parenteral nutrition as soon as possible to optimize nutritional status

- Administer perioperative antibiotics, completing prescribed course

- Manage postoperative pain with regional analgesia and opioid therapy; standardized postoperative pain protocols are recommended

DOCUMENTATION

See the Documentation section under General Considerations.

GASTROSCHISIS

DEFINITION

Gastroschisis is a full-thickness defect in the abdominal wall through which the uncovered intestines protrude (Poenaro, 2012).

PRESENTATION

Apparent at birth, this defect is not encapsulated in a sac. It protrudes, typically to the right of the umbilical ring. The exposed bowel appears edematous, matted, and covered in a fibrous peel. The abdominal cavity is small and underdeveloped (Martin & Fishman, 2009a).

DIAGNOSIS

Gastroschisis is usually prenatally diagnosed with elevated AFP level or found on a second trimester fetal US (Martin & Fishman, 2009a). The defect appears most often in young mothers and those of low gravidity (Fillingham & Rankin, 2008).

PREOPERATIVE ASSESSMENT AND NURSING CARE

■ Use careful handling to avoid injury to the bowel wall

■ Place the lower two thirds of the infant in a bowel bag with 20 mL of warmed sterile saline

■ Place the infant on his side to prevent injury to the bowel or kinking of mesenteric vessels

■ Monitor for IWL

■ Assess bowel frequently for adequate perfusion

▪ The bowel should be pink throughout; report any areas on the bowel that are dusky or discolored.

■ Provide gastric decompression, fluid resuscitation, and antibiotic prophylaxis

SURGICAL PROCEDURE

■ Primary repair—This method involves stretching of the abdominal cavity to return contents, and closing the peritoneum and abdominal wall.

■ Staged repair—This occurs when the infant's abdominal contents are too large or the infant is too unstable or premature to tolerate a primary repair with full return of bowel into the abdominal cavity.

▪ An extra-abdominal prosthetic sac, that is, silo, is utilized that supports the defect at a 90° angle and assists with reduction of the defect by gravity.

▪ Various techniques are available to achieve the return of bowel to the abdomen; these include a silo with a spring-loaded ring placed under the fascia or a mesh sac that is sutured.

▪ Gradual reduction of the defect occurs over several days; optimal timing of the closure is 5 to 7 days to decrease the risk of infection.

POSTOPERATIVE ASSESSMENT AND NURSING CARE

- Primary repair
  - For risk of increased intra-abdominal pressure, assess for adequate lung volumes and blood gases to assure sufficient ventilation.
  - For abdominal compartment syndrome risk, monitor for adequate urine output as well as distal pulses.
    - With abdominal compartment syndrome, there is a concern for increased abdominal pressure causing decreased renal perfusion as well as decreased perfusion and blood flow to distal extremities.
- Staged repair
  - Assess the silo for dislodgement during daily reduction of the bowel back into the abdominal cavity.
  - Care should be taken to maintain a moist base at the level where the silo enters the abdominal wall, which can be achieved with a Vaseline gauze or Xeroform.
  - To measure for additional drainage and fluid losses (so that IV fluids can be adjusted), collect and measure fluid on the gauze dressing placed around the base of the silo.
- For primary and staged repairs:
  - Conduct frequent assessments of respiratory and cardiovascular status since intra-abdominal pressure rises in both primary and staged repairs.
  - Maintain constant vigilance over the infant since there are major concerns of venous stasis, respiratory compromise, infection, and nutrition.
  - Report signs of increased respiratory distress.
  - Report decreased perfusion to the legs as well as decreased urine output, which is indicative of compromised perfusion related to increased abdominal pressure.

■ Provide ventilatory support, antibiotic prophylaxis, and central line for parenteral nutrition since infants remain NPO until bowel function is restored.

■ Manage postoperative pain with regional analgesia and opioid therapy; standardized postoperative pain protocols are recommended.

■ Educate providers and parents that one third of infants with gastroschisis will experience growth delay in infancy, and that prolonged intestinal dysmotility is common (Phillips, Raval, Redden, & Weiner, 2008; South, Marshall, Bose, & Laughon, 2008).

DOCUMENTATION

See the Documentation section under General Considerations.

HIRSCHSPRUNG DISEASE

DEFINITION

Hirschsprung disease is a functional bowel obstruction caused by a lack of ganglion cells in the intestine. It typically involves the sigmoid colon and rectum. Hirschsprung disease results from a failure of development in neural cell migration along the bowel lumen and results in aganglionosis, an absence of ganglion cells (neurons necessary for bowel function). This occurs in a cranial-to-caudal direction; the point of cessation of neural cell development results in a transition zone. Peristalsis below this level is ineffective; the affected colon and rectum cannot relax, which results in obstruction of stool. Hirschsprung disease occurs in 1 in approximately 5,000 to 8,000 live births and in males more often than females. The majority involves the rectum or sigmoid colon region, although 10% have total colonic aganglionosis. Most cases are sporadic, but 10% to 20% have a familial history. There is a 5% to 10% incidence of trisomy 21 and a small association, approximately 15%, with meconium plug syndrome (Lovvern, Glenn, Pacetti, &

Carter, 2011; Pursley, Hansen, & Puder, 2009; Song, Upperman, & Niklas, 2012).

PRESENTATION

An infant with Hirschsprung disease presents with a failure to pass meconium in the first 48 hours, feeding intolerance, and/or abdominal distension. It may present with constipation or diarrhea, depending on the length of intestine involved. Paradoxical diarrhea is due to liquid stool passing around obstipated stool. Approximately 5% to 10% of cases present as toxic megacolon, a life-threatening condition. Toxic megacolon presents as an enterocolitis with fever, emesis, abdominal distension, foul-smelling stool, and septic shock. Mortality is significantly higher in this presentation (Lovvern et al., 2011; Song et al., 2012).

DIAGNOSIS

A contrast enema shows a transitional zone between proximal dilated bowel and the contracted colon and rectum. Definitive diagnosis is made by suction rectal biopsy. A positive biopsy shows an absence of ganglion cells.

PREOPERATIVE ASSESSMENT AND NURSING CARE

- Discontinue enteral feedings
- Provide gastric decompression to decrease gastric distension and risk of aspiration of bilious emesis
- Establish IV access
- Collect laboratory studies including a CBC, chemistries, coagulation studies, and blood type and cross match (in anticipation of surgery and subsequent blood loss)
- Initiate IV hydration and correct any fluid and electrolyte abnormalities due to gastric losses
- Administer antibiotics
- Assist in preparation for suction rectal biopsy, often performed at the patient's bedside

■ Conduct rectal irrigations; if irrigations maintain an adequate stooling pattern and examination is stable, then enteral feeds may be restarted until evaluation is complete and surgery occurs.

SURGICAL PROCEDURE

■ Surgical correction is based on the clinical condition of the infant and the level of intestinal involvement.

   ■ Emergent colostomy is performed if toxic megacolon presents.

   ■ If stable, a laparoscopic-assisted endorectal pull-through is performed.

   ■ A primary transanal pull-through or staged reconstruction is performed in some cases; this involves creation of a colostomy with delayed reanastomosis in 3 to 6 months.

■ Serial intraoperative biopsies occur to identify the level of intestine with functioning ganglion cells.

POSTOPERATIVE ASSESSMENT AND NURSING CARE

■ Continue gastric decompression

■ Maintain NPO

   ■ Continue maintenance IV fluids with electrolytes and begin parenteral nutrition as soon as possible to optimize nutritional status until the return of bowel function.

   ■ Bowel function typically resumes 24 hours following pull-through procedures.

   ■ In severe cases where there is significant bowel loss resulting in short bowel syndrome (SBS), long-term nutritional management may be indicated.

■ Administer perioperative antibiotics, completing the prescribed course

■ Manage postoperative pain with regional analgesia and opioid therapy; standardized postoperative pain protocols are recommended

- Continue gastric decompression until the return of bowel function, which may occur over several days
- Assess stoma and perform stoma care if indicated

DOCUMENTATION

See the Documentation section under General Considerations.

IMPERFORATE ANUS

DEFINITION

Imperforate anus is a condition of anorectal malformation in which the anus is not patent. This condition often occurs with urogenital or rectal fistula. It occurs in one in 2,500 to 5,000 live births and is slightly more common in males. The positioning of the rectum may be low, intermediate, or high; a high-placed rectum has a greater chance of associated anomalies. Occasionally a correlation exists with VACTERL association or trisomy 21 (Lovvern et al., 2011; Pursley et al., 2009).

PRESENTATION

Imperforate anus is identified on physical exam as the absence of an anus.

DIAGNOSIS

The abdominal x-ray may show dilated bowel loops consistent with a distal obstruction. A perianal US is performed to evaluate where the rectum terminates. In males, a contrast study of the urethra is performed to evaluate for a rectourethral fistula.

PREOPERATIVE ASSESSMENT AND NURSING CARE

- Discontinue enteral feedings
- Provide gastric decompression to decrease gastric distension and risk of aspiration of bilious emesis

■ Establish IV access

■ Collect laboratory studies including a CBC, chemistries, coagulation studies, and blood type and cross match (in anticipation of surgery and subsequent blood loss)

■ Initiate IV hydration and correct any fluid and electrolyte abnormalities due to gastric losses

■ Correct fluid, electrolyte, and acid–base abnormalities

■ Administer antibiotics until presence of a fistula is ruled out

SURGICAL PROCEDURE

■ Varies depending on the level of rectum and presence of fistula

  ■ Anoplasty, or repair of the rectum

  ■ Dilation of fistulas

  ■ Colostomy with reanastomosis in 3 to 6 months

POSTOPERATIVE ASSESSMENT AND NURSING CARE

■ Continue gastric decompression until the return of bowel function, which may occur over several days

■ Maintain NPO

■ Continue maintenance IV fluids with electrolytes and begin parenteral nutrition as soon as possible to optimize nutritional status until the return of bowel function

  ■ Bowel function typically resumes 24 hours following a pull-through procedure

■ Administer perioperative antibiotics, completing the prescribed course

■ Manage postoperative pain with regional analgesia and opioid therapy; standardized postoperative pain protocols are recommended

■ Assess stoma and perform stoma care if indicated

DOCUMENTATION

See the Documentation section under General Considerations.

INTESTINAL ATRESIA

DEFINITION

Intestinal atresia, which occurs in 0.7 to 1.8 per 10,000 live births (Best et al., 2012), is a congenital structural obstruction of the intestine. The defect typically occurs in the jejunum but may also occur in the ileum, or in both (Stollman et al., 2009). Unlike duodenal atresia that occurs early in gestation, ileal and jejunal atresia are believed to occur later in gestation as the result of ischemic necrosis and bowel resorption due to a mesenteric vascular accident or segmental volvulus. Intestinal atresia defects are usually not associated with other non-GI anomalies, although they sometimes occur with abdominal wall defects and malrotation. Intestinal atresia has been reported in some neonates with cystic fibrosis (Stollman et al., 2009).

PRESENTATION

Polyhydramnios occurs frequently in proximal atresia but is rare in distal atresia. Atresia presents with early feeding intolerance, bilious emesis typically in the first 48 hours after birth, abdominal distention (more significant with distal atresia), and visible bowel loops on examination. Neonates with intestinal atresia tend to be small for gestational age.

DIAGNOSIS

Abdominal x-rays show distended loops of bowel and a paucity of air distal to the obstruction. Contrast enemas may demonstrate a microcolon since that portion of bowel has been unused. Several classifications of intestinal atresias occur with varying degrees of mesentery involvement and bowel length that greatly affect morbidity and mortality.

PREOPERATIVE ASSESSMENT AND NURSING CARE

■ Discontinue enteral feedings

■ Provide gastric decompression to decrease gastric distension and risk of aspiration of bilious emesis

■ Establish IV access

■ Collect laboratory studies including a CBC, chemistries, coagulation studies, and blood type and cross match (in anticipation of surgery and subsequent blood loss)

■ Initiate IV hydration and correct any fluid and electrolyte abnormalities due to gastric losses

SURGICAL PROCEDURE

■ The goal of surgical repair is to restore intestinal continuity.

■ The segment of atresia is resected and, when possible, an end-to-end anastomosis is performed.

■ There is often a size disparity in the bowel ends due to dilation of the proximal end, which limits immediate anastomosis as an option.

■ Bowel resection of the dilated portion or temporary creation of a stoma may occur.

POSTOPERATIVE ASSESSMENT AND NURSING CARE

■ Continue gastric decompression until the return of bowel function, which may occur over several days

■ Monitor for excessive amounts of gastric drainage and the need for fluid replacement if excessive

■ Continue maintenance IV fluids with electrolytes and begin parenteral nutrition as soon as possible to optimize nutritional status

■ Administer perioperative antibiotics, completing the prescribed course

■ Manage postoperative pain with regional analgesia and opioid therapy; standardized postoperative pain protocols are recommended

■ Assess stoma appearance if applicable, including color and drainage

■ Perform stoma care; typically a stoma is covered with moist dressing (i.e., xeroform gauze) during the initial PODs and then transitioned to an ostomy appliance once the output increases

DOCUMENTATION

See the Documentation section under General Considerations.

MALROTATION/VOLVULUS

DEFINITION

Malrotation is the failure of rotation and fixation of the midgut during early gestation. Malrotation predisposes the bowel to twist, resulting in a volvulus, a condition that may acutely decrease enteric blood supply and result in bowel ischemia and infarction.

PRESENTATION

Malrotation symptoms are present in (approximately) 50% of infants during the first months of life (Pursley et al., 2009; Song et al., 2012). Early signs of malrotation are feeding intolerance and bilious emesis; however, the infant may be asymptomatic. Symptoms indicative of a volvulus are more acute and may include abdominal distension, bilious emesis, bloody emesis or stools, and abdominal erythema. As the condition progresses, infants often have symptoms of systemic signs of shock, hypotension, anuria, acidosis, and leukocytosis. A volvulus is a surgical emergency; failure to provide prompt medical and surgical intervention may result in significant bowel loss or death.

DIAGNOSIS

Abdominal x-ray in the patient with a malrotation, with or without volvulus, demonstrates evidence of bowel obstruction, typically a dilated duodenum and stomach. The gold standard radiographic study is an upper GI that will demonstrate the malrotation and obstruction. Neonates with systemic signs consistent with a volvulus require immediate surgical intervention; the procedure is not delayed for the completion of an upper GI study.

PREOPERATIVE ASSESSMENT AND NURSING CARE

- Discontinue enteral feedings
- Provide gastric decompression to decrease gastric distension and risk of aspiration of bilious emesis
- Establish IV access
- Collect laboratory studies including a CBC, chemistries, coagulation studies, and blood type and cross match (in anticipation of surgery and subsequent blood loss)
- Initiate IV hydration and correct any fluid and electrolyte abnormalities due to gastric losses
- Provide volume resuscitation
- Administer antibiotic therapy

SURGICAL PROCEDURE

- A laparotomy and Ladd's procedure, involving the division of Ladd's bands to relieve the duodenal obstruction, is performed to reposition the bowel and correct the malrotation.
- During the procedure there is widening of the mesenteric base to allow improved blood flow to the bowel.
  - An appendectomy is also performed at the same time.
- With a volvulus, any necrotic bowel is resected and a stoma is created.

POSTOPERATIVE ASSESSMENT AND NURSING CARE

- Continue gastric decompression until the return of bowel function, which may occur over several days
- Maintain NPO
- Continue maintenance IV fluids with electrolytes and begin parenteral nutrition as soon as possible to optimize nutritional status until the return of bowel function
- Administer perioperative antibiotics, completing the prescribed course
- Manage postoperative pain with regional analgesia and opioid therapy; standardized postoperative pain protocols are recommended
- In severe cases the infant may have significant bowel loss resulting in SBS; long-term nutritional management may be indicated
- Assess the stoma and perform stoma care if indicated

DOCUMENTATION

See the Documentation section under General Considerations.

MECONIUM ILEUS

DEFINITION

Meconium ileus is the functional obstruction of the small intestine due to excessively thick meconium from abnormally viscous intestinal secretions and a lack of pancreatic enzymes. Ninety percent of neonates with meconium ileus have cystic fibrosis.

PRESENTATION

Symptoms of meconium ileus include abdominal distension, bilious emesis, and failure to pass meconium. In severe cases, symptoms may worsen to include abdominal erythema, edema, and respiratory distress due to abdominal distension. Occasionally, intrauterine perforation has occurred.

DIAGNOSIS

Meconium ileus most frequently occurs in the ileum. The abdominal radiograph demonstrates an echogenic abdominal mass, "soap-bubble" appearance of air trapped in meconium with dilated loops of bowel. A contrast enema typically shows a microcolon and pellets of thickened meconium at the distal end of the obstruction. Occasionally, a meconium ileus may lead to intrauterine perforation, which would be seen as microcalcifications.

PREOPERATIVE ASSESSMENT AND NURSING CARE

- Discontinue enteral feedings
- Provide gastric decompression to decrease gastric distension and risk of aspiration of bilious emesis
- Establish IV access
- Collect laboratory studies including a CBC, chemistries, coagulation studies, and blood type and cross match (in anticipation of surgery and subsequent blood loss)
- Initiate IV hydration and correct any fluid and electrolyte abnormalities due to gastric losses
- Administer antibiotic therapy
- Assist with administering a hyperosmolar enema (i.e., Gastrografin), which draws fluid into the bowel lumen to dilute viscous meconium and ease passage of the meconium

SURGICAL PROCEDURE

- Surgical repair typically includes an enterotomy (small incision in bowel) through which saline or mucomyst is instilled.
- In severe cases, resection of the obstructed bowel segment and creation of stoma is performed.

POSTOPERATIVE ASSESSMENT AND NURSING CARE

■ Continue gastric decompression until the return of bowel function, which may occur over several days

■ Maintain NPO

■ Continue maintenance IV fluids with electrolytes and begin parenteral nutrition as soon as possible to optimize nutritional status until the return of bowel function

■ In severe cases where there is significant bowel loss resulting in SBS, long-term nutritional management may be indicated

■ Administer perioperative antibiotics, completing the prescribed course

■ Manage postoperative pain with regional analgesia and opioid therapy; standardized postoperative pain protocols are recommended

■ Assess the stoma and perform stoma care if indicated

■ Administer rectal or ostomy irrigation with saline or mucomyst if indicated

DOCUMENTATION

See the Documentation section under General Considerations.

MECONIUM PLUG SYNDROME

DEFINITION

Meconium plug syndrome is the failure to pass stool, resulting in a meconium plug. The plug often forms in the distal segment of the colon or rectum. It results from excessively thick meconium causing a functional obstruction of the bowel. Immature ganglion cells are the likely etiology. Approximately 5% of newborns with meconium plug syndrome are associated with Hirschsprung disease (Fanaroff, 2013; Lovvern et al., 2011).

PRESENTATION

Symptoms of meconium plug syndrome include bilious emesis, hyperactive bowel sounds, abdominal distension, and failure to pass stool, although they may pass a small amount of gray meconium. In severe cases, this condition may progress to perforation and the infant may develop systemic symptoms of sepsis.

DIAGNOSIS

The plug most frequently occurs in the distal segment of the colon or rectum. Abdominal x-ray demonstrates multiple distended bowel loops. An intraluminal plug is often visualized by a water-soluble enema, which often dislodges the plug.

PREOPERATIVE ASSESSMENT AND NURSING CARE

- ■ Discontinue enteral feedings
- ■ Provide gastric decompression to decrease gastric distension and the risk of aspiration of bilious emesis
- ■ Establish IV access
- ■ Collect laboratory studies including a CBC, chemistries, coagulation studies, and blood type and cross match (in anticipation of surgery and subsequent blood loss)
- ■ Initiate IV hydration and correct any fluid and electrolyte abnormalities due to gastric losses

SURGICAL PROCEDURE

- ■ A majority of infants will pass the plug spontaneously without surgical intervention.
- ■ Rectal dilation or contrast enema may be a curative treatment.
- ■ In rare instances of bowel perforation, the infant will require surgical repair and the creation of a stoma.

POSTOPERATIVE ASSESSMENT AND NURSING CARE

■ Continue gastric decompression until the return of bowel function, which may occur over several days

■ Maintain NPO

■ Continue maintenance IV fluids with electrolytes and begin parenteral nutrition as soon as possible to optimize nutritional status until the return of bowel function

■ In severe cases where there is significant bowel loss resulting in SBS, long-term nutritional management may be indicated

■ Administer perioperative antibiotics, completing the prescribed course

■ Manage postoperative pain with regional analgesia and opioid therapy; standardized postoperative pain protocols are recommended

■ Assess the stoma and perform stoma care if indicated

DOCUMENTATION

See the Documentation section under General Considerations.

NECROTIZING ENTEROCOLITIS

DEFINITION

NEC is an acquired disorder characterized by hemorrhage, ischemia, and sometimes necrosis of the mucosal and submucosal layers of the intestinal tract.

PRESENTATION

Infants present with abdominal distention, increased gastric residuals, emesis, hypotension, and bloody stools. Infants may also present with symptoms of sepsis, including lethargy, temperature instability, apnea, and poor feedings. NEC commonly presents in extremely low-birth-weight (ELBW) infants during the first couple of weeks after birth, and before the initiation of enteral feedings (Gordon, Christensen, Weitkamp, & Maheshwari, 2009). The etiology of NEC is not fully understood but is thought to be multifactorial (Gregory et al., 2011; Moss, 2008). Contributing factors to NEC include conditions that alter mesenteric blood flow, resulting in ischemia, from PDA, hypovolemia, hypotension, hypothermia, polycythemia, infection, and enteral feeds (Patel et al., 2015).

Occasionally, an SIP may occur without evidence of NEC. Etiology of this event may be related to an immature intestinal barrier, increased gastric pH, use of umbilical artery catheters, and administration of medications for closure of the patent ductus arteriosis (indomethacin or ibuprofen).

The age at onset of NEC is inversely related to gestational age, with a mean age of 3 to 4 days for term infants and 3 to 4 weeks for infants born at less than 28 weeks gestation (Wilson-Castello, 2013). The incidence of developing NEC for infants born weighing less than 1,500 g ranges between 7% and 10%. The mortality rate of affected infants ranges from 25% to 30%; up to 50% receive surgical intervention (Chappin, 2012; Moss, 2008). One third of the patients present with a milder form of disease that resolves with medical therapy alone, and approximately 50% of cases require surgical intervention (Chappin, 2012; Moss, 2008). Initial injury to the intestinal mucosa may be caused by hypoxia, ischemia, intestinal inflammation, and/or bacterial infection, so care is directed at minimizing injury.

DIAGNOSIS

Initial laboratory findings of metabolic and respiratory acidosis, electrolyte abnormalities, neutropenia, and thrombocytopenia are likely. Radiologic diagnosis is also reliable. Kidneys, ureters, and bladder (abdominal x-ray) as well as left lateral decubitus x-rays need to be obtained to assess for small bubbles of gas in the lumen of the intestine (pneumatosis). If those bubbles of gas rupture into the mesenteric vascular bed, a pneumoperitoneum will be found on radiographic images.

PREOPERATIVE ASSESSMENT AND NURSING CARE

■ Assessment and documentation of apnea episodes, abdominal girths, emesis, or other subtle signs of sepsis need to be evaluated closely for etiology

■ Check for increased gastric residuals if indicated (Torrazza et al., 2015)

■ Decompress the stomach with low intermittent suction through a sump tube

■ Promptly initiate antibiotic therapy as this is crucial to the treatment of NEC

■ Intubate and support the infant's respiratory status

■ Infants can experience apnea or increasing respiratory distress due to compression of the diaphragm from abdominal distension

■ Assess for hypotension

  ■ Support blood pressure and maintain adequate perfusion with the use of fluid resuscitation and vasoactive infusions

■ Insert a central line to allow adequate nutrition while the infant is unable to receive enteral feeds while the bowel heals

■ Follow serial abdominal x-rays every 6 to 8 hours (or more frequently) to assess for progression of the pneumotosis to intestinal perforation

■ Monitor blood work frequently to assess for anemia, thrombocytopenia, and abnormal coagulation

■ Send the blood clot for blood type and cross match since infants with NEC frequently need treatment for bleeding or blood loss, and sometimes a coagulopathy (with PRBCs, FFP, and cryoprecipitate)

SURGICAL PROCEDURE

■ The most common surgical interventions performed on infants with NEC are laparotomies and placement of peritoneal drains (Hansen et al., 2009).

■ The type of operation performed for perforated NEC does not influence survival or other clinically important early outcomes in preterm infants (Moss et al., 2006; Raval, Hall, Pierro, & Moss, 2013).

■ Placement of a peritoneal drain may be the best choice as either a temporary measure or definitive treatment in smaller or more unstable neonates (Moss, Dimmitt, Barnhart, Sylvester, Brown, Powell et al., 2006).

■ The drain is less invasive, does not require the infant to be placed under anesthesia, and can be placed at the bedside.

■ During a laparotomy, necrotic bowel is resected and an ostomy is created.

POSTOPERATIVE ASSESSMENT AND NURSING CARE

■ Ensure the infant receives adequate parenteral nutrition to facilitate healing

■ Maintain gastric decompression until the return of bowel function

■ Monitor fluid status closely

■ Infant may require aggressive fluid resuscitation to maintain adequate blood pressure and perfusion due to fluid losses during surgery.

■ Assess the abdomen's appearance and girth

■ Assess the peritoneal drain site or ostomy bud for color and adequate perfusion; report changes to the drain site or ostomy bud as soon as they are noted

■ Manage postoperative pain with regional analgesia and opioid therapy; standardized postoperative pain protocols are recommended

■ Resume enteral feedings once the infant has received 10 to 14 days of bowel rest, treatment with antibiotics, and bowel function has recovered

■ Educate providers and parents that although more than 70% of patients with NEC survive, long-term GI complications include intestinal strictures and SBS

DOCUMENTATION

See the Documentation section under General Considerations.

OMPHALOCELE

DEFINITION

An omphalocele is an abdominal wall defect most commonly found at the level of the umbilicus (Martin & Fishman, 2009b).

PRESENTATION

This defect occurs from failure of the abdominal organs to completely return to the abdomen during week 10 of development, causing incomplete closure of the anterior abdominal wall. The defect is covered with a peritoneal sac that may be intact or have ruptured in utero. Bowel is trapped within the umbilical ring; larger defects may include the liver as well as bowel. Multiple and often life-threatening syndromes and anomalies occur greater than 50% of the time with an omphalocele diagnosis (Montrowl, 2014).

DIAGNOSIS

Omphaloceles are usually prenatally diagnosed with elevated AFP level or found on second trimester fetal US.

PREOPERATIVE ASSESSMENT AND NURSING CARE

■ Protect the eviscerated organs, decompress the gut, and provide hydration to account for insensible losses
■ If the sac is intact, moisten sterile gauze with warmed sterile saline and loosely wrap around the defect

- Apply a dry gauze dressing around the outside over the moist dressing
- If the sac has ruptured, place the infant in a bowel bag, a clear polyurethane sac that provides a barrier, thus decreasing loss of fluid and heat

SURGICAL PROCEDURE

- Primary repair—For small defects, the contents of the omphalocele are returned into the abdominal cavity and there is closure of the defect via a skin-flap.
- Staged repair—A silo (see Gastroschisis section for information on silos) is used to suspend the contents of large defects above the patient. Reduction maneuvers are then carried out daily to return the organs to the small abdominal cavity.
  - Complete return of the organs into the abdominal cavity is generally achieved over 7 to 10 days.
- Delayed repair—Performed when the infant is extremely premature, there is a giant omphalocele, or when respiratory failure makes a primary repair not feasible.
  - The sac is treated with a drying antiseptic agent (to prevent infection); examples include povidone-iodine and silver sulfadiazine.
  - Application of these agents dries the sac, creating an eschar covering that protects the abdominal contents.
  - Tissue granulates and skin eventually cover the entire defect.
  - With growth and stabilization of the infant, surgical repair is accomplished with an abdominal wall closure.

POSTOPERATIVE ASSESSMENT AND NURSING CARE

- Monitor for major concerns including respiratory compromise, infection, and nutrition
- Conduct frequent assessments of respiratory and cardiovascular status for changes associated with increased intra-abdominal pressure

- Manage postoperative pain with regional analgesia and opioid therapy; standardized postoperative pain protocols are recommended
- Increase ventilator settings as needed to compensate for increased intra-abdominal pressure and monitor blood gases
- Administer antibiotic prophylaxis
- Place a central line for TPN nutrition since infants remain NPO until bowel function is restored

DOCUMENTATION

See the Documentation section under General Considerations.

REFERENCES

Best, K. E., Tennant, P. W., Addor, M. C., Bianchi, F., Boyd, P., Calzolari, E., … Rankin, J. (2012). Epidemiology of small intestinal atresia in Europe: A register-based study. *Archives of Diseases in Child Fetal Neonatal Education*, 97(5), 353–358.

Chappin, M. (2012). Necrotizing enterocolitis. In C. A. Gleason & S. Devaskar (Eds.), *Averys diseases of the newborn* (9th ed., pp. 1022–1029). Philadelphia, PA: Elsevier Saunders.

Choudhry, M. S., Rahman, N., Boyd, P., & Lakhoo, K. (2009). Duodenal atresia: Associated anomalies, prenatal diagnosis and outcome. *Pediatric Surgery International*, 25, 727–730.

Cragan, J. D., Martin, M. L., Moore, C. A., & Khoury, M. J. (1993). Descriptive epidemiology of small intestinal atresia in Atlanta, Georgia. *Teratology*, 48(5), 441–450.

Fanaroff, A. (2013). Selected disorders of gastrointestinal tract. In A. Fanaroff & J. Fanaroff (Eds.), *Klaus and Fanaroff's care of the high risk neonate* (6th ed., pp. 151–200). Philadelphia, PA: Elsevier Saunders.

Fillingham, A., & Rankin, J. (2008). Prevalence, prenatal diagnosis and survival of gastroschisis. *Prenatal Diagnosis*, 28(13), 1232–1237. doi: 10.1002/pd.2153

Gordon, P., Christensen, R., Weitkamp, J.-H., & Maheshwari, A. (2009). Mapping the new world of necrotizing enterocolitis (NEC): Review and opinion. *EJ Neonatology Research, 2*(4), 145–172.

Gregory, K. E., DeForge, C. E., Natale, K. M., Phillips, M., & Van Marter, L. J. (2011). Necrotizing enterocolitis in the premature infant: Neonatal nursing assessment, disease pathogenesis, and clinical presentation. *Advances in Neonatal Care, 11*(3), 155–164.

Hansen, A. R., Modi, B. P., Ching, Y. A., & Jaksic, T. (2009). Necrotizing enterocolitis. In A. R. Hansen & M. Puder (Eds.), *Manual of neonatal surgical intensive care* (2nd ed., pp. 245–263). Shelton, CT: BC Decker.

Kay, S., Yoder, S., & Rothenberg, S. (2009). Laparoscopic duodenoduodenostomy in the neonate. *Journal of Pediatric Surgery, 44*(5), 906–908.

Lovvern, H. N., Glenn, J. B., Pacetti, A. S., & Carter, B. S. (2011). Neonatal surgery. In S. L. Gardner, B. S. Carter, M. Enzman-Hines, & J. A. Hernandez (Eds.), *Merenstein & Gardner's handbook of neonatal intensive care* (7th ed., pp. 812–847). St. Louis, MO: Mosby Elsevier.

Martin, C. R., & Fishman, S. J. (2009a). Gastroschisis. In A. R. Hansen & M. Puder (Eds.), *Manual of neonatal surgical intensive care* (2nd ed., pp. 224–237). Shelton, CT: BC Decker.

Martin, C. R., & Fishman, S. J. (2009b). Omphalocele. In A. R. Hansen & M. Puder (Eds.), *Manual of neonatal surgical intensive care* (2nd ed., pp. 238–244). Shelton, CT: BC Decker.

Montrowl, S. J. (2014). Gastrointestinal systems. In C. Kenner & J. W. Lott (Eds.), *Comprehensive neonatal nursing care* (5th ed., pp. 189–228). New York, NY: Springer Publishing Company.

Moss, R. L., Dimmitt, R. A., Barnhart, D. C., Sylvester, K. G., Brown, R. L., Powell, D. M, … Silverman, B. L. (2006). Laparotomy versus peritoneal drainage for necrotizing enterocolitis and perforation. *New England Journal of Medicine, 354*(21), 2225–2234.

Moss, R. L., Kalish, L. A., Duggan, C., Johnston, P., Brandt, M. L., Dunn, J. C. Y., & Sylvester, K. G. (2008). Clinical parameters do not adequately predict outcome in necrotizing enterocolitis: A multi-institutional study. *Journal of Perinatology, 28,* 665–674.

Patel, R. V., Kandefer, S., Walsh, M. C., Bell, E. F., Carlo, W. A., Laptook, A. R., & Stoll, B. J. (2015). Causes and timing of death in extremely premature infants from 2000 through 2011. *New England Journal of Medicine*, 372(4), 331–340.

Phillips, J. D., Raval, M. V., Redden, C., & Weiner, T. M. (2001). Gastroschisis, atresia, dysmotility: Surgical treatment strategies for a distinct clinical entity. *Journal of Pediatric Surgery, 43*(12), 2208–2212. doi: 10.1016/j.jpedsurg.2008 .08.065

Poenaro, D. (2012). Abdominal wall problems. In C. A. Gleason & S. Devaskar (Eds.), *Averys diseases of the newborn* (9th ed., pp. 1007–1015). Philadelphia, PA: Elsevier Saunders.

Pursley, D., Hansen, A. R., & Puder, M. (2009). Obstruction. In A. R. Hansen & M. Puder (Eds.), *Manual of neonatal surgical intensive care* (2nd ed., pp. 264–286). Shelton, CT: BC Decker.

Raval, M. V., Hall, N. J., Pierro, A., & Moss, R. L. (2013). Evidence-based prevention and surgical treatment of necrotizing enterocolitis: A review of randomized controlled trials. *Seminars in Pediatric Surgery, 22*, 117–121.

Song, C., Upperman, J. A., & Niklas, V. (2012). Structural anomalies of the gastrointestinal tract. In C. A. Gleason & S. Devaskar (Eds.), *Averys diseases of the newborn* (9th ed., pp. 979–993). Philadelphia, PA: Elsevier Saunders.

South, A. P., Marshall, D. D., Bose, C. L., & Laughon, M. M. (2008). Growth and neurodevelopment at 16 to 24 months of age for infants born with gastroschisis. *Journal of Perinatology, 28*, 702–706.

Stollman, T. H., de Blaauw, I., Wijnen, M. H., van der Staak, F. H., Rieu, P. N., Draaisma, J. M., & Wijnen, R. M. (2009). Decreased mortality but increased morbidity in neonates with jejunoileal atresia; a study of 114 cases over a 34-year period. *Journal of Pediatric Surgery, 44*, 217–221.

Torrazza, R. M., Parker, L. A., Li, Y., Talaga, E., Shuster, J., & Neu, J. (2015). The value of routine gastric residuals in very low birth weight infants. *Journal of Perinatology, 35*, 57–60.

Wilson-Castello, D., Kliegman, R. M., & Fanaroff, A. A. (2013). Necrotizing enterocolitis. In A. Fanaroff & J. Fanaroff (Eds.), *Klaus and Fanaroff's care of the high risk neonate* (6th ed., pp. 151–200). Philadelphia, PA: Elsevier Saunders.

SURGICAL DISORDERS OF THE LOWER ABDOMEN AND GENITALS

Stephanie Packard and Tricia Grandinetti

HYDROCELE

DEFINITION

Hydrocele occurs when a collection of fluid moves from the abdomen to the scrotal sac.

PRESENTATION

Surgery is rarely required. A majority of hydroceles will resolve spontaneously as the processus vaginalis closes, generally between 1 and 2 years of age (Clarke, 2010; Parker, 2014).

DIAGNOSIS

Transillumination of the scrotum will reveal a fluid-filled sac when a hydrocele is present.

PREOPERATIVE ASSESSMENT AND NURSING CARE

■ Evaluate hydroceles daily to differentiate between the presence of fluid (hydrocele) or bowel (hernia)

SURGICAL REPAIR

Hydroceles that persist beyond 2 years of age require high ligation of the processus vaginalis. This surgery entails drainage of fluid from the scrotal sac and closure of the processus vaginalis (Greene, Lee, & Puder, 2009).

POSTOPERATIVE ASSESSMENT AND NURSING CARE

■ In the rare event that a hydrocele requires repair in the neonatal period, follow recommendations for postoperative care of the inguinal hernia.

DOCUMENTATION

- Vital signs
- Assessment of surgical incision; include signs of infection and drainage
- Pain scores
- Parental teaching

INGUINAL HERNIA

DEFINITION

Inguinal hernia is the escape of a bowel segment or other abdominal contents through the inguinal canal, which appears as a bulge in the groin.

PRESENTATION

Inguinal hernias occur in both male and female infants. They usually present in the first 6 months of life and are nine times more prevalent in male infants. The incidence of inguinal hernias is greater in preterm infants; the risk of incarceration is 12% for males and 17% for females (Greene, Lee, & Puder, 2009). In female infants, hernias can contain an ovary, with or without portions of the fallopian tube (15%–20% of the time) (Goldstein & Potts, 1958). When the ovary is present within the hernia, the risk of incarceration dramatically increases (Boley, Cahn, Lauer, Weinburg, & Kleinhaus, 1991; Kapur, Caty, & Glick, 1998). Thirty-one percent of incarcerated hernias occur in infants younger than 2 months of age (Cloherty, 2012). Inguinal hernias rarely, if ever, resolve spontaneously.

DIAGNOSIS

- It is important to differentiate between a hydrocele, inguinal hernia, and incarcerated hernia because the first resolves on its own over time, the second requires surgical correction, and the third (respectively) requires emergent surgical intervention.

▨ Diagnostic studies to help differentiate between a hydrocele, inguinal hernia, and incarcerated hernia include x-ray and/or US.

■ The hernia presents as a firm, smooth mass in the scrotum or inguinal canal that may be exacerbated by increased abdominal pressure.

■ An incarcerated hernia cannot be returned to the abdominal cavity.

▨ Symptoms of incarceration include scrotal swelling or firmness, redness, tenderness or pain, emesis, and irritability.

▨ This condition can rapidly evolve into strangulation of the bowel and gangrenous hernia contents if not surgically corrected.

■ Incarceration of the ovary occurs in approximately 43% of cases (Bronsther, Abrams, & Elboim, 1972).

▨ As the ovary swells, it becomes incarcerated and less likely to reduce, unlike a bowel containing hernia.

▨ Any irreducible ovary should always be treated as an emergency, even if it is nontender (Boley et al., 1991).

PREOPERATIVE ASSESSMENT AND NURSING CARE

■ Perform daily reduction and assessment of the hernia by applying gentle pressure to determine if the intestines can be easily passed back through the processus vaginalis.

■ If the hernia is *not* reducible, this may indicate incarceration, which is a surgical emergency.

■ Symptoms of incarcerated hernia include well-defined, tender, nonreducible scrotal mass; pain; emesis; fever; tachycardia; edema; and erythema (Greene, Lee, & Puder, 2009).

■ These symptoms dictate the need for an emergency surgical consult.

■ All inguinal hernias are at risk for becoming incarcerated; therefore, surgical evaluation and correction are recommended as soon as possible, depending on the patient's age, weight, and condition.

■ Provide parental teaching that includes monitoring for signs of intestinal herniation and incarceration.

SURGICAL REPAIR

Surgical correction of the hernia is performed laparoscopically or via an open incision. The hernia is placed back into the abdominal cavity after being separated from the surrounding tissue, and is followed by the closure of the processus vaginalis (Clarke, 2010; Parker, 2014).

POSTOPERATIVE ASSESSMENT AND NURSING CARE

- Place the infant in a supine or side-lying position. Ideally, keep the head turned to the side as this may minimize disruption to the suture line
- Monitor the incision site and/or suture line closely
- Report signs of infection
- Determine the timeline for removal if sutures are present
  - Often, dissolvable sutures are used.
  - Check with the surgeon or the operative note to confirm suture material and plan.
- Assess pain for a minimum of every 4 hours
  - Comfort may be achieved with acetaminophen alone, but consider narcotics on a patient-specific basis.
- Observation in an ICU for 24 hours is recommended for premature infants due to increased risk for apnea secondary to anesthesia exposure

DOCUMENTATION

- Vital signs
- Assessment of surgical incision, including signs of infection and drainage
- Pain scores
- Parental teaching

TESTICULAR TORSION

DEFINITION

Testicular torsion is a twisting of the spermatic cord; this structure is connected to the internal reproductive organs that contain blood vessels, nerves, muscles, and a tube for carrying semen. It is the result of incomplete attachment of the gubernaculum to the testis that allows for torsion and infarction.

PRESENTATION

- Approximately 70% of testicular torsion cases diagnosed in the newborn period occur prenatally (Feins & Papadakis, 2009).
- The findings include an enlarged swollen scrotum with a firm scrotal mass; the infant may experience varying levels of discomfort.
  - Prenatal torsion is marked by minimal to no discomfort; the infant is generally asymptomatic, afebrile, and comfortable.
  - Postnatal torsion presents with considerable tenderness and swelling of a previously normal testicle.
    - Red or blue discoloration may be present.

DIAGNOSIS

A diagnosis of testicular torsion is made by physical examination and can be confirmed by US. If the torsion is acute it will be extremely tender to palpation.

PREOPERATIVE ASSESSMENT AND NURSING CARE

Assess the scrotum daily to determine if the testicles have descended into the scrotal sac

- With torsion, the testicle is firm, nontender to painful, indurated, and swollen with a bluish or dusky cast of the affected side of the scrotum.

- Without prompt identification and surgical treatment, the blood supply to the testicle is compromised and a testicle can die in as little as 4 to 6 hours.

- Testicular torsion is a surgical emergency; thus, if detected on examination, the surgical team must be notified immediately.

SURGICAL REPAIR

- If there is any suspicion of torsion, emergency exploration and detorsion should be performed within 4 to 6 hours of presentation.

- If the testis is viable, it is detorsed and secured or pexed into the scrotum.

- Due to the chance of contralateral torsion, the contralateral testis is prophylactically secured at the time of surgery.

POSTOPERATIVE ASSESSMENT AND NURSING CARE

- Admit premature infants to the ICU for 24 hours of observation with exposure to anesthesia and increased risk for apnea

- Monitor sutures and/or the incision line closely; observe the surgical site for signs of bleeding and infection

- Place the infant in a supine or side-lying position
  - Ideally, keep the head turned to the side as this may minimize the disruption of suture lines.

- Assess pain for a minimum of every 4 hours
  - Comfort may be attainable with acetaminophen alone, but consider narcotics on a patient-specific basis.

- Remove dressings within 48 hours or as directed by the surgeon

DOCUMENTATION

- Vital signs
- Assessment of incision site
- Pain scores

- Dressing drainage amount
- Parental teaching

UNDESCENDED TESTES

DEFINITION

Undescended testicle or cryptorchidism is a testicle that hasn't moved into the scrotal sac before birth.

PRESENTATION

Usually just one testicle is undescended, although 10% of the time both testicles are undescended. An undescended testicle is uncommon in general, but quite common among males born prematurely. In most cases, the undescended testicle moves into its proper position spontaneously; however, in some cases it is necessary to correct surgically before 1 year of age.

DIAGNOSIS

Diagnosis is by physical examination with the absence of testes in the scrotal sac.

PREOPERATIVE ASSESSMENT AND NURSING CARE

- Assess for spontaneous resolution with the appearance of the testicles in the scrotal sac

SURGICAL REPAIR

- Surgical correction of the undescended testicle is called orchiopexy. It is the anchoring of the testes in the scrotum. This procedure is performed by laparoscope or open surgery.

POSTOPERATIVE ASSESSMENT AND NURSING CARE

- Admit premature infants to the ICU for 24 hours of observation due to exposure to anesthesia and increased risk for apnea

- Monitor incision and sutures (if present) closely for signs of bleeding and infection
- Place the infant in a supine or side-lying position
  - Ideally, position the head to the side as this may minimize disruption to the suture line
- Assess pain for a minimum of every 4 hours
- Achieve comfort with acetaminophen alone, but consider narcotics on a patient-specific basis
- Remove dressing(s) within 48 hours or as directed by the provider

DOCUMENTATION

- Vital signs
- Assessment of incision site
- Pain scores
- Dressing drainage amount
- Parental teaching

REFERENCES

Boley, S. J., Cahn, D., Lauer, L., Weinburg, G., & Kleinhaus, S. (1991). The irreducible ovary: A true emergency. *Journal of Pediatric Surgery, 26*(9), 1035–1038.

Bronsther, B., Abrams, M. W., & Elboim, C. (1972). Inguinal hernias in children: A study of 1,000 cases and a review of the literature. *Journal of the American Medical Women's Association, 10,* 522.

Clarke, S. (2010). Pediatric inguinal hernia and hydrocele: An evidence-based review in the era of minimal access surgery. [Review]. *Journal of Laparoendoscopic Advanced Surgical Techniques, 20*(3), 305–309. doi:10.1089/lap.2010.9997

Cloherty, J. P. (2012). *Manual of neonatal care* (7th ed.). Philadelphia, PA: Wolters Kluwer Health/Lippincott Williams & Wilkins.

Feins, N. R., & Papadakis, K. (2009). Testicular torsion. In A. R. Hansen & M. Puder (Eds.), *Manual of neonatal surgical intensive care* (2nd ed., pp. 436–439). Shelton, CT: People's Medical Publishing House.

Goldstein, R., & Potts, W. J. (1958). Inguinal hernias in female infants and children. *Annals of Surgery, 148*(5), 819–822.

Greene, A. K., Lee, S., & Puder, M. (2009). Inguinal hernia. In A. R. Hansen & M. Puder (Eds.), *Manual of neonatal surgical intensive care* (2nd ed., pp. 310–318). Shelton, CT: People's Medical Publishing House.

Hansen, A. R., & Puder, M. (2009). *Manual of neonatal surgical intensive care* (2nd ed.). Shelton, CT: People's Medical Publishing House.

Kapur, P., Caty, M. G., & Glick, P. L. (1998). Pediatric hernias and hydroceles. *Pediatric Clinics of North America*, *45*(4), 773–789.

Parker, L. A. (2014). Genitourinary system. In C. Kenner & J. W. Lott (Eds.), *Comprehensive neonatal nursing care* (5th ed.). New York, NY: Springer Publishing Company.

Skin Care

Carolyn Lund

OVERVIEW

Neonatal skin care is an important clinical concern for neonatal nurses. Goals of skin care for newborn infants include protecting skin integrity, reducing exposure to potential toxicity from topical agents, and promoting healthy skin barrier function. An understanding of the unique anatomic and physiologic differences in premature, full-term newborn, and young infant skin is fundamental to providing effective care to these populations.

PHYSIOLOGIC AND ANATOMIC VARIATIONS IN NEWBORN, YOUNG INFANT, AND PREMATURE INFANT SKIN

Newborn skin undergoes an adaptation process during the transition from the aquatic environment of the uterus to the aerobic environment after birth. The skin assists in thermoregulation, serves as a barrier against toxins and micro-organisms, is a reservoir for fat storage and insulation, and is a primary interface for tactile sensation and communication.

STRATUM CORNEUM AND EPIDERMIS

The stratum corneum, which provides the important barrier function of the skin, contains 10 to 20 layers in the adult and in the full-term newborn. Although full-term newborns reportedly have skin barrier function comparable to that of adult skin, as indicated by a measurement called transepidermal water loss (TEWL), there is now some evidence that the stratum corneum does not function as well as adult skin during the first year of life. Infant skin is 30% thinner than adult skin, the basal layer of the epidermis is 20% thinner than that of the adult, and the keratinocytes in this layer have a higher cell turnover rate, which may account for the faster wound healing that has been observed in neonates.

The premature infant has far fewer cell layers in the stratum corneum, with the specific number determined by gestational age. At less than 30 weeks gestation, there may be as few as two or three layers, and the extremely premature infant of 23 to 24 weeks gestation has almost no stratum corneum and negligible barrier function. The deficient stratum corneum results in excessive fluid and evaporative heat losses during the first weeks of life, leading to increased risk of dehydration and significant alterations in electrolyte levels, such as hypernatremia. Techniques used to reduce these losses include the use of polyethylene coverings immediately after delivery and use of high levels of relative humidity (> 70% RH) in incubators. Maturation of the skin barrier, particularly for infants of 23 to 25 weeks gestation, occurs over time, with evidence of mature barrier function delayed until about 30 to 32 weeks postconceptional age.

DERMIS

The dermis of the full-term newborn is thinner and not as well developed as the adult dermis. The collagen and elastin fibers are shorter and less dense, and the reticular layer of the dermis is absent, which makes the skin feel very soft.

Premature infant skin exhibits decreased cohesion between the epidermis and dermis, which places these babies at risk for skin injury from removal of medical adhesives. When extremely aggressive adhesives are used, the bond between adhesive and epidermis may be stronger than that between epidermis and dermis, resulting in stripping of the epidermal layer and loss of or significantly diminished skin barrier function.

SKIN pH

Skin surface typically has an acidic pH, due to a number of chemical and biologic processes involving the stratum corneum. This "acid mantle" of the skin (pH < 5) contributes to the immune function of the stratum corneum by inhibiting the growth of pathogenic microorganisms and supporting the proliferation of commensal, or "healthy," bacteria on the skin.

Full-term newborns are born with an alkaline skin surface (pH > 6), but within the first 4 days after birth the pH falls to less than 5. Skin surface pH in premature infants of varying gestational ages has been reported to be more than 6 on the first day of life; however, it decreases to 5.5 by the end of the first week and 5.1 by the end of the first month. Bathing and other topical treatments transiently alter skin pH, and diapered skin has a higher pH due to the combined effects of urine contact and occlusion. The higher pH of diapered skin reduces the barrier function of the stratum corneum, rendering it more susceptible to mechanical damage from friction.

RISK OF TOXICITY FROM TOPICAL AGENTS

Toxicity from topically applied substances has been reported in numerous case reports due to the increased permeability of both preterm and full-term newborn skin. This is due to a number of factors including the fact that newborn skin is 20% to 40% thinner than adult skin, and the ratio of body surface to weight is nearly five times greater in newborns than in older children and adults, which places newborns at increased risk for percutaneous absorption and toxicity. Examples of toxicity from percutaneous absorption include encephalopathy and death among premature infants bathed with hexachlorophene, and alterations in iodine levels and thyroid function related to routine use of povidone iodine in neonatal intensive care units (NICUs).

SKIN CARE PRACTICES

Evidence-based skin care practices for neonates are provided in the third edition of the *Neonatal Skin Care: Evidence-Based Clinical Practice Guideline*, published by the Association of Women's Health, Obstetric and Neonatal Nurses (AWHONN, 2013). This guideline includes recommendations for 12 aspects of neonatal skin care, ranging from bathing to the use of disinfectants to diaper dermatitis. A brief summary of selected aspects is included here for neonatal nurses.

BATHING

The newborn's first bath should occur when his or her temperature and vital signs are stable; the World Health Organization (WHO) recommends waiting at least 6 hours. Clear water or water and a mild baby wash product with a neutral or mildly acidic pH (5.5–7) may be used, but soap-based products should be avoided because they can be drying or irritating to the skin. Leaving residual vernix caseosa intact has several benefits, including protecting the infant from infection, moisturization, development of the acid mantle, and temperature regulation; it can be left in place to wear off with normal care and handling. Consider an "immersion" or tub bath even with the umbilical cord still in place, as this has been shown to be more soothing and results in less temperature loss. For routine bathing, it is not necessary to bathe a newborn more than every other day.

UMBILICAL CORD CARE

Cleanse the umbilical cord during bathing with clear water, and dry the infant to remove excess water. Leave the umbilical cord stump clean, dry, and uncovered by keeping the diaper folded underneath the cord. Educate parents to use "natural drying" by keeping the cord area clean and dry, without the use of topical agents. This is also the recommendation of the WHO. In some developing countries, however, a single application of chlorhexidine gluconate has been shown to reduce infection.

DIAPER DERMATITIS

Maintaining a healthy skin environment in the diaper area is the primary goal. In the newborn period, changing the diaper when wet or soiled, as often as every 1 to 3 hours, is beneficial. Avoid rubbing the perineal skin, and use soft cloths, water, or a gentle disposable diaper wipe that has been tested on newborn skin.

If diaper dermatitis occurs, determine the underlying cause. The most common type is irritant contact diaper dermatitis caused by fecal enzymes. This type is seen in the perianal skin, and can range from bright red to excoriated or denuded. Skin affected in this way can benefit from an immersion bath once daily, as well as application of petrolatum-based ointment either as a preventive strategy or to protect reddened skin with each diaper change. For more severe skin excoriation, use a skin barrier product, such as those containing zinc oxide; the barrier should be applied in a very thick coating over the excoriated skin, and reapplied with every diaper change. Consider if there is an underlying cause, such as diarrhea, that is infectious, from opiate withdrawal or from significant malabsorption of nutrients due to a surgical condition; a change in diet or other medical interventions may be indicated.

Another type of diaper dermatitis involves *Candida albicans*; this may also be called a yeast or fungal diaper dermatitis. This type of diaper dermatitis is characterized by "beefy" red skin, with "satellite" lesions scattered at the edges; the skin may or may not be denuded. An antifungal ointment or cream is applied topically three to four times a day; if the rash does not respond in several days, it may be necessary to select another antifungal preparation.

EMOLLIENTS

Emollients are topical substances composed of fat or oil, sometimes combined with water. The routine use of emollients in newborn skin care is not clear, although application of an emollient to skin that is dry or cracked is recommended. Large studies of very premature infants weighing less than 1,000 g reported no differences in mortality when a petrolatum-based ointment was applied twice daily, compared with using this emollient only on an "as needed" basis for dry skin; they also reported an increase in bloodstream infections in the smallest infants weighing less than 750 g with the routine use of this ointment. For this reason, the routine use of emollients in premature infants weighing less than 1,000 g is not recommended.

In some cultures, the routine use of an emollient, usually in the form of oil, is used during infant massage. Although some oils such as sunflower seed oil have been shown to be beneficial, others such as olive oil or grape seed oil may be more irritating according to some laboratory investigations. The role of these oils in the NICU is not well studied, and concerns about using them with infants who have central venous catheters, for example, have been raised.

DISINFECTANTS

Disinfecting skin surfaces prior to invasive procedures such as insertion of central venous catheters, umbilical catheters, intravenous catheters, chest tubes, or venipuncture reduces the risk of infection. Current skin disinfectants used in this manner include 70% isopropyl alcohol, 10% povidone iodine, and chlorhexidine gluconate, with concentrations ranging from 0.5% to 3.15%, some in aqueous solutions and many combined with 70% isopropyl alcohol. When evaluating different products used for skin disinfection, efficacy of skin sterilization, systemic toxicity, and skin irritation or chemical burns should be considered.

Chlorhexidine gluconate-containing solutions have been shown to reduce the risk of bloodstream infection in adults with central venous catheters, but there is no study to date to demonstrate this in the NICU population. Povidone iodine is next in terms of efficacy, with isopropyl alcohol the least effective for skin decontamination.

Systemic toxicity has been reported with povidone iodine use in premature infants, affecting thyroid function transiently; if this solution is used, it should be removed completely using sterile water or saline to reduce skin exposure and absorption. Toxicity to chlorhexidine products has been seen with exposure to the eyes and ear structures. In adults, there have been reports of anaphylactic reactions when using chlorhexidine gluconate impregnated urinary catheters or with large areas of exposure during repeated surgical procedures.

Chemical burns and skin irritation have been reported with alcohol-containing disinfectants. A number of reports involve the peri-umbilical skin that has been disinfected with chlorhexidine gluconate in extremely low-birth-weight premature infants but safety data are lacking. Disinfectants should be used with caution in this population.

MEDICAL ADHESIVES

Medical adhesives such as tape, electrodes, and transparent adhesive dressings are applied and removed many times a day in the typical NICU. These secure critical life support equipment such as endotracheal tubes, intravenous and arterial catheters, and chest tubes, as well as numerous monitoring devices and probes. Skin injury from medical adhesives is a known problem in the NICU population. As mentioned previously, one reason is immature skin with decreased cohesion between the epidermis and dermis layers.

There are a number of different types of adhesive products, including cloth tape, plastic perforated tape, transparent adhesive dressings, hydrocolloid adhesives, hydrogel adhesives, and silicone adhesives. Depending on the critical need to adhere, different adhesives are selected for different indications. For example, hydrogel adhesives may work well for electrocardiogram electrodes, but are not suitable to secure an endotracheal tube. Silicone adhesives work well as a border around dressings, and to secure electroencephalogram electrodes to the scalp and hair, and are very gentle when removed. However, silicone tapes do not adhere well to plastic tubes and cannulas.

Another strategy to reduce skin injury from adhesives is the use of silicone-based skin protectants that do not contain alcohol; these are commonly used on skin surrounding ostomy sites. They have been reported as beneficial in several small studies in premature infants. The use of bonding agents such as tincture of benzoin to increase the stickiness of adhesives is not recommended, because the bond that these agents forms between the adhesive and the epidermis may be stronger than the fragile cohesion between the epidermis and dermis and can result in epidermal stripping when removed.

Silicone-based adhesive removal products are being seen in the literature, and are described as very beneficial for infants with genetic skin disorders such as epidermolysis bullosa. It is possible that these, too, may benefit premature infants but more research in this area is encouraged. Alcohol- or organic-based skin removers contain hydrocarbon derivatives or petroleum distillates that have a potential for systemic toxicity, and should not be used.

CONCLUSION

Newborn skin has unique properties that are important to understand when providing skin care. Both full-term and premature newborns require careful consideration during such daily care practices as bathing, skin disinfection, umbilical cord care, adhesive and emollient use, and management of diaper dermatitis. Optimal approaches for neonatal skin care that are evidence based have been shown to be practical in both the neonatal intensive care unit as well as "well baby" nursery settings, while also improving the overall skin condition for newborns and young infants.

REFERENCE

Association of Women's Health, Obstetric and Neonatal Nurses. (2013). *Neonatal skin care: Evidence-based clinical practice guideline* (3rd ed.). Washington, DC: Author.

ADDITIONAL CHAPTER RESOURCES

Heimall, L. M., Storey, B., Stellar, J. J., & Davis, K. F. (2012). Beginning at the bottom: Evidence-based care of diaper dermatitis. *MCN. American Journal of Maternal Child Nursing, 37*(1), 10–16.

Lund, C. (2014). Medical adhesives in the NICU. *Newborn & Infant Nursing Reviews, 14*(4), 160–165.

World Health Organization. (2006). *Pregnancy, childbirth, postpartum and newborn care: A guide for essential practice.* Geneva, Switzerland: Author.

Developmental Care

Xiaomei Cong

OVERVIEW

Neonatal developmental care aims to support the infant's physiologic stabilization, behavioral functioning, and emotional and social well-being, and to facilitate the infant's growth and development in the long term. Based on each infant's maturity, abilities, sensitivities, and status of subsystem functioning, developmental care integrates a supportive environment, individualized assessment and intervention, family- and infant-centered care, and a collaborative clinical practice model to provide personalized and consistent caregiving. Interventions include monitoring light and sound in the nursery, providing supportive handling and positioning, enhancing cue-based care, reducing the infant's pain and stress, protecting sleep rhythms, and promoting the involvement of parents.

KANGAROO MOTHER CARE

Kangaroo mother care (KMC), also called skin-to-skin contact between the mother and infant, is the upright prone positioning of the diaper-clad infant, skin-to-skin, chest-to-chest between maternal breasts. KMC was developed and initiated in Bogota, Colombia, in the late 1970s and was first reported in 1983 by two pediatricians, Rey and Martinez (Ludington, Anderson, Swinth, Thompson, & Hadeed, 1994). Mothers' bodies can be used to resemble marsupial caregiving because infants are placed between breasts in the pouch-like valley between the mammary mounds. KMC is a vital component of developmental care, especially for preterm infants hospitalized in the neonatal intensive care unit (NICU), which provides multisensory stimulation to the infant—including emotional, tactile, proprioceptive, vestibular, olfactory, auditory, visual, and thermal stimulation—in a unique interactive style. Benefits of KMC for infants include promoting physiologic stability, attachment, breastfeeding, sleep, and neurobehavioral maturation, as well as reducing pain and stress (Cong et al., 2012). Benefits for parents include promoting parent–infant interaction and bonding; optimizing physical and psychological well-being; and reducing parental stress, anxiety, and postpartum depression (Cong et al., 2015).

Continuous KMC (24 hours per day) has been implemented as an ideally alternative measure for preterm infants in low-income settings and also in some high-income countries. Intermittent KMC (at least 1 hour per session) has been recommended for NICU infants to take into account the infant's adaptation and promote sleep (Davanzo et al., 2013). KMC can be practiced by both mothers and fathers with their newborns immediately after birth, and regularly and safely with stable preterm infants. It can also be used in parents who have difficulties with parent–infant bonding, breastfeeding, or terminal care situations.

STEP-BY-STEP KMC PROCEDURE

READINESS OF INFANT

1. Readiness of infant for KMC does not depend on gestational age, postnatal age, or neurodevelopmental maturation levels, but is based on infant stability.

2. Stable neonates including preterm and/or low-birth-weight infants are eligible for KMC. Stability is assessed based on vital signs.

3. Very sick infants may not be eligible for KMC, including infants who are receiving mechanical ventilations and/or treatment with vasopressor medications, having umbilical artery catheter and venous catheter or chest tube, and having major surgery within

24 hours. Other respiratory support, such as oxygen supplementation or nasal continuous positive airway pressure (CPAP), may not be a contraindication for KMC.

READINESS OF PARENTS

1. Parents need to be given adequate information about KMC and show their willingness to hold their infant skin to skin.
2. Parental emotional readiness needs to be assessed. KMC is still recommended to practice, even if the mother expresses inappropriate emotions, such as depression, anxiety, withdrawal, hopelessness, guilt, or uninvolvement, because KMC has many emotional benefits to mothers.

PREPARATION OF KMC

1. Prepare and set up equipment: extra blankets for mother and infant; recliner or chair/rocker with footstool; and privacy screen when needed.
2. Encourage the parent to wear a shirt/blouse that opens in front or put on a hospital gown when needed. Ordinary daily hygiene is satisfactory for parents providing KMC.
3. Before KMC begins, if possible, perform any needed procedures that may interrupt KMC.
4. Secure all infant catheter lines and tubes.
5. Dress the infant in a diaper. Hat and booties are optional depending on the infant's body weight and postnatal age.

TRANSFER TO KMC POSITION

1. Use either the standing transfer technique (mother receives her infant while standing beside the incubator/crib) or the sitting transfer technique (mother receives infant while sitting in the recliner), depending on the parent's comfort and condition.

2. Place the infant upright on the parent's chest between the breasts or on either breast, and keep the infant with arms and legs contained in the midline.

3. Place a blanket over the infant's back.

4. Close the parent's cover gown over the infant to protect from side drafts and slipping.

5. Maintain infant stability during transfer, including oxygenation, heart rate, and thermoregulation; secure ventilator tubing; and prevent extubation.

DURING KMC

1. Mother or father sits in a recliner with footrest/stool support. Place the diaper-clad infant on the parent's chest, skin to skin, in a prone and an upright position at an incline of 30° to 40°. Maintain the infant's legs and arms in a flexed and midline position and the head and neck in a slight sniffing position to prevent airway obstruction. Cover the infant and avoid fixation of the head.

2. Encourage the parent to give KMC for at least 1 hour to allow the infant to complete a sleep cycle and allow the infant to continue to sleep as long as possible.

3. Encourage the parent to keep his or her hands clasped behind the infant's back and allow the infant to sleep. If possible, give a hand mirror to the parent so the mother or father can look at the infant's face and see his or her facial expression. The parent can softly talk, read, or sing to her or his infant during KMC.

4. Maintain all routine monitoring including cardiorespiratory, pulse oximetry, and temperature during KMC per nursery protocol. Monitor and document any sign of distress. The infant can be fed during KMC either by mouth or by gavage.

5. Keep a quiet, calm, and low-light environment for KMC.

6. Assess the parent's comfort level and needs during KMC.

POST-KMC

1. A lactating mother may pump her breasts immediately after KMC because KMC significantly increases mother's milk production.

2. Document the infant's physiologic and behavioral responses, including vital signs, oxygen saturation, temperature, sleep states, and crying, and how the infant tolerates KMC.

3. Document the parent's responses and comments regarding KMC.

4. Discuss with parents and provide additional education about KMC.

REFERENCES

Cong, X., Cusson, R. M., Walsh, S., Hussain, N., Ludington-Hoe, S. M., & Zhang, D. (2012). Effects of skin-to-skin contact on autonomic pain responses in preterm infants. *Journal of Pain*, 13(7), 636–645.

Cong, X., Ludington-Hoe, S. M., Hussain, N., Cusson, R. M., Walsh, S., Vazquez, B., ... Vittner, D. (2015). Parental oxytocin responses during skin-to-skin contact in pre-term infants. *Early Human Development*, 91(7), 1–406.

Davanzo, R., Brovedani, P., Travan, L., Kennedy, J., Crocetta, A., Sanesi, C., ... De Cunto, A. (2013). Intermittent kangaroo mother care: A NICU protocol. *Journal of Human Lactation*, 29(3), 333–338.

Ludington, S., Anderson, G. C., Swinth, J., Thompson, C., & Hadeed, A. J. (1994). Kangaroo care. *Neonatal Network*, 13(4), 61–62.

POSITIONING

Supportive positioning is one of the developmental care strategies used to optimize infant musculoskeletal development and neurobehavioral-emotional functioning. Without normal newborn flexion and protection from the mother's womb, premature infants need supports in adaptation to an inappropriate environment challenged by gravity, ventilators, and other equipment. The aims of positioning are to improve infant neurophysiologic status, promote flexed postures to support conservation of infant body heat and energy, facilitate motor skills such as hand to face/mouth movements and mobility, support self-regulatory behaviors, and prevent head deformities, external rotation of hips and growth, and developmental delays (Aucott, Donohue, Atkins, & Allen, 2002).

Many positioning techniques have been practiced in nurseries, such as swaddling, containing, nesting, and using positioning aids. These techniques can also be used to relieve infant stress during painful procedures by delineating the infant's boundaries, maintaining flexed positions, and providing constant stimulation to the proprioceptive, thermal, and tactile sensory systems.

Importantly, as infants approach term and discharge to home, the sudden infant death syndrome (SIDS) safe sleeping guidelines by the American Academy of Pediatrics (AAP) need to be implemented unless contradicted (Task Force on Sudden Infant Death Syndrome, American Academy of Pediatrics, & Moon, 2011). Parents need to be educated regarding SIDS prevention and learn positioning techniques when preparing for discharge home.

GENERAL PRINCIPLES OF NEONATAL POSITIONING PRACTICE

1. Safety is the key for positioning practice. Avoid any positioning aids to occlude and distort the infant's nares and mouth. These aids should be easily removed in emergency situations.

2. Promote flexed and symmetric postures appropriate for gestational maturation: flexion of the limbs and trunk, as well as flexion and adduction of the shoulder and hip.

3. Facilitate midline orientation and neutral alignment of the head, neck, and trunk, and neutral alignment of ankles with dorsiflexion. Prevent postural deformity.

4. Prevent head deformities and torticollis.

5. Support posture and movement during any procedures and activities. Promote a calm state whenever possible.

6. Positioning practice (i.e., how much, how long) is based on the infant's cues and needs.

7. Avoid boundaries being too tight as it may restrict the infant's spontaneous movements.

8. Promote family involvement. Educate parents on the use of positioning techniques and safety knowledge including SIDS prevention.

PRONE POSITIONING

Prone positioning has been used to improve gas exchange in infants with acute respiratory disease; it is also preferred for preterm infants with low muscle tone and for infants with feed intolerance. It is important to provide boundaries in prone positioning because sick or very preterm infants do not have the muscle strength to maintain a comfortable flexed position.

While in the prone position:

1. Place the infant's arms and legs flexed with the hands close to the shoulders or face for self-comforting.

2. Position the head to one side with the chin slightly tucked, but regularly alternate to the other side to prevent head/neck deformity.

3. Prevent excessive hip abduction with positioning aids and maintain the position by using a nest or swaddling.

4. For ventilated or CPAP infants, an alternate, one quarter turn prone position can be used when the infant is stable: The uppermost arm and leg are flexed using a roll for support, the other arm and leg are positioned in a recovery position, and both knees and feet are placed in a neutral position with appropriate positioning aids.

SIDE-LYING POSITIONING

Side-lying positioning has effects on minimizing hip and shoulder abduction and rotation, as well as promoting midline behaviors. It can be used for stable infants who do not have to be in a prone position and tolerate milk feeding.

While in a side-lying position:

1. Keep the head in midline with the shoulder neutral and align with the trunk.

2. Support the back so it is slightly curved/rounded. Maintain the hip and legs, and keep the knees tucked and flexed.

3. Place the lower arm and shoulder forward to prevent the infant from turning to the prone position.

4. Leave the infant's hands free and allow the hands/fingers to touch the face and mouth for self-comforting.

5. Use positioning aids to maintain the appropriate position such as using a sling, roll, or swaddling, but avoid overprotection.

6. Apply to treat unilateral lung disease by positioning the "good" lung uppermost.

SUPINE POSITIONING

Supine positioning is a safe sleep measure for all stable healthy infants based on the AAP recommendations. It is also recommended for infants with relaxed muscles, with unilateral and bilateral intercostal catheters, as surgically required, or when ready for discharge. According to AAP, the supine position is safe for infants with reflux or gastroesophageal reflux disease (GERD) for every sleep period if the infant has no large vomiting spells during the previous 48 hours.

While in the supine position:

1. Support the head in midline with soft neck flexion and maintain the midline position for the whole body for preterm infants.

2. Support the shoulders so they are slightly forward; flex the arms, hips, legs, and knee; and support the infant for foot bracing.

3. Use positioning aids, such as rolls and a nest, to maintain the appropriate position for preterm infants.

4. Regularly check pressure areas (every 3–4 hours).

5. Be aware of and prevent head flattening on one side (plagiocephaly) and/or twisted neck (torticollis). Support and encourage the

infant's head rotation to both the right and left sides. Talk to the infant from both sides. Place pictures or toys at both sides.

6. Educate parents and encourage earlier transition to supine sleep to prepare for home discharge.

CONTAINMENT POSITIONING STRATEGIES FOR PRETERM INFANTS IN THE NICU

Containment is commonly used to support preterm infants in a flexed and midline position to minimize the sequelae of prematurity. NICU caregivers often provide swaddling, nesting, hand containment, and facilitated tucking to help infants achieve optimal positioning, decrease stress/pain and physical unrest, improve sleep and self-regulation, and promote neuromuscular development (Peyrovi, Alinejad-Naeini, Mohagheghi, & Mehran, 2014). Family members should be educated and encouraged to do all types of containment that will improve parental involvement, interaction, and bonding with their infants.

1. **Swaddling:** Swaddling is a traditional baby wrapping custom by which infants are wrapped tightly but comfortably in sheets, blankets, or other aids to maintain the upper and lower limbs in flexion, with hands positioned near the mouth. Blankets or other wrapping material used for swaddling should come no higher than the infant's shoulders and allow the infant's head position from side to side. Based on the AAP SIDS Guidelines (2011), no bumpers or toys should be in the sleeping area, such as a bed or cot. Swaddling can be used to reduce stress/pain during procedures and also can assist newborns with cerebral defects and withdrawal symptoms.

2. **Nesting:** Nesting is commonly implemented in the NICU so that boundaries are placed around the infant's body. Caregivers can use blankets and/or cloth rolls to create boundaries all the way around the infant so the preterm infant is "nested" in. The "nest" provides a comfortable and secure environment for the infant and supports the flexed position to optimize neuromuscular development.

3. **Facilitated tucking:** Facilitated tucking is effective in promoting physiologic and behavioral stability and has been used for soothing preterm infants during suctioning, nasogastric/oral gastric (NG/OG) placement, and other stressful/painful procedures. The infant is placed in a side-lying position with the shoulders, arms, and legs in flexed positions near the midline of the body. Hands are placed near the infant's mouth. Facilitated tucking can also be used with nesting and containment.

REFERENCES

Aucott, S., Donohue, P. K., Atkins, E., & Allen, M. C. (2002). Neurodevelopmental care in the NICU. *Mental Retardation Developmental Disabilities Research Reviews*, 8(4), 298–308.

Peyrovi, H., Alinejad-Naeini, M., Mohagheghi, P., & Mehran, A. (2014). The effect of facilitated tucking position during endotracheal suctioning on physiological responses and coping with stress in premature infants: A randomized controlled crossover study. *Journal of Maternal Fetal Neonatal Medicine*, 27(15), 1555–1559.

Task Force on Sudden Infant Death Syndrome, American Academy of Pediatrics, & Moon, R. Y. (2011). SIDS and other sleep-related infant deaths: Expansion of recommendations for a safe infant sleeping environment. *Pediatrics*, 128(5), 1030–1039.

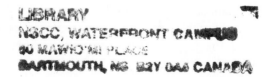

The Neonatal Intensive Care Unit Environment

Leslie B. Altimier

OVERVIEW

Infants born as early as 22 weeks gestation now have a chance of survival in part due to technologic advances. This progress comes with great costs as premature infants are in the neonatal intensive care unit (NICU) for many weeks or months, and many have impaired short- and long-term outcomes. These tiny patients are at a high risk for a variety of developmental problems including cognitive deficits, poor academic achievement, and behavior disorders (Taylor, 2010). More focus is now directed to preterm and low-birth-weight infants who have mental health issues such as attention deficit and attention deficit hyperactive disorders, anxiety disorders, and emotional disorders (Hack et al., 2009; Heinonen, Raikkonen, & Pesonen, 2010; Johnson, Hollis, & Kochlar, 2010; Vanderbilt & Gleason, 2010). A significant proportion of prematurely born children are now showing behaviors consistent with autism (Limperopoulos, 2008, 2009, 2010). Although the cause of these findings remains unclear, it is thought that early environmental influences on the brain during critically sensitive developmental periods account for these adverse outcomes (Browne, 2011).

Neuroprotection has been defined as strategies capable of preventing cell death. Neuroplasticity refers to the ability of the brain to make short-term or long-term modifications to the strength and number of its synaptic neuronal connections in response to incoming stimuli associated with activity and experience. Neuroplasticity is a lifelong property of the human brain, although it is most prominent from birth until late childhood. It is thought that neuroplasticity peaks during early life because it is a period of rapid brain growth with the generation of excessive new synapses (synaptogenesis) and the activity-dependent and experience-dependent pruning of synapses. Neuroprotective strategies are interventions used to support the developing brain or to facilitate the brain after a neuron injury in a way that allows it to heal through developing new connections and pathways for functionality and by decreasing neuronal death.

NEUROPROTECTIVE CARE

Neurosupportive care is not about protection from or prevention of harm, but is a proactive and purposeful continuation of the normal neurodevelopmental trajectory based on ecologically salient/ expected sensory inputs that lead to physiological regulation and a secure attachment, parallel processes that are based on the same limbic circuitry. As we strive to continue to improve our morbidity and mortality rates, we are challenged to enhance neuroprotective strategies for prematurely born infants that focus on the interpersonal experiences of the preterm infant and his or her family in the NICU (Bergman, 2015). Infants have demonstrated markedly improved outcomes when the stress of environmental overstimulation is reduced. This can be accomplished by incorporating neuroprotective strategies into the care of neonates as well as the design of an NICU (Altimier, 2015b).

Neuroprotective developmentally supportive care includes creating a healing environment that manages stress and pain while offering a calming and soothing approach to help keep the whole family involved in the infant's care and development (Altimier, 2011, 2015b; Altimier & Phillips, 2013; Altimier & White, 2014). Neuroprotective developmental care is grounded in support by research from a number of disciplines including nursing, medicine, neuroscience, and psychology (Altimier & Phillips, 2013; Liaw, Yang, Chang, Chou, & Chao, 2009). Improvements in health outcomes and lengths of stays, as well as hospital costs, have been documented when neuroprotective education and subsequent change of care practices were implemented (Altimier, Eichel, Warner, Tedeschi, & Brown, 2005; Hendricks-Munoz,

Prendergast, Caprio, & Wasserman, 2002; Ludwig, Steichen, Khoury, & Krieg, 2008).

Skin-to-skin contact (SSC) is called out separately to emphasize its overlap and critical importance in relationship to each and every core measure. SSC is a fundamental component of neuroprotective and patient–family-oriented care for hospitalized preterm infants. SSC became codified through the World Health Organization (WHO) into what is frequently called kangaroo mother care (KMC), a full-care strategy (Bergman, 2015).

NEONATAL INTEGRATIVE DEVELOPMENTAL CARE MODEL

The Neonatal Integrative Developmental Care (IDC) Model (Philips Healthcare) identifies seven distinct developmental core measures (Neuroprotective Practices) of neonatal care: healing environment, partnering with families, positioning and handling, safeguarding sleep, minimizing stress and pain, protecting skin, and optimizing nutrition (Altimier & Phillips, 2013) (see Figure 11.1).

Each neuroprotective core measure will be reviewed along with a thorough definition, standard/guideline/policy/procedure, idealized infant characteristics, identified goals for each infant to achieve, and evidence-based neuroprotective interventions to incorporate into practice.

CORE MEASURE # 1: HEALING ENVIRONMENT

The NICU is where an extraordinary period of growth and development will take place for premature infants. Because the infant is no longer protected in the uterus, his or her physiologic and neuroprotective needs have dramatically changed. The healing environment encompasses the physical environment (space, privacy, and safety) as well as the sensory environment (touch and temperature; positioning and handling; smell, taste, sound, and light) (Altimier, 2015b) (Figure 11.2).

The optimal environment for any newborn, but particularly for the premature infant, is SSC with the mother (or father). The defining feature is direct contact between maternal skin and infant skin. Essentially, this is a *place* of care, the "normal environment."

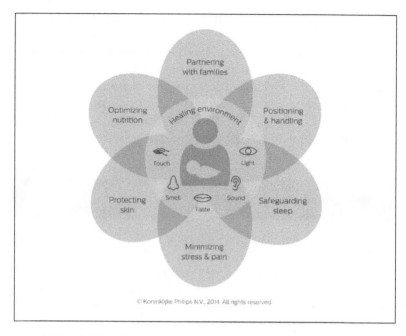

FIGURE 11.1. The Neonatal Integrative Developmental Care Model.

The key feature of SSC is direct contact between maternal skin and infant skin. Incubator care is highly "abnormal" to the epigenes, DNA, and the developing brain of an infant (Bergman, 2015). SSC provides the right environment (place) for the epigenes, DNA, neural circuits, and physiologic regulation to do their normal and healthy things, making this the "optimal environment" for any newborn, especially premature infants.

DEFINITION

The healing environment encompasses the physical environment of space, privacy, and safety, as well as the sensory environment. The physical environment involves not only space, but also characteristics of space, which affect position, movement, and motor development. The sensory system includes the tactile (touch), vestibular (movement, proprioception, and balance), gustatory (taste), olfactory (smell), auditory (noise), and visual (light) systems. All sensory stimuli carry social and emotional connections and characteristics. Adverse environmental

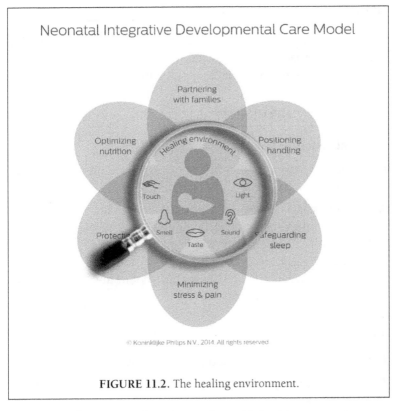

FIGURE 11.2. The healing environment.

sensory insults can significantly interfere with health, appropriate neurodevelopment, and neuroprocessing, resulting in lifelong alterations in brain development and function (Graven & Browne, 2008).

STANDARD

A policy/procedure/guideline on the healing environment, including physical space, privacy, and safety, as well as the protection of the infant's sensory system, exists and is followed throughout the infant's stay.

INFANT CHARACTERISTICS

Characteristics include stability of the infant's autonomic, sensory, motor, and state regulation systems.

GOALS

An environment will be maintained that promotes healing by minimizing the impact of the artificial, oftentimes harsh, extrauterine NICU environment on the developing infant's brain.

NEUROPROTECTIVE INTERVENTIONS

Physical space

■ Provide appropriate environmental modifications or construction/renovation of new NICU facilities.

■ The physical design should meet the neurodevelopmental needs of the infant and provide adequate private space and facilities that support family-centered care (FCC), while at the same time meet the needs of the NICU staff. The latest recommended standards for NICU design should always be utilized (White, Smith, & Shepley, 2013).

Tactile

■ Facilitate early, frequent, and prolonged SSC

■ Provide gentle, yet firm, touch in all handling and caregiving interactions

■ Provide a neutral thermal environment (NTE) for the infant utilizing SSC or incubator humidity during the first 2 weeks after birth

■ Provide midline, flexion, containment, and comfort when positioning the infant

■ Incorporate noninvasive monitoring and testing whenever possible

■ Minimize routine labs and procedures

Vestibular

■ Facilitate early, frequent, and prolonged SSC

■ Change the infant's position slowly and gradually with no sudden movements

- Provide supportive and circumferential boundaries when positioning
- Utilize facilitative tucking and containment principles during care
- Provide balanced clustering of care
- Coordinate exams and care between multiple health care staff

Gustatory

- Facilitate early, frequent, and prolonged SSC
- Position the infant with hands near the face/mouth
- Provide colostrum or expressed breast milk (EBM) oral care per protocol
- Provide nonnutritive sucking (NNS) opportunities (especially during tube feedings)
- Provide positive oral feeding experiences—promote breastfeeding and nuzzling
- Minimize adhesives around the mouth and nose

Olfactory

- Facilitate early, frequent, and prolonged SSC
- Maintain a scent-free and fragrance-free unit (evaluate cleaners in unit)
- Provide the mother's scent when possible via breast pad or soft cloth
- Open alcohol/chloraprep/mastisol pads away from the infant (outside incubator/away from infant and mother)
- Provide NNS with the mother's milk (when possible) during tube feedings

Auditory

- Facilitate early, frequent, and prolonged SSC (promoting the mother's and father's voices along with appropriate vestibular support)
- Monitor sounds to maintain a noise level of less than 50 decibels (dB) (less than 45 dB in a single-family room)

■ Silence alarms as quickly as possible

■ Facilitate "approach behavior" through calm, quiet voice prior to interactions

■ Cover and protect the incubator/bed

■ Eliminate extraneous sounds

■ Consider ceiling tiles with high noise reduction coefficients (NRC)

■ Evaluate noisy equipment in the unit and fix or eliminate when possible

Visual

■ Facilitate early, frequent, and prolonged SSC (promoting the mother's and father's voices along with appropriate vestibular support)

■ Provide adjustable light levels up to a maximum of 60 foot candles (ftc)

■ Avoid purposeful visual stimulation prior to 38 weeks gestational age (GA)

■ Promote enface visual opportunities with parents

■ Cover the infant's eyes during exams and procedures

■ Cover and protect the incubator/bed

■ Utilize eye-patches when exposed to phototherapy lights or direct lighting

■ Cycle lighting per unit protocol at greater than 31 weeks

CORE MEASURE # 2: PARTNERING WITH FAMILIES

Because of the high rates of developmental consequences among prematurely born children, attention is shifting to modifiable aspects of the NICU environment, including parental partnerships, which can optimize developmental outcomes. In NICUs across the nation, true collaboration and shared decision making with families in the care of their baby has not yet become the standard of care. The overwhelming and often traumatic experience of being the parent of a critically ill infant can preclude such collaboration. Family presence and participation in bedside rounds has been lauded as a key component of the partnership and knowledge exchange between health care providers and families, which is at the core of FCC (American Academy of Pediatrics, 2003). For most parents, the experience of participation on medical rounds helps them be less worried and anxious about their child. Nurses frequently comment that parents appear less anxious after rounds (Grzyb, Coo, & Dow, 2014). The medical fragility and prolonged hospitalization of survivors can also negatively impact the parent–infant bond (Harris, 2014) (Figure 11.3).

Neuroprotective care with zero separation from parents will ensure neurodevelopment is supported to normal standards (as in optimal development assumed for term infants), not merely

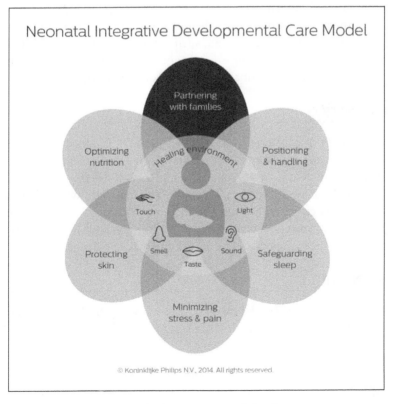

FIGURE 11.3. Partnering with families.

protected from the effects of toxic stress (Bergman, 2014). Early bonding with both physical and psychological components leads to secure attachment, which includes parental relationships and parenting behaviors as well as the unfolding ability of the infant, child, and adult to form and maintain meaningful and enduring relationships (Busse, Stromgren, Thorngate, & Thomas, 2013). A baby's interaction with his or her mother makes a huge difference in the infant's brain development.

The social and practical constructs that will enable parents to practice zero separation are a nonnegotiable condition for neurosupportive care. Reciprocal tactile stimulation between mother and infant may contribute to increased maternal responsiveness and infant attachment (Bystrova, Ivanova, & Edhborg, 2009). SSC helps fathers in their attachment, confidence, caregiving, and interactions with premature infants. When the quality and/or quantity of parental care toward infants is limited, such as with preterm infants in the NICU setting, these adverse experiences can lead to changes in brain architecture and function (Gudsnuk & Champagne, 2011).

DEFINITION

The concept of partnering with families in the NICU includes a philosophy of care, which acknowledges that over time the family has the greatest influence over an infant's health and well-being. Compassionately delivered FCC, with zero separation, where SSC is the norm is currently seen as the ideal model of care to encourage parental involvement, attachment, and bonding, as well as create partnerships with the health care team (Altimier, 2015a; Bergman, 2015).

STANDARD 1

A policy/procedure/guideline on partnering with families exists and is followed throughout the infant's stay.

STANDARD 2

There is a specific mission statement addressing partnering with families.

INFANT CHARACTERISTICS

Characteristics include the infant's response to parental relationships and interactions.

GOALS

■ Parents will be viewed not as "visitors" but as vital members of the caregiving team with zero separation encouraged (24-hour/day access).

■ Parents will be supported as the primary and most important caregivers for their infant.

■ Infants will develop secure attachment with parents.

NEUROPROTECTIVE INTERVENTIONS

■ Facilitate early, frequent, and prolonged SSC

■ Encourage zero separation

■ Promote active participation via medical rounds and shift-to-shift report

■ Acknowledge where the family is in regards to stages of grief and loss and provide individualized and appropriate resources as needed

■ Actively observe and listen to families' feelings and concerns (both verbal and nonverbal)

■ Communicate the infant's medical and developmental needs in a culturally appropriate and understandable way

■ Encourage and support breastfeeding and breast milk expression

■ Assist parents in becoming competent in caring for their baby

■ Encourage parents as they develop confidence in their own abilities to continue providing SSC for their baby after going home

■ Educate parents on infant attachment, developmental, and safety issues

■ Provide social networking opportunities for parents of premature infants in the NICU (Altimier & Phillips, 2013)

CORE MEASURE # 3: POSITIONING AND HANDLING

Developmentally appropriate or neuroprotective care includes both positioning and handling activities. In utero, the infant is contained in a circumferential enclosed space with 360° of well-defined boundaries. Conversely, the spontaneous resting posture of a third-trimester NICU infant often is flat, extended, asymmetrical with the head to one side (usually the right), and with the extremities abducted and externally rotated (Hunter, 2010). Over time, neuronal connections can be reinforced that favor this flattened, externally rotated, and asymmetrical resting posture as baseline for these infants (Figure 11.4).

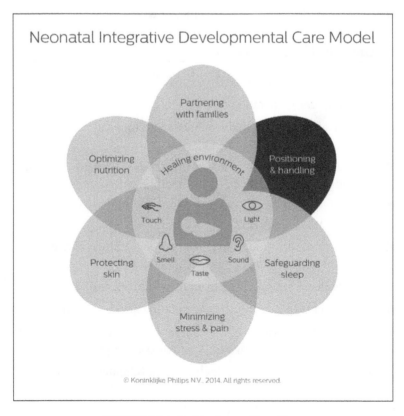

FIGURE 11.4. Positioning and handling.

Common musculoskeletal consequences of NICU positioning include abnormal spinal curvatures; excessive abduction and external rotation in the hips (called a "frog leg" posture); "W" arm positioning in which the shoulders are elevated, abducted, and externally rotated; and skull deformities (Hunter, Lee, & Altimier, 2015). These body misalignments can lead to motor delays and functional limitations that may follow an infant from the NICU into childhood and subsequently extend across the life span (Sweeney & Gutierrez, 2002).

Prolonged medical positioning and necessary intervention can lead to deformational infant head shapes and tightness of neck musculature. Inadequate positioning in the NICU setting can affect the infant's early muscle and bone formation (Danner-Bowman & Cardin, 2015). The pliability of a newborn's head is the antecedent of changes in head shape, particularly in premature infants whose cranial bones are even softer and thinner than those of term infants (Hunter, Lee, & Altimier, 2015). In premature infants, the head is the body part that takes the greatest amount of pressure whether in supine, prone, or side-lying positions (Marcellus, 2004). In addition to tremendous pressure, skull softness, and rapid growth of the brain within, lying in certain positions for extended periods of time increases the risk of deformational head shaping (Danner-Bowman & Cardin, 2015).

Careful, thoughtful positioning has been shown to preserve musculoskeletal integrity and facilitate developmental progression (Altimier & Phillips, 2013; Byrne & Gargber, 2013). Secure therapeutic positioning promotes improved rest, supports optimal growth, and helps to normalize neurobehavioral organization. Containment increases the infant's feelings of security and self-control and decreases stress (Colson, Meek, & Hawdon, 2008).

Positioning and handling can be extended to include SSC. The overriding factor related to positioning and handling includes the safe technique for SSC, which is the protection of the airway, with secure containment that will allow parents to sleep while doing SSC. Additionally, when an infant is more upright, the contents of the abdominal cavity can shift away from the upper abdomen, creating an increase in negative subdiaphragmatic pressure, favoring the outward recoil of the chest (Ammari et al., 2009).

DEFINITION

NICU positioning has traditionally been a neuromotor developmental intervention to minimize positional deformities and improve muscle tone, postural alignment, movement patterns, and ultimately developmental milestones. Each body position that an infant experiences while in the NICU affects alignment and shaping of the musculoskeletal system. Therapeutic positioning in the NICU is a fundamental mainstay and can influence not only neuromotor and musculoskeletal development, but also physiologic function and stability, skin integrity, thermal regulation, bone density, head shaping, sleep facilitation, and brain development.

STANDARD

A policy/procedure/guideline on positioning and handling exists and is followed throughout the infant's stay.

INFANT CHARACTERISTICS

■ Autonomic stability during handling
■ Ability to maintain tone and flexed postures with and without supports

GOALS

■ Autonomic stability will be maintained throughout positioning changes and handling activities as well as during periods of rest and sleep.
■ Preventable positional deformities will be eliminated or minimized by maintaining infants in a midline, flexed, contained, and comfortable position throughout their NICU stay.
■ The caregiver sees herself or himself in partnership with the baby so that caregiving procedures are performed "with" the infant rather than "to" the infant.
■ Infants will be provided with developmentally appropriate stimulation/play, only as they mature (i.e., mobiles, swings).

NEUROPROTECTIVE INTERVENTIONS

■ Facilitate early, frequent, and prolonged SSC

■ Utilize a validated and reliable positioning assessment tool (i.e., Infant Positioning Assessment Tool (IPAT)] routinely to ensure appropriate positioning and encourage accountability

■ Anticipate, prioritize, and support the infant's individualized needs during each caregiving interaction to minimize stressors known to interfere with normal development

■ Maintain a midline, flexed, contained, and comfortable position at all times utilizing appropriate positioning aids and boundaries

■ Provide appropriate ventral support when positioned prone to ensure flexed shoulders/hips

■ Provide appropriate gel-filled positioning supports to protect fragile skin and support musculoskeletal development

■ Assess the infant sleep–wake cycle to evaluate appropriate timing of positioning and handling

■ Reposition the infant with care and minimally every 4 hours

■ Implement minimal handling protocols when warranted

■ Provide four-handed support during positioning and caring activities

■ Provide swaddling when bathing and weighing

■ Promote hand to mouth/face contact

■ Educate parents about the principles of positioning, containment, and handling, as well as the necessities of minimizing unnecessary inappropriate touch and handling

CORE MEASURE # 4: SAFEGUARDING SLEEP

Sleep is an extremely important issue for the infant in the NICU and is critical to brain health (Hobson, 1995). At approximately 28 weeks gestation, individual sleep patterns begin to emerge, characterized by rapid eye movement (REM) and nonrapid eye movement (NREM) sleep periods. These periods become more consistent by 36 to 38 weeks GA. REM sleep dominates in the initial sleep cycles; REM and NREM are nearly equal as the infant approaches term, and by 8 months of age NREM sleep occupies nearly 80% of sleep time. A complete rest–activity cycle is 60 to 90 minutes long. During SSC, preterm infants using frontal electroencephalograms (EEGs) demonstrate regular patterns of sleep and normal cycling, compared to infants separated from their parents (Figure 11.5).

In SSC, there are clear sleep cycles, with a rapid onset of quiet sleep, followed by active sleep. Autonomic indices demonstrate the

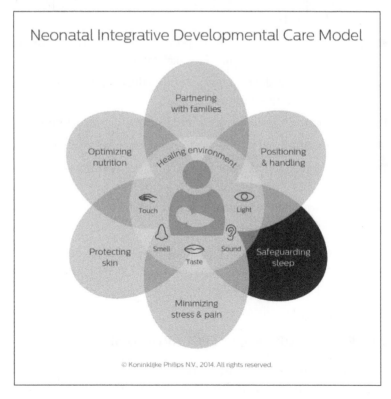

FIGURE 11.5. Safeguarding sleep.

presence of anxious arousal while infants are in a crib, with greatly prolonged time to sleep onset. In cribs, quiet sleep is greatly reduced by more than 85% and sleep cycles are eliminated. SSC releases oxytocin and the peptide cholecystokinin (CCK) in both the mother and the infant, making both relax, fall asleep, and feel safe, all of which are necessary for quality sleep (Bergman, 2015; Karner & Cortese, 2009; Klaus & Klaus, 2010). SSC even for 1 hour shortly after birth impacts state organization and the time spent sleeping (Ferber & Makhoul, 2004; Ludington-Hoe et al., 2006). Additionally, maternal scent stimulates the infant's olfactory system, promoting sleep cycling, which further emphasizes the necessity of SSC.

The premature infant has challenges in safeguarding sleep, because of the care procedures and interventions required to support life. Continuous bright lights in the NICU can disrupt sleep–wake states. Any event, process, or drug that disrupts REM sleep will disrupt the organization of the eye cells, structures, and connections. Patients of any age who are trying to sleep find direct light unpleasant. Premature infants are photophobic; however, they will open their eyes with dim lights. If the light levels never change, infants never experience the diurnal rhythm necessary for development. Reducing light levels may facilitate rest and subsequent energy conservation, as well as promote organization and growth (Altimier, 2015b; Altimier & White, 2014; White, 2015). Many of our care practices, however, could be adjusted to some extent to avoid interrupting a sleep cycle if we could determine at what point in the cycle a baby is. In the absence of this information, most clinical interventions are scheduled at the convenience of staff and, when possible, should be performed at the most optimal time for the baby, which is around their sleep cycles.

DEFINITION

REM and NREM sleep cycling are essential for early neurosensory development, learning and memory, and preservation of brain plasticity for the life of the individual (Graven, 2006). Sleep deprivation (both REM and NREM) results in a loss of brain plasticity, which is manifested by smaller brains, altered subsequent learning, and long-term effect on behavior and brain function (Axelin et al., 2010). Facilitation and protection of sleep and sleep cycles are essential to long-term learning and continuing brain development through the preservation of brain plasticity (Weisman et al., 2011).

STANDARD

A policy/procedure/guideline on safeguarding sleep and back-to-sleep practices exists and is followed throughout the infant's stay.

INFANT CHARACTERISTICS

- Infant demonstrates sleep–wake states, cycles, and transitions
- Infant's maturity and readiness for back-to-sleep protocol

GOALS

- Infant sleep–wake states will be assessed before initiating all caregiving activities.
- Prolonged periods of uninterrupted sleep will be protected.
- Infants will be transitioned to the back-to-sleep protocol when developmentally appropriate.

NEUROPROTECTIVE INTERVENTIONS

- Facilitate early and prolonged SSC
- Utilize a valid and reliable sleep state scale
- Approach the infant using a soft voice followed by gentle firm touch
- Promote noise control in a quiet environment to ensure uninterrupted sleep; single-family rooms with families present can enhance sleep
- Soothing auditory stimuli, such as maternal voice and heartbeat, and other soothing sounds are showing value

■ Protect the infant's eyes from direct light exposure and maintain low levels of ambient light (utilize incubator covers) for light control

■ Educate parents on how to read their infant's behavioral cues related to sleep and how to promote sleep cycling

■ Cluster care and individualize caregiving activities around sleep–wake states

■ Provide some daily exposure to light, preferably including shorter wavelengths, for entrainment of the circadian rhythm

■ Avoid high doses of sedative and depressing drugs which can depress the endogenous firing of cells, thus interfering with visual development, REM, and NREM sleep cycles

■ Protect sleep and sleep cycles, especially REM sleep

■ Pay close attention to infant signs of stress during care

■ Provide developmental care appropriate for the age and maturation of the infant

■ Assure the infant is able to maintain a normal sleep pattern during back-to-sleep well before discharge and role model this behavior

■ Provide tummy time/prone-to-play time routinely for infants that are back-to-sleep

■ Educate parents about the importance and rationale for back-to-sleep time and tummy time (inform parents to communicate this importance to other family members and caregivers) (Altimier & Phillips, 2013)

CORE MEASURE # 5: MINIMIZING STRESS AND PAIN

The NICU is often a stressful environment for infants, parents, and staff (Grunau, Whitfield, & Petrie-Thomas, 2009). Early life stress is known to permanently affect neurobiologic, hormonal, and physiologic systems. Preterm infants are particularly at risk for adverse effects of early stress, since their physiologic systems are immature during their time in the NICU. Their brains are in a period of rapid development and their stress systems are sensitive to programming while they are exposed to repeated painful procedures in the NICU (Volpe, 2009). Seemingly typical handling and caregiving by the NICU staff such as bathing, weighing, and diaper changes have been perceived as stressful to the infant (Comaru & Miura, 2009). These stresses occur for the infant during a critical period of development and may contribute to short- and long-term morbidity (DiMaggio & Gibbins, 2005). NICU stressors and painful interventions may raise cortisol levels, limiting neuroplastic reorganization, and therefore the learning and memory of motor skills (Brummelte et al., 2012). Even a single adverse sensation or situation is enough to increase cortisol; high cortisol levels signal stress, even when the infant appears to be resting and calm (Figure 11.6).

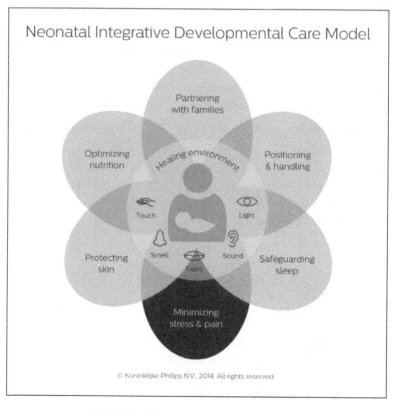

Neonatal Integrative Developmental Care Model

Partnering with families

Optimizing nutrition

Healing environment

Positioning & handling

Touch

Light

Protecting skin

Smell

Sound

Safeguarding sleep

Taste

Minimizing stress & pain

FIGURE 11.6. Minimizing stress and pain.

Minimizing stress in preterm infants may have many neurologic benefits such as reducing the likelihood of programming abnormal stress responsiveness, which will help preserve existing neuroplastic capacity (Pitcher et al., 2011). Infant massage has been shown to decrease cortisol levels (Mendes & Procianoy, 2008). Infant stress is also rapidly reduced by SSC. Just 20 minutes of SSC reduces cortisol levels by 60% in infants greater than 25 weeks GA (Morelius, Theodorsson, & Nelson, 2005). Maternal and neonatal stress levels synchronously decrease during SSC. Breastfeeding and SSC in tandem may be the most profound analgesic available, with no side effects. A simple gentle nurturing touch from parents to their infants can influence pain sensitivity, affect, and growth in neonates.

DEFINITION

Sources of stress for infants include the physical environment, caregiver interventions, medical and surgical procedures, pain, distress, pathologic processes, temperature changes, handling and multiple modes of stimulation, and, most importantly, the separation from parents. Consequences of neonatal stress include increased energy expenditure, decreased healing and recovery, altered growth, impaired physiologic stability, and altered brain development and organization.

STANDARD

A policy/procedure/guideline on the assessment and management of stress and pain exists and is followed throughout the infant's stay.

INFANT CHARACTERISTICS

Characteristics include behavioral cues indicating stress or self-regulation.

GOALS

The goal is to promote self-regulation and neurodevelopmental organization.

NEUROPROTECTIVE INTERVENTIONS

■ Facilitate early and prolonged SSC

■ Utilize a validated and reliable pain assessment tool

■ Provide individualized care in a manner that anticipates, prioritizes, and supports the needs of infants to minimize stress and pain

■ Provide nonpharmacologic support (positioning, containment, swaddling, pacifier, and sucrose) with all minor invasive interventions

■ Involve parents in supporting their infant during painful procedures if they choose by providing SSC or by assisting with containment

■ Educate parents on how to read their infant's behavioral cues related to stress and pain and how to provide comforting interventions (Altimier & Phillips, 2013)

CORE MEASURE # 6: PROTECTING SKIN

Infants in the neonatal intensive care unit are at risk for skin compromise due to immature skin, compromised perfusion, fluid retention, compromised immune system, medical diagnosis, and so on, as well as the presence of dressings, tapes, adhesives, and various medical devices that are essential to their care (Visscher & Narendran, 2014). At the moment of birth, the skin is sterile; within 24 hours, it has been colonized with its own bacteria (Allwood, 2011). An acid mantle with a pH of less than 5 is created by the skin to protect it from microorganisms. Maintaining skin integrity is an important health care goal because of the essential role of the skin in protecting the infant and providing innate immunity. Achievement of this goal requires constant vigilance and awareness of factors that can negatively impact the skin (Figure 11.7).

Protecting skin becomes of particular importance when dealing with neonates at the limits of viability (22–24 weeks), where

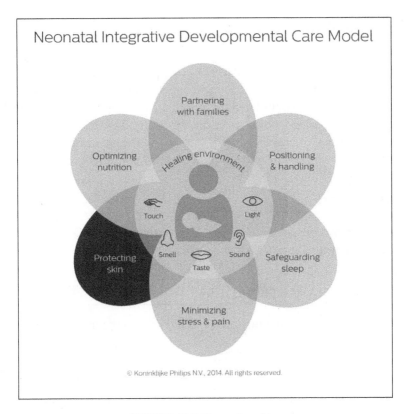

Neonatal Integrative Developmental Care Model

Partnering with families

Optimizing nutrition

Healing environment

Positioning & handling

Touch

Light

Protecting skin

Smell

Sound

Safeguarding sleep

Taste

Minimizing stress & pain

FIGURE 11.7. Protecting skin.

the brain and body certainly benefit, but the skin is fragile. SSC minimizes transepidermal water loss (TEWL), which improves the skin-barrier function (Chiou & Blume-Peytavi, 2004). Maternal breasts warm up and conduct heat to the infant, as well as regulate the infant's temperature. Father's chests warm infants, too. Both mom and baby, while in the NICU, are colonized with NICU organisms (bacteria and viruses). The mother develops antibodies to these organisms and transfers these protective antibodies back to her infant via breast milk and during SSC, which in turn helps protect the infant from hospital-acquired infections.

DEFINITION

Functions of the skin include thermoregulation; fat storage and insulation; fluid and electrolyte balance; barrier protection against penetration and absorption of bacteria and toxins; sensation of touch, pressure, and pain; and conduit of sensory information to the brain. Skin care practices outlining bathing practices, emollient usage, humidity practices, and use of adhesives for babies in each stage of development should be incorporated into unit practices and policies.

STANDARD

A policy/procedure/guideline on skin care exists and is followed throughout the infant's stay.

INFANT CHARACTERISTICS

Characteristics include maturity and integrity of the infant's skin.

GOALS

■ Maintain skin integrity of the infant from birth to discharge

■ Reduce TEWL of extremely low-birth-weight (ELBW) infants

■ Provide developmentally appropriate infant massage

NEUROPROTECTIVE INTERVENTIONS

■ Facilitate early and prolonged SSC

■ Utilize a validated and reliable skin assessment tool (i.e., Braden Q) on admission and routinely according to hospital protocol

■ Provide appropriate humidity via SSC with the mother or incubator to facilitate stratum corneum maturation during the first 2 weeks of life

■ Implement evidence-based catheter insertion practices

■ Minimize use of adhesives and use caution when removing adhesives to prevent epidermal stripping

■ Utilize products that protect the skin from adhesive damage

■ Provide appropriate positioning utilizing gel-filled products to protect skin and prevent skin breakdown

■ Avoid soaps and routine use of emollients

■ Provide full body swaddled bathing no more than every 72 to 96 hours

■ Use water only for bathing infants who are less than 1,000 g

■ Use pH neutral cleansers for bathing infants who are greater than 1,000 g

■ Educate parents on protecting skin, swaddled bathing, and delivery of developmentally appropriate infant massage (Altimier & Phillips, 2013).

CORE MEASURE # 7: OPTIMIZING NUTRITION

Breast milk is the optimal nutrition for NICU infants; any breast milk the infant receives is valuable. Breastfeeding is not an intervention, but rather a neurobehavioral consequence of being in a safe habitat (Alberts & Ronca, 2012). SSC provides a safe habitat for the infant, thus promoting breast milk production and breastfeeding. Breastfeeding supports the early anchoring of the healthy microbiome, ensures direct immune protection, and is per se a regulator of cardiorespiratory stability. SSC promotes initiation of prefeeding behaviors, exclusivity of breastfeeding, longer duration of breastfeeding, better recognition of mother's milk, and higher milk production (Klaus & Klaus, 2010; Mcinnes & Chambers, 2008). Evidence from the Cochrane Review on early SSC shows that breastfeeding is the primary outcome of SSC; infants that have been provided with SSC are discharged breastfeeding more successfully than infants who have not been provided SSC (Conde-Agudelo & Diaz-Rossello, 2014). The semirecumbent position of SSC helps to release primitive neonatal reflexes that stimulate breastfeeding (Figure 11.8).

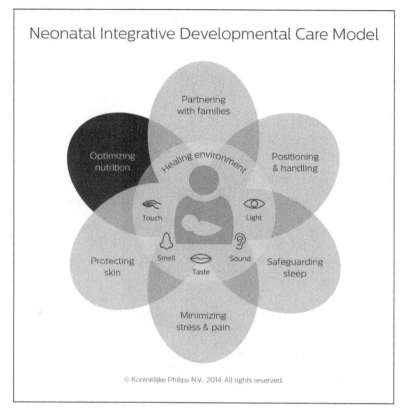

FIGURE 11.8. Optimizing nutrition.

NNS or "dry" sucking without fluid, such as on a fist or pacifier, is present but disorganized in infants younger than 30 weeks; sucking rhythm generally improves by 30 to 32 weeks postconception. Because NNS does not interrupt breathing, it is usually (but not always) established before an infant has the neurologic maturation to coordinate sucking with swallows and breathing. Benefits of NNS have been summarized as increased oxygenation, faster transition to nipple feeding, and better bottle-feeding performance (Hunter, Lee, & Altimier, 2015).

Neurosupportive feeding focuses on the infant. Neurologic maturation, medical issues, ongoing physiologic status, current stage of feeding readiness and skills, and psychosocial and interactive skills have redefined feeding success in the NICU. Quantity becomes secondary to the safety and quality of the feed.

DEFINITION

Breastfeeding is the single most powerful and well-documented preventive modality available to health care providers to reduce the risk of common causes of infant morbidity. Even when adequate breast milk is available, most premature neonates learn to eat via nipple feeding. Nipple feeding is a complex task for premature infants and requires a skilled caregiver in assisting the infant in achieving a safe, functional, and nurturing feeding experience. Infant-driven feeding scales that address feeding readiness and quality of nippling, as well as developmentally supportive caregiver interventions, are beneficial when initiating oral feedings in the premature neonate (Holloway, 2014; Ludwig & Waitzman, 2007; Waitzman, Ludwig, & Nelson, 2014).

STANDARD 1

A policy/procedure/guideline on optimizing nutrition (cue-based/infant-driven breast- or bottle-feeding), which includes infant readiness; quality of nippling and caregiver techniques is followed throughout the infant's stay.

STANDARD 2

A policy/procedure/guideline on SSC exists and is followed throughout the infant's stay.

INFANT CHARACTERISTICS

■ Physiologic stability with handling and feeding
■ Feeding readiness cues

- Coordinated suck/swallow/breathing (SSB) throughout bottle or breastfeeding
- Endurance to maintain nutritional intake and support growth

GOALS

- Feeding will be safe, functional, nurturing, and neurosupportive.
- Optimized nutrition will be enhanced by individualizing all feeding care practices.
- Oral aversions will be prevented by assuring it is a positive experience for the infant
- Infants of breastfeeding mothers will be competent at breastfeeding prior to discharge

NEUROPROTECTIVE INTERVENTIONS

- Facilitate early, frequent, and prolonged SSC
- Utilize validated and reliable infant-driven feeding scales
- Support mother's EBM supply
- Provide the taste and smell of breast milk with gavage feedings
- Minimize negative perioral stimulation (adhesives, suctioning, etc.)
- Utilize indwelling gavage tubes rather than intermittent tubes
- Promote NNS at the mother's pumped breast during gavage feeds
- Hold the infant and use NNS with an appropriate-sized pacifier during gavage feeds when the mother is not available
- Individualize care by incorporating cue-based/infant-driven feeding practices
- Once orally feeding, focus on the quality of feeding experience versus quantity of feeds
- Utilize caregiver techniques when nippling infant to avoid twisting, jiggling, excessive chin and neck support, and so on

- Promote the side-lying position close to the parent/caregiver when bottle feeding
- Educate parents about infant feeding cues
- Support breastfeeding mothers in feeding infants at the breast

CONCLUSION

Learning the principles of neurodevelopment and understanding the meaning of preterm behavioral cues make it possible for the NICU caregiver to provide individualized, developmentally appropriate, neuroprotective care to each infant and family in the NICU environment. The seven core measures of the Neonatal IDC Model provide specific and structured guidance in optimizing care for infants and families in the NICU environment. Acknowledging challenges that the physical NICU environment has on the infant's sensory system is critical in order to mitigate risks to the developing infant. Partnering with families and encouraging SSC promotes parent–infant attachment and sets the stage for emotional stability. Providing gentle containment, supportive boundaries, and midline, flexed positions help to simulate the womb positioning that was lost prematurely. By safeguarding sleep, minimizing stress and pain, protecting skin, and optimizing nutrition, NICU caregivers can enhance the experience of infants and families in their care, increasing the likelihood of achieving optimal physical, cognitive, and emotional outcomes.

REFERENCES

Alberts, J., & Ronca, A. (2012). The experience of being born: A natural context for learning to suckle. *International Journal of Pediatrics, 2012*, Article ID 129328. doi:10.1155/2012/129328

Allwood, M. (2011). Skin care guidelines for infants aged 23–30 weeks' gestation: A review of the literature. *Neonatal, Paediatric & Child Health Nursing, 14*(1), 20–27.

Altimier, L. (2015). Neuroprotective core measure 1: The healing environment. *Newborn and Infant Nursing Reviews, 15*(3), 89–94. doi:10.1053/j.nainr.2015.06.014

Altimier, L. (2015a). Compassionate family care framework: A new Collaborative Compassionate Care model for NICU families and caregivers. *Newborn & Infant Nursing Reviews, 15*(1), 33–41. doi:10.1053/j.nainr.2015.01.005

Altimier, L. (2015b). Neuroprotective core measure 1: The healing environment. *Newborn and Infant Nursing Reviews, 15*(3), 89–94. doi:10.1053/j.nainr.2015.06.014

Altimier, L., & Phillips, R. (2013). The neonatal integrative developmental care model: Seven neuroprotective core measures for family-centered care. *Newborn & Infant Nursing Reviews, 13*(1), 9–22.

Altimier, L., & White, R. (Eds.). (2014). *The neonatal intensive care unit (NICU) environment* (5th ed.). New York, NY: Springer Publishing Company.

Altimier, L., Eichel, M., Warner, B., Tedeschi, L., & Brown, B. (2005). Developmental care: Changing the NICU physically and behaviorally to promote patient outcomes and contain costs. *Neonatal Intensive Care, 18*(4), 12–16.

American Academy of Pediatrics, A. (2003). Family-centered care and the pediatrician's role. *Pediatrics, 112*, 691–696.

Ammari, A., Schulze, K., Ohira-Kist, K., Kashyap, S., Fifer, W., Myers, M., & Sahni, R. (2009). Effects of body position on thermal, cardiorespiratory and metabolic activity in low birth weight infants. *Early Human Development, 85*(8), 497–501.

Axelin, A., Kirjavainen, J., Salantera, S., & Lehtonen, L. (2010). Effects of pain management on sleep in preterm infants. *European Journal of Pain, 14*, 752–758. doi:10.1016/j.ejpain.2009.11.007

Bergman, N. (2014). The neuroscience of birth—And the case for zero separation. *Curationis, 37*(2), 1–4. doi:10.4102/curationis.v37i2.1440

Bergman, N. (2015). Skin-to-skin contact as a neurosupportive measure. *Newborn & Infant Nursing Reviews, 15*(3), 145–150.

Biran, V., Phan Duy, A., Decobert, F., Bednarek, N., Alberti, C., & Baud, O. (2014). Is melatonin ready to be used in preterm infants as a neuroprotectant? *Developmental Medicine and Child Neurology, 56*, 717–723.

Born, J., & Wagner, U. (2009). Sleep, hormones, and memory. *Obstetrics and Gynecology Clinics of North America, 36*(4), 809. doi:10.1016/j.ogc.2009.10.001

Browne, J. (2011). Developmental care for high-risk newborns: Emerging science, clinical application, and continuity from newborn intensive care unit to community. *Clinics in Perinatology, 38*, 719–729. doi:10.1016/j.clp.2011.08.003

Brummelte, S., Grunau, R., Chau, V., Poskitt, K., Brant, R., Vinall, J., . . . Miller, S. (2012). Procedural pain and brain development in premature newborns. *Annals of Neurology, 71*(3), 385–396. doi:10.1002/ana.22267

Busse, M., Stromgren, K., Thorngate, L., & Thomas, K. (2013). Parents' responses to stress in the neonatal intensive care unit. *Critical Care Nurse [serial online], 33*(4), 52–60. doi:10.4037/ccn2013715

Byrne, E., & Garber, J. (2013). Physical therapy intervention in the neonatal intensive care unit. *Physical & Occupational Therapy in Pediatrics, 33*(1), 75–110. Retrieved from http://informahealthcare.com/potp. doi:10.3109/01942638.201 2.750870

Bystrova, K., Ivanova, V., & Edhborg, M. (2009). Early contact versus separation: Effects on mother–infant interaction one year later. *Birth, 36*(2), 97–109.

Chiou, Y., & Blume-Peytavi, U. (2004). Stratum corneum maturation. A review of neonatal skin function. *Skin Pharmacology and Physiology, 17*(2), 57–66.

Cohen-Engler, A., Hadash, A., Shehadeh, N., & Pillar, G. (2012). Breastfeeding may improve nocturnal sleep and reduce infantile colic: Potential role of breast milk melatonin. *European Journal of Pediatrics, 171*, 729–732.

Colson, S., Meek, J., & Hawdon, J. (2008). Optimal positions for the release of primitive neonatal reflexes stimulating breastfeeding. *Early Human Development, 84*(7), 441–449. doi:10.1016/j.earlhumdev.2007.12.003

Comaru, T., & Miura, E. (2009). Postural support improves distress and pain during diaper change in preterm infants. *Journal of Perinatology, 29*, 504–507.

Conde-Agudelo, A., & Diaz-Rossello, J. (2014). Kangaroo mother care to reduce morbidity and mortality in low birthweight infants. *The Cochrane Database of Systematic Reviews, 4*, CD002771.

Danner-Bowman, K., & Cardin, A. (2015). Core measure 3: Positioning & handling—A look at preventing positional plagiocephaly. *Newborn and Infant Nursing Reviews, 15*(3). doi:org/10.1053/j.nainr.2015.06.009

DiMaggio, T., & Gibbins, S. (2005). Neonatal pain management in the 21st century. In H. Taeusch (Ed.), *Avery's diseases of the newborn* (8th ed., pp. 438–446). Philadelphia, PA: Elsevier.

Ferber, S., & Makhoul, I. (2004). The effect of skin-to-skin contact (kangaroo care) shortly after birth on the neurobehavioral responses of the term newborn: A randomized controlled trial. *Pediatrics, 113*(4), 858–865.

Graven, S. (2006). Sleep and brain development. *Clinics in Perinatology, 33*(3), 693–706.

Graven, S., & Browne, J. (2008). Sensory development in the fetus, neonate, and infant: Introductions and overview. *Newborn & Infant Nursing Reviews, 8*(4), 169–172.

Grunau, R., Tu, M., & Whitfield, M. (2010). Cortisol, behavior, and heart rate reactivity to immunization pain at 4 months corrected age in infants born very preterm. *Clinical Journal of Pain, 26*(8), 698–704.

Grzyb, M., Coo, H., & Dow, K. (2014). Views of parents and health-care providers regarding parental presence at bedside rounds in a neonatal intensive care unit. *Journal of Perinatology, 34,* 143–148.

Gudsnuk, K., & Champagne, F. (2011). Epigenetic effects of early developmental experiences. *Clinics in Perinatology, 38*(4), 703–717.

Hack, M., Taylor, H., Schluchter, M., Andreias, L., Drotar, D., & Klein, N. (2009). Behavioral outcomes of extremely low birth weight children at age 8 years. *Journal of Developmental & Behavioral Pediatrics, 30*(2), 122–130. doi:10.1097/DBP.0b013e31819e6a16

Harris, G. (2014). Family-centered rounds in the neonatal intensive care unit. *Nursing for Women's Health, 18*(1), 19–27. doi:10.1111/1751-486X.12090

Heinonen, K., Raikkonen, K., & Pesonen, A. (2010). Behavioural symptoms of attention deficit/hyperactivity disorder in preterm and term children born small and appropriate for age: A longitudinal study. *BioMed Center Pediatrics, 10,* 91.

Hendricks-Muñoz, K., Prendergast, C., Caprio, M., & Wasserman, R. (2002). Developmental care: The impact of wee care developmental care training on short-term infant outcome and hospital costs. *Newborn & Infant Nursing Reviews, 2*(1), 39–45.

Hobson, J. (1995). *The development of sleep.* New York, NY: Scientific American Library.

Holloway, E. (2014). The dynamic process of assessing infant feeding readiness. *Newborn & Infant Nursing Reviews, 14*(3), 119–123.

Hunter, J. (2010). Therapeutic positioning: Neuromotor, physiologic, and sleep implications. In C. K. J. McGrath (Ed.), *Developmental care of newborns and infants* (pp. 285–312). Glenview, IL: National Association of Neonatal Nurses.

Hunter, J., Lee, A., & Altimier, L. (2015). Neonatal intensive care unit. In J. Case-Smith & J. C. O'Brien (Eds.), *Occupational therapy for children and adolescents* (7th ed., pp. 595–635). St. Louis, MO: Mosby.

Hunter, J., Lee, A., & Altimier, L. (Eds.). (2015). *Neonatal intensive care unit* (7th ed.). St. Louis, MO: Mosby.

Johnson, S., Hollis, C., & Kochlar, P. (2010). Psychiatric disorders in extremely preterm children: Longitudinal finding at age 11 years in the EPICure study. *Journal of the American Academy of Child & Adolescent Psychiatry, 49*(5), 453–463, e451.

Karner, S., & Cortese, S. (2009). The kangaroo method as early intervention in premature infant nursing: Providing warmth, safety and security. *Pflege Zeitschrift, 62*(1), 14–17.

Klaus, M., & Klaus, P. (2010). Academy of breastfeeding medicine founder's lecture 2009: Maternity care re-evaluated. *Breastfeeding Medicine: The Official Journal of the Academy of Breastfeeding Medicine, 5*(1), 3–8. doi:10.1089/bfm.2009.0086

Liaw, J., Yang, L., Chang, L., Chou, H., & Chao, S. (2009). Improving neonatal caregiving through a developmentally supportive care training program. *Applied Nursing Research, 22*(2), 86–93. doi:10.1016/j.apnr.2007.05.001

Limperopoulos, C. (2009). Autism spectrum disorders in survivors of extreme prematurity. *Clinics in Perinatology, 36*(4), 791–805.

Limperopoulos, C. (2010). Extreme prematurity, cerebellar injury, and autism. *Seminars in Pediatric Neurology, 17*(1), 25–29.

Limperopoulos, C., Bassan, H., Sullivan, N., Soul, J., Robertson, R., Moore, M., . . . du Plessis, A. (2008). Positive screening for autism in ex-preterm infants: Prevalence and risk factors. *Pediatrics, 121*(4), 758–765. doi:10.1542/peds .2007-2158

Ludington-Hoe, S. (2010). Kangaroo care is developmental care. In C. K. J. McGrath (Ed.), *Developmental care of newborns and infants: A guide for health professionals* (pp. 349–388). Glenview, IL: National Association of Neonatal Nurses.

Ludington-Hoe, S., Johnson, M., Morgan, K., Lewis, T., Gutman, J., Wilson, P., & Scher, M. (2006). Neurophysiologic assessment of neonatal sleep organization: Preliminary results of a randomized, controlled trial of skin contact with preterm infants. *Journal of the American Academy of Child & Adolescent Psychiatry, 45*(12), 1455–1455.

Ludwig, S., Steichen, J., Khoury, J., & Krieg, P. (2008). Quality improvement analysis of developmental care in infants less than 1500 grams at birth. *Newborn & Infant Nursing Reviews, 8*(2), 94–100.

Ludwig, S., & Waitzman, K. (2007). Changing feeding documentation to reflect infant-driven feeding practice. *Newborn & Infant Nursing Reviews, 7*(3), 155–160.

Marcellus, L. (2004). Determination of positional skin-surface pressures in premature infants. *Journal of Neonatal Nursing: Neonatal Network, 23*(1), 25–30.

McInnes, R., & Chambers, J. (2008). Supporting breastfeeding mothers: Qualitative synthesis. *Journal of Advanced Nursing, 62*(4), 407–427. doi:10.1111/j.1365–2648.2008.04618.x

Mendes, E., & Procianoy, R. (2008). Massage therapy reduces hospital stay and occurrence of late-onset sepsis in very preterm neonates. *Journal of Perinatology, 28*, 815–820.

Mörelius, E., Theodorsson, E., & Nelson, N. (2005). Salivary cortisol and mood and pain profiles during skin-to-skin care for an unselected group of mothers and infants in neonatal intensive care. *Pediatrics, 116*(5), 1105–1113. doi:10.1542/peds.2004

Pitcher, J., Schneider, L., Drysdale, J., Ridding, M., & Owens, J. (2011). Motor system development of the preterm and low birthweight infant. *Clinics in Perinatology, 38*, 605–625. doi:10.1016/j.clp.2011.08.010

Sweeney, J., & Gutierrez, T. (2002). Musculoskeletal implications of preterm infant positioning in the NICU. *Journal of Perinatal and Neonatal Nursing, 16*, 58–70.

Tarullo, A. R., Balsam, P. D., & Fifer, W. P. (2011). Sleep and infant learning. *Infant and Child Development, 20*, 35–46.

Taylor, H. (Ed.). (2010). *Academic performance and learning disabilities.* New York, NY: Cambridge University Press.

Vanderbilt, D., & Gleason, M. (2010). Mental health concerns of the premature infant through the lifespan. *Child and Adolescent Psychiatric Clinics of North America, 19*(2), 211–228.

Visscher, M., & Narendran, V. (2014). Neonatal infant skin: Development, structure and function. *Newborn & Infant Nursing Reviews, 14*(4), 135–141. doi:10.1053/j.nainr.2014.10.004

Volpe, J. J. (2009). Brain injury in premature infants: A complex amalgam of destructive and developmental disturbances. *Lancet Neurology, 8*(1), 110–124.

Waitzman, K., Ludwig, S., & Nelson, C. (2014). Contributing to Content Validity of the Infant-Driven Feeding Scales© through Delphi surveys. *Newborn & Infant Nursing Reviews, 14*(3), 88–91.

Weisman, O., Magori-Cohen, R., Louzoun, Y., Eidelman, A., & Feldman, R. (2011). Sleep–wake transitions in premature neonates predict earlydevelopment. *Pediatrics, 128*, 706–714.

White (2015). Core measure 4: Safeguarding sleep—Its value in neuroprotection of the newborn. *Newborn & Infant Nursing Reviews, 12*(3), 114–115. doi:10.1053/j.nainr.2015.06.012

Palliative Care

Charlotte Wool and Anita Catlin

OVERVIEW

Integral to the care of medically fragile neonates is the reality that not all will survive. Perinatal palliative care is an interdisciplinary, comprehensive, coordinated approach to supporting families facing the possibility of perinatal death (Wool, 2013). Perinatal death refers to fetal deaths after 20 weeks gestation and live births with only brief survival (Barfield & The Committee on Fetus and Newborn, 2011). One aspect of palliative care, called end-of-life care, supports a peaceful, dignified death for the infant and the provision of loving support to the family and health care providers (National Association of Neonatal Nurses [NANN], 2010). This chapter defines and discusses perinatal and neonatal palliative care.

BACKGROUND AND INCIDENCE

The technology behind expanded prenatal testing has developed rapidly (Hickerton, Aitkin, Hodgson, & Delatycki, 2012), resulting in increased detection of anomalies and the subsequent need to provide care to families facing an unexpected fetal diagnosis. Today, the majority of diagnoses for several life-limiting disorders occur in the prenatal period (Irving, Richmond, Wren, Longster, & Embleton, 2011). Palliative care may begin in the prenatal period and then continue for infants born with life-limiting conditions or who develop life-limiting conditions during their neonatal hospitalization.

The World Health Organization (WHO; 2014) estimates 1.2 million children are in need of palliative care at the end of life worldwide. Congenital anomalies occur in approximately 3% of all live births and are the leading causes of infant mortality (MacDorman, Kimeyer, & Wilson, 2012). Preterm-related causes of death together account for 35% of all infant deaths, more than any other single cause (Centers for Disease Control and Prevention, 2013). More than 29,000 infants under 1 year of age die each year in the United States, and 66% of these deaths occur during the neonatal period (Xu, Kochanek, & Tejada-Vera, 2009), many in the neonatal intensive care unit (NICU) (Brandon, Docherty, & Thorpe, 2007).

Palliative care is focused on interventions aimed at improving quality of life and maximizing comfort. WHO (2014) states that, in the case of life-limiting conditions, palliative care should begin at the same time that curative care begins. Curative and comfort interventions may coexist (Catlin & Carter, 2002).

RECOMMENDED INTERVENTIONS

■ Palliative care should be offered at any period in which the infant's life may be limited—prenatally, at the time of birth, after the birth, initially in the labor and delivery suite, in the NICU, and at home following discharge.

■ When a prenatal diagnosis is made, palliative care should be offered while the fetus is in utero. Parents should be supported throughout the decision-making process. Options for terminating or continuing the pregnancy should be offered in a balanced manner and family decisions should be supported by the health care team.

■ When continuing the pregnancy is chosen, an advocate or coordinator of care for a family should be identified prenatally to assist with (a) helping families navigate the health care system, (b) coordinating care conferences between the health care team and family, (c) answering questions, and (d) assisting parents with a birth plan that is appropriate. A birth plan is a written document available to all stakeholders outlining parental wishes about the pregnancy, labor, birth, and postnatal period.

■ Provision of care and services should be coordinated among interdisciplinary team members. Recommendations should be made as a team through consensus to avoid fragmentation in communication and care. Should any party wish to change the agreed upon plan, the interdisciplinary team must all meet to reassess whether changes should be made.

■ Parents are part of the caregiving team and should participate in the decision-making process. Family conferences are essential to caregivers' understanding of families' needs, hopes, and goals for their infant.

■ Appropriate family support services should be provided, including those of perinatal social workers, hospital chaplains, and clergy; hospital palliative care team members to provide emotional and spiritual support; a child life specialist or family support specialist to support the infant's siblings; and a lactation consultant to assist mothers who want to breastfeed their infant or donate breast milk at the end of life and to help mothers manage cessation of lactation (Moore & Catlin, 2003).

■ Initial training, availability of written protocols, annual competencies, and support services should be available for all staff members. Debriefing for staff is essential after a difficult death.

ASSESSMENT

The International Council of Nurses (2015) views the nurse's role as fundamental to a palliative approach that aims to reduce suffering and improve the quality of life for dying patients and their families through early assessment, identification, and management of pain and physical, social, psychological, spiritual, and cultural needs. Nurses and other caregivers determine when intensive therapies no longer offer hope for a cure or recovery, and they then shift the focus of treatment toward solely the provision of comfort for the infant and family.

Comprehensive assessment in the physical, psychological, social, spiritual, and cultural domains should recur on a regular basis. Recommendations support decision making using the same ethical criteria that is applied to other medical interventions. That is, using the best interest standard, which weighs the benefits and burdens of a particular intervention in light of pathophysiologic parameters, the goals of treatment, and the parents' preferences (American Academy of Hospice and Palliative Medicine [AAHPM], 2013).

A document for the health care team to use and refer to should be created to avoid fragmentation of care and provide continuity of care.

DIAGNOSIS AND PLANNING

Diagnostic information should be offered in a timely and compassionate manner. Since prognosis may be uncertain and an infant may live longer than expected, a treatment plan can be developed prenatally. A treatment plan is a written document available to all stakeholders stating fetal/neonatal diagnoses and anticipated treatments necessary to keep the infant comfortable as assessment dictates (i.e., breathing, pain, feeding). Palliative care is appropriate for neonates with a wide range of life-limiting conditions, including severe prematurity and its accompanying complications, birth-related trauma or complex congenital anomalies, and whether the condition will result in death during the infant's first few hours of life or after several years.

Written information should be given to parents that complements palliative care interventions, such as (a) referrals to community resources, counselors, community members, and other parents; (b) what to expect during the dying process; and (c) who to contact when death occurs.

When an infant with a potentially life-limiting condition is being transported to a tertiary care center, parents should be informed that palliative care may be the focus of care, as parents may believe that transport means cure when in fact transport may be indicated to confirm a diagnosis.

When a decision has been made to pursue palliative care interventions, the proper focus of palliative care should be maintained.

■ Active orders should be reviewed to determine whether they should be continued when palliative care is initiated.

■ Pain and distressing symptoms, such as gasping or seizures, should be treated in consultation with a neonatal pharmacist, with the least invasive route considered the desired method of delivery (i.e., buccal, dermal, or rectal delivery if intravenous access is no longer desired or available).

- Comfort measures including holding and kangaroo care should be encouraged.
- A validated instrument to measure infant pain and sedation should be used.

End-of-life care should give attention to the following concerns:

- Care should be provided in a private location within or near nursing staff, with the goal of keeping the family members together.
- If possible the environment should have a "home away from home" feel to facilitate comfort and privacy.
- Alarms and pagers of those in attendance should be turned off. Light levels should be adjusted for family comfort.
- Routine measurement of vital signs and lab analyses should cease.
- Pain assessments to identify infant distress should be performed frequently.
- Pain medication should be offered frequently in standardized doses based upon the infant's weight.
- No painful assessments (e.g., heel sticks, measurement of blood gases) should be made.
- Appropriate access to medications (intravenous, rectal, buccal, or topical) should be given.
- Offering small amounts of oral fluids such as drops of breast milk and lip lubrication as a comfort measure is appropriate.
- Infants should be bathed, dressed, and held.
- Infants should be taken outside into the sunlight if possible.
- Spiritual support should be offered to the family.
- Family and friends should be welcomed, and visiting restrictions should be waived.
- Memory-making activities should be encouraged, including taking family photographs (by lay or professional photographers), making handprints and footprints, cutting locks of hair, and holding special spiritual or religious ceremonies.

■ If the family is not available, nurses should hold and comfort the infant.

■ Family should be accompanied by staff when leaving the hospital.

TRANSITIONS TO HOME AND PRIMARY CARE

When palliative care includes the removal of life-sustaining technology in the hospital or a home, support from a hospice or palliative care organization should be provided. Before life-sustaining technology is removed, a plan should be in place for the eventuality that the infant continues to breathe independently. When ventilator support of an infant is discontinued, caregivers should attend to the following concerns:

■ The infant's parents should decide who will be present.

■ Vasopressors should be discontinued.

■ The infant should be weaned from neuromuscular blocking agents prior to the removal of life-sustaining technology.

■ Nurses should explain as much of the process to the parents as the parents wish to hear.

■ The infant should be held by a parent or family members, or, if the parents and family do not wish to hold the infant, by a staff member. (Some parents may find it difficult to hold a dying infant.)

■ Gentle suction may be performed, and the endotracheal tube may be removed.

■ Tape and additional lines may be removed.

■ Medication such as morphine should be given if respiratory discomfort exists; oxygen therapy may be used as a comfort measure based upon assessment and parental wishes.

■ Medications to treat respiratory distress or to prevent discomfort should be given in standardized dosages based upon the infant's weight and may be repeated if necessary. (Bolus medications in larger than normal doses are not appropriate.)

Hospital personnel should have a relationship with a local hospice or palliative care organization in order to offer seamless continuity of care. Where local hospices do not provide pediatric care, pediatric home health agencies and a primary care pediatrician may oversee the palliative care needs. Infants who are discharged with life-limiting illnesses should have a plan of care, including necessary resources and a portable nonresuscitation plan to avoid unnecessary resuscitation.

The provision of whether the infant who continues to live will receive artificial nutrition and hydration should be discussed. Artificial feeding and hydration are viewed as a life-extending technology and may or may not be appropriate in palliative care (Diekema & Botkin, 2009). The family and staff members must be aware that the infant who receives only oral measures as comfort may not expire for 1 to 3 weeks (Hellmann, Williams, Ives-Baine, & Shah, 2012). Families may appreciate this time without artificial feeding as a time to get to know their infant and enjoy care without tubes and lines (Hellmann et al., 2012; Vesely & Beach, 2013). Local pediatric inpatient hospices, if they exist, can support parents and the baby during this difficult period (Vesely & Beach, 2013). Insertion of a feeding tube has the potential to extend life and prevent the natural dying process. Research on adult patients at the end of life report that adults are more comfortable when they are not fed. When adults are being fed at the same time that organs are shutting down, they often develop complications such as pulmonary edema, cardiac failure, painful abdominal distention, diarrhea, and aspiration pneumonia (Winter, 2000). When not receiving nutrients, the body releases endorphins that provide analgesia (Carter & Leuthner, 2003).

BEREAVEMENT

Bereavement interventions can be offered by nursing staff and identified community services. Support may include:

■ Giving the parents a gift such as a stuffed teddy bear to take home (which allows them to leave the hospital without empty arms)

■ Calling the family the next day

■ Sending the family a card, e-mail, or letter from the staff; if possible, personalize the message and send it signed by the team

■ Contacting the family on anniversaries of the infant's birth or death, as the family wishes (by telephone, card, text, or e-mail)

■ Introducing the family to a member of a local or online support group or organization

■ Providing a brochure about bereavement, including support contacts

■ Paying attention to sibling needs and supportive services

■ Archiving infant photographs for a period to allow parents to consider if they wish to have them

■ Conducting follow-up meetings where family members can ask questions or express their perceptions of the care they received

■ Holding an annual memorial event for bereaved families in memory of their babies

EVALUATION

Consequences of palliative care include increased patient and family coping, relief of suffering, advance care planning, healing within relationships, increased quality of life, effective closure, and improved bereavement outcomes (Meghani, 2004).

Written documentation reflects the need for physician management, skilled nursing care, and interdisciplinary support. Appropriate diagnoses and accurate procedural coding ensures reimbursement of palliative care measures. Assessment of quality indicators through regular and systematic measurements from patients (i.e., patient satisfaction) and other stakeholders (outcomes related) should be conducted.

This chapter contains portions of the National Association of Neonatal Nursing Position Statement #3051, 2015, Palliative Care for Neonates, used with permission.

REFERENCES

American Academy of Hospice and Palliative Medicine. (2013). *Statement on artificial nutrition and hydration near the end of life*. Retrieved from http://aahpm.org/positions/anh

Barfield, D., & The Committee on Fetus and Newborn. (2011). Standard terminology for fetal, infant, and perinatal deaths. *Pediatrics, 128*(1), 177–181.

Brandon, D., Docherty, S. L., & Thorpe, J. (2007). Infant and child deaths in acute care settings: Implications for palliative care. *Journal of Palliative Medicine, 10*(4), 910–918.

Carter, B. S., & Leuthner, S. R. (2003). The ethics of withholding/withdrawing nutrition in the newborn. *Seminars in Perinatology, 27*(6), 480–487.

Catlin, A., & Carter, B. (2002). Creation of a neonatal end of life palliative care protocol. *Journal of Perinatology, 22*, 184–195.

Centers for Disease Control and Prevention. (2013). *Preterm birth*. Retrieved from http://www.cdc.gov/reproductivehealth/maternalinfanthealth/pretermbirth.htm

Diekema, D. S., & Botkin, J. R. (2009). Forgoing medically provided nutrition and hydration in children. *Pediatrics, 124*(2), 813–822.

Hellmann, J., Williams, C., Ives-Baine, L., & Shah, P. S. (2012). Withdrawal of artificial nutrition and hydration in the Neonatal Intensive Care Unit: Parental perspectives. *Archives of Disease in Childhood-Fetal and Neonatal Edition*, fetal-neonatal-2012. doi: 10.1136/fetalneonatal-2012-301658

Hickerton, C. L., Aitkin, M., Hodgson, J., & Delatycki, M. B. (2012). Did you find that out in time?: New life trajectories of parents who choose to continue a pregnancy where a genetic disorder is diagnosed or likely. *American Journal of Medical Genetics Part A, 158A*, 373–383.

International Council of Nurses. (2015). *Nurses' role in providing care to dying patients and their families* [Position statement]. Retrieved from http://www.icn.ch/images/stories/documents/publications/position_statements/A12_Nurses_Role_Care_Dying_Patients.pdf

Irving, C., Richmond, S., Wren, C., Longster, C., & Embleton, N. D. (2011). Changes in fetal prevalence and outcome for trisomies 13 and 18: A population-based study over 23 years. *Journal of Maternal, Fetal, and Neonatal Medicine, 24*, 137–141.

MacDorman, M. F., Kimeyer, S. E., & Wilson, E. C. (2012). Fetal and perinatal mortality, United States, 2006. *National Vital Statistics Report, 60*(8), 23.

Meghani, S. H. (2004). A concept analysis of palliative care in the United States. *Journal of Advanced Nursing, 46*(2), 152–161.

Moore, D. B., & Catlin, A. (2003). Lactation suppression: Forgotten aspect of care for the mother of a dying child. *Pediatric Nursing, 29*(5), 383–384.

National Association of Neonatal Nurses (NANN). (2015). Palliative and End-of-Life Care for Newborns and Infants. Position Statement #3063. NANN: Chicago, IL.

Vesely, C., & Beach, B. (2013). One facility's experience in reframing nonfeeding into a comprehensive palliative care model. *Journal of Obstetric, Gynecologic, & Neonatal Nursing, 42*(3), 383–389.

Winter, S. M. (2000). Terminal nutrition: Framing the debate for the withdrawal of nutritional support in terminally ill patients. *American Journal of Medicine, 109*(9), 723–726.

Wool, C. (2013). State of the science on perinatal palliative care. *Journal of Obstetric, Gynecologic, and Neonatal Nursing, 42,* 372–382.

World Health Organization. (2014). Global atlas of palliative care at the end of life. Retrieved from file://storage/home/My%20Documents/Global_Atlas_of_Palliative_Care.pdf

Xu, J., Kochanek, K. D., & Tejada-Vera, B. (2009). Deaths: Preliminary data for 2007. *National Vital Statistics Report, 58*(1), 1–51.

Transition to Home and Primary Care

Marina Boykova and Carole Kenner

OVERVIEW

The transition from hospital to home for infants and their families who experienced a neonatal intensive care stay consists of two major components:

- Transition to primary health care settings for medical and developmental follow-up care
- Transition to independent caregiving and parenting

These two major transitions can influence the infant's health to a great extent.

The provision of care postdischarge should be carefully coordinated using an integrated team approach. This section focuses on postdischarge care.

FOLLOW-UP AND POSTDISCHARGE CARE FOR HIGH-RISK INFANTS

BEFORE DISCHARGE

Before high-risk infants can be discharged, they have to meet the following criteria:

- They must be physiologically stable and have mature respiratory control.

■ Oral feedings should be sufficiently established to support appropriate growth.

■ They must be able to maintain normal body temperature in a homelike environment without supplemental heat (American Academy of Pediatrics [AAP], 2008).

Most preterm infants achieve physiologic milestones by 34 to 36 weeks postconceptual age, but feeding and oxygen milestones are achieved last (Bakewell-Sachs, Medoff-Cooper, Escobar, Silber, & Lorch, 2009). Apneic episodes are common in preterm infants; observation up to 10 days without apnea before discharge is recommended (Lorch, Srinivasan, & Escobar, 2011; Nivamat, 2012). Feedings and weight gain are also challenging issues postdischarge (Radtke, 2011; Silberstein et al., 2009; Westerberg et al., 2010). For infants who are in the neonatal intensive care unit (NICU), a weight gain of 15 to 30 g/d must continue for several days (up to 1 week), and it should occur in an open environment (crib) (LaHood & Bryant, 2007; Sherman, Aylward, & Lauriello, 2013). Hearing screening should be performed before discharge in any infant who was hospitalized for more than 5 days. The auditory brainstem response (ABR, automated or not) is preferable so the auditory neuropathy is not missed (Delaney & Ruth, 2012). Also, the first ophthalmic examination should be done in the hospital before discharge: infants between 4 and 6 weeks of chronologic age or between 31 and 33 weeks postmenstrual age should be evaluated for the signs of retinopathy. Age-appropriate immunizations also should be performed before discharge in infants with a prolonged hospital stay (Sherman et al., 2013).

TIMING OF THE FIRST FOLLOW-UP

Some of the high-risk infants should be examined weekly or semimonthly in the immediate period after discharge (American Academy of Pediatrics [AAP] & American College of Obstetricians and Gynecologists [ACOG], 2012). The appointments with primary care providers for high-risk infants should occur in accordance with the needs of the infant (AAP & ACOG, 2012). For preterm infants and infants with an early discharge from the maternity unit (< 48 hours after delivery), AAP (2012) as well as the Canadian Pediatric Society (Whyte, 2010) recommend that the first appointment with the primary care provider should occur in the first 2 to 4 days after discharge.

MONITORING GROWTH OF AN INFANT

The weight gain of 15 to 30 g/d should continue during the first 3 to 4 months of life and then decline to 5 to 15 g/d by age 12 to 18 months (Sherman et al., 2013). Breast-milk fortification, iron, vitamins, folate, and vitamin D supplementation are often necessary for adequate weight gain and growth (LaHood & Bryant, 2007). The University of Iowa, for example, has guidelines for use of these fortifiers. See http://www .uichildrens.org/iowa-neonatology-handbook/feeding/human-milk.

Caloric intake should be monitored as well. For larger and healthier infants, 108 kcal/kg/d can be sufficient for adequate growth. For preterm infants, 120 to 130 kcal/kg/d can be required with increased protein intake (Casey, 2008; Sherman et al., 2013). The infants with specific conditions or dependence on technology will have differing needs than the average NICU graduate. Such infants include late preterm infants (34–37 weeks of gestation), term infants that have had surgery, and infants with chronic lung diseases (CLDs) or congenital heart defects (CHDs) that require surgeries later after initial discharge. Depending on the exact condition, the infant may require more calories due to the work of breathing or digestive problems. With CLD, the infant may require 120 to 150 kcal/kg/d plus increased protein intake, fluid restriction, and electrolyte management, as well as control of vital functions at the home environment by using certain equipment (Sherman et al., 2013). An infant with CHD will often require fluid restriction and may need increased caloric intake as well (for more specific information about CHD, see Chapter 2). In highrisk infants, periodic evaluation of electrolyte status, acid–base balance, and blood tests should be performed; it is important to monitor for low levels of hemoglobin, hematocrit, potassium, and calcium as well as for other components in order to prevent possible development of various problems (such as apnea, anemia, or osteopenia).

Length, head circumference, and weight should always be considered together for proper infant health assessment. Frontal-to-occipital head circumference in preterm infants should be increasing by 0.7 to 1 cm/wk (in term infants 0.5 cm) in the immediate postnatal period; by 12 to 18 months of age the increase in head circumference should decline to 0.1 to 0.4 cm/month (Sherman et al., 2013). The increase in crown-to-heel length should be approximately 0.8 to 2.2 cm/wk in preterm infants (0.7–0.75 in term babies), and by the age of 12 to 18 months it should decline to 0.75 to 1.5 cm/month (Sherman et al., 2013).

MONITORING DEVELOPMENT OF AN INFANT

The neurodevelopmental, behavioral, and sensory status of the high-risk infants should be assessed several times during the first year "to ensure early identification of problems and referral for the appropriate interventions" (AAP & ACOG, 2012). Purdy and Melwak (2012) have suggested the following "red flags" for high-risk infant follow-up:

- Apgar score at 5 minutes of less than 4
- Intraventricular hemorrhage more than Grade II, hydrocephalus
- Hypoxic–ischemic encephalopathy, abnormal neurologic exam (tremors, hypo/hypertonia), seizures
- Hyperbilirubinemia close to exchange transfusion levels
- Severe infections (sepsis, meningitis)
- Hypoglycemia requiring treatment
- Persistent pulmonary hypertension, extracorporeal membrane oxygenation, use of inhaled nitric oxide
- Discharge on apnea monitor and caffeine
- Infant of substance-abusing mother
- Congenital birth defects (such as trisomy 21 or Down syndrome)

Infants who underwent major and minor surgeries (for conditions such as diaphragmatic hernia, major heart defects, pyloric stenosis, and even inguinal hernia) may have developmental delays as well

(Walker, Holland, Halliday, & Badawi, 2012). Several risk factors can be identified for developmental delays in such surgical patients: genetic predisposition, prematurity, premorbid status, age at the time of surgery, duration of the procedure, and type of anesthetic/analgesic agents used (Walker et al., 2012).

FREQUENCY OF INFANT HEALTH CHECKS

Frequency of follow-up visits with primary care practices should be consistent with the AAP's guidelines on preventive care (AAP, 2008; AAP & ACOG, 2012); however, high-risk infants may require more follow-up. Physical examination and measurements, developmental surveillance, and psychosocial and behavioral assessments are recommended at the infancy period at 1, 2, 4, 6, 9, and 12 months. In early childhood, these visits should take place at 15, 18, 24, and 30 months of age, and then at 3 and 4 years of age. Developmental screening using validated and standardized tools is recommended at 9, 18, and 24 or 30 months of age (AAP, 2008). Infants born with birth weight less than 1,500 g, as well as infants with hypoxic–ischemic encephalopathy, seizures, hypoxic cardiorespiratory failure, and multiple congenital anomalies, should have standard neurodevelopmental tests at 1 and 2 years of corrected age. Sherman et al. (2013) also recommend evaluation at the corrected age of 6 months (chronologic age minus weeks born prematurely) in order to identify possible indicators of severe handicaps. The Centers for Disease Control and Prevention (CDC) has information on developmental milestones through the first 5 years of life at http://www.cdc.gov/ncbddd/actearly/milestones/index.html. The CDC also lists early intervention (EI) services by state at http://www.cdc.gov/ncbddd/actearly/parents/states.html.

Ophthalmic examinations should be performed. Infants less than 1,500 g or younger than 32 weeks, as well as infants with an unstable clinical course, should have retinal screening (AAP Section on Ophthalmology, American Academy of Ophthalmology, & American Association for Pediatric Ophthalmology and Strabismus, 2006). According to these recommendations, the first fundal examination for infants older than 22 weeks of gestation should occur between 4 and 6 weeks of chronologic age or between 31 and 33 weeks postmenstrual age (which might happen in the NICU). Follow-up appointments should occur in 1- to 3-week intervals.

Hearing screenings are also needed. After discharge, an infant should be evaluated at 1 and 3 months of age; infants with identified hearing loss should be enrolled in EI programs by 6 months of age (American Academy of Pediatrics [AAP] & Joint Committee on Infant Hearing, 2007). Very early enrollment, in the first 3 months, is beneficial for infants with hearing loss in terms of language development (Vohr et al., 2008). Evaluation by an audiologist every 6 months for the first 3 years of life is recommended (Delaney & Ruth, 2012).

PRIMARY CARE TRANSITION ISSUES

Continuity and coordination of care postdischarge is of vital importance for infant health and development. Appropriate information about primary care providers and referral options should be given to parents at the time of discharge, in order to enhance their adherence with recommendations for infant's health checks, continuation of needed treatments, or discontinuation of medicines, for example. Often, several health care specialists should be involved in the postdischarge care of a high-risk infant. These specialists are nutritionists, dieticians, developmental specialists, speech/language and occupational therapists, pediatric surgeons, pulmonologists, and neurologists. Parents should be provided with information on how to get referral to these health care providers. In addition, immunizations are important, including the prophylactic administration of palivizumab to reduce the frequency and severity of the respiratory syncytial virus (RSV) infection (seasonal prevalence October/November–March/May). Sherman and colleagues discuss important issues in follow-up care of high-risk infants and provide regular updates that can be found at http://emedicine.medscape.com/article/1833812-overview#a1

REFERENCES

American Academy of Pediatrics (AAP). (2008). *Recommendations for preventive pediatric health care*. Retrieved from http://www.aap.org/en-us/professional-resources/practice-support/financing-and-payment/Documents/Recomendations_Preventive_Pediatric_Health_Care.pdf

American Academy of Pediatrics (AAP) & American College of Obstetricians and Gynecologists (ACOG). (2012). *Guidelines for perinatal care* (7th ed.). Elk Grove Village, IL: AAP.

American Academy of Pediatrics (AAP) & Joint Committee on Infant Hearing. (2007). Principles and guidelines for early hearing detection and intervention programs. *Pediatrics, 120*(4), 898–921.

American Academy of Pediatrics (AAP) Section on Ophthalmology, American Academy of Ophthalmology, & American Association for Pediatric Ophthalmology and Strabismus. (2006). Screening examination of premature infants for retinopathy of prematurity. *Pediatrics, 117*(2), 572–576.

Bakewell-Sachs, S., Medoff-Cooper, B., Escobar, G. J., Silber, J. H., & Lorch, S. A. (2009). Infant functional status: The timing of physiologic maturation of premature infants. *Pediatrics, 123*(5), e878–e886.

Casey, P. H. (2008). Growth of low birth weight preterm children. *Seminars in Perinatology, 32*(1), 20–27.

Delaney, A., & Ruth, R. (2012). *Newborn hearing screening.* Retrieved from http://emedicine.medscape.com/article/836646-overview

LaHood, A., & Bryant, C. A. (2007). Outpatient care of the premature infant. *American Family Physician, 76*(8), 1156–1164.

Lorch, S. A., Srinivasan, L., & Escobar, G. J. (2011). Epidemiology of apnea and bradycardia resolution in premature infants. *Pediatrics, 128*(2), e366–e373.

Nivamat, D. J. (2012). *Apnea of prematurity.* Retrieved from http://emedicine.medscape.com/article/974971-overview

Purdy, I. B., & Melwak, M. A. (2012). Who is at risk? High-risk infant follow-up. *Newborn and Infant Nursing Reviews, 12*(4), 221–226.

Radtke, J. V. (2011). The paradox of breastfeeding-associated morbidity among late preterm infants. *Journal of Obstetric, Gynecologic, and Neonatal Nursing, 40*(1), 9–24. doi:10.1111/j.1552-6909.2010.01211.x

Sherman, M. P., Aylward, G. P., & Lauriello, N. F. (2013). *Follow-up of the NICU patient.* Retrieved from http://emedicine.medscape.com/article/1833812-overview#a1

Silberstein, D., Geva, R., Feldman, R., Gardner, J. M., Karmel, B. Z., Roszen, H., & Kuint, J. (2009). The transition to oral feeding in low-risk premature infants: Relation to infant neurobehavioral functioning and mother–infant feeding interaction. *Early Human Development, 85*(3), 157–162.

Vohr, B., Jodoin-Krauzyk, J., Tucker, R., Johnson, M. J., Topol, D., & Ahlgren, M. (2008). Early language outcomes of early-identified infants with permanent hearing loss at 12 to 16 months of age. *Pediatrics, 122*(3), 525–544.

Walker, K., Holland, A. J., Halliday, R., & Badawi, N. (2012). Which high-risk infants should we follow-up and how should we do it? *Journal of Paediatrics and Child Health, 48*(9), 789–793.

Westerberg, A. C., Henriksen, C., Ellingvag, A., Veierod, M. B., Juliusson, P. B., Nakstad, B., … Drevon, C. A. (2010). First year growth among very low birth weight infants. *Acta Paediatrica, 99*(4), 556–562.

Whyte, R. (2010). Safe discharge of the late preterm infant. *Paediatrics and Child Health, 15*(10), 655–666. Retrieved from http://www.ncbi.nlm.nih.gov/pubmed/22131865

CARE FOR PARENTS POSTDISCHARGE

PARENTAL PREPAREDNESS AND EDUCATION

Preparing parents for the transition to home while still in the hospital is vital to the infant's and family's health following discharge. Before discharge, parents, especially mothers, must be evaluated for their own readiness to take over the care of their infant. Appropriate parental teaching about feedings, medicine administration (e.g., inhalers), and home use of oxygen and humidifiers (if prescribed) should be done before discharge. Parents should also receive teaching regarding cardiopulmonary resuscitation and car seat safety. The Children's Hospital of Philadelphia has a good video and information on car seat safety for a newborn and child up to the age of 2 years available at http://www.chop.edu/centers-programs/car-seat-safety-kids/car-seat-safety-by-age/newborn-2-years#.Vwb6OnqRy6Y. The information about major developmental milestones for an infant should be given as well.

PARENTAL EMOTIONAL AND PSYCHOSOCIAL WELL-BEING AFTER DISCHARGE

High-risk and preterm births, infant hospitalization, and specific needs of initially sick or prematurely born infants produce tremendous stress on parents. Parents of high-risk infants often suffer from posttraumatic stress disorder (PTSD). Symptoms include recurrent memories, flashbacks of traumatic events, changes in thinking or mood with very negative tones, avoidance behaviors, trouble sleeping, overreaction to situations, outbursts of anger, and distractibility; such emotions and behaviors are usually centered on situations that bring back bad memories related to infant hospitalization. Parents with PTSD should receive appropriate professional support if needed.

Parents of NICU infants often suffer from depression that has been shown to affect infant development. It is recommended to screen parents for depressive symptoms and other emotional disorders (Hynan, Mounts, & Vanderbilt, 2013). Parents often have prominent anxiety and worries about their infant after discharge that are related to possible illnesses, repeated readmissions, and the development of their infants in the future. Parenting of an infant who survived a life-threatening condition is a challenging task. Attention should be given to the style of parenting in these parents, as they might be prone for overprotective behaviors, compensatory parenting, and vulnerable child syndrome. Parenting disturbances might influence infant development (or even cause the child to have behavioral problems in the future) and the use of health care services postdischarge (overuse of emergency departments, for instance). In severe cases, a parent may require professional support from a counselor or a psychologist.

Health professionals postdischarge should also consider the social consequences of having a medically fragile infant. Parents might suffer from social isolation due to infant vulnerability and parental willingness to protect their infant from possible infections (such as RSV infection). In some instances, social stigmatization may occur depending on the cultural characteristics of the family and surrounding communities. It is important to provide parents with the information about parental support groups available.

Health professionals also should be careful with stigmatization produced by themselves and should not put labels on such parents and infants (such as former preemie, parent of preemie), but rather treat these vulnerable families with dignity and support. Establishing trustful relationships and honest communication are the keys. Contacting parents in the nearest period after discharge, even by telephone call, will help to develop trust, decrease parental anxiety and worry, and possibly prevent unneeded use of health care (for instance, overuse of emergency rooms). Regular contacts with parents are recommended as the means of improving care for infants and parents postdischarge.

Parents postdischarge often report physical exhaustion, sleep deprivation, and tiredness related to caring for an infant with specific needs, numerous appointments, and many treatments. Information about respite care should be given to parents if necessary. There is also a resource for parents who have infants and children with disabilities called Parent Training and Information Centers, which can be found at http://www.parentcenterhub.org/find-your-center. In addition, it is important to remember the financial consequences of having a medically vulnerable infant. With the increasing costs of health care, parents should be advised on the availability of helpful resources in order to decrease their health care costs and out-of-pocket expenses (such as their ability to cover some expenses with Medicaid). Providing parents with such information will also help improve parental adherence with recommendations for infant health check-ups and promote the use of specialized services (speech/language therapy, occupational/physical therapy, EI programs).

In summary, the following strategies can be recommended to help parents and families during the transition to home:

- Discharge teaching and information giving
- Clear communication and coordinated continuity of care postdischarge
- Adequate social and professional support
- Timely health and developmental screening
- Home care

CONCLUSION

This chapter highlights the common issues regarding follow-up care for high-risk infants and parents who are making the transition from the NICU to home and to community-based primary care practices. The recommended screening and follow-up care are outlined.

REFERENCES

Hynan, M. T., Mounts, K. O., & Vanderbilt, D. L. (2013). Screening parents of high-risk infants for emotional distress: Rationale and recommendations. *Journal of Perinatology, 33,* 748–753.

This chapter is adapted from Boykova, M., Kenner, C., & Ellerbee, S. (2013). *Postdischarge care of the newborn, infant, and families.* In C. Kenner & J. W. Lott (Eds.), Comprehensive neonatal nursing care (5th ed., pp. 786–810). New York, NY: Springer Publishing Company.

Common Procedures, Diagnostic Tests, and Lab Values

Common Procedures

Patricia Johnson

OVERVIEW

This chapter outlines the most common procedures done in a neo-natal intensive care unit. The content presents basic information on each procedure.

BLOOD DRAWS

Patricia Johnson

DEFINITION

Blood draws in the newborn are performed to obtain serum or whole blood specimens for laboratory testing.

Blood may be drawn by arterial stick, heel stick, venipuncture, or from a central catheter. Before obtaining any specimen, the patient's identity should be confirmed by institutional protocol, that is con-firm correct patient by name band and number.

CLINICAL INDICATIONS FOR VENIPUNCTURE

This procedure is most commonly used when obtaining over 1 mL of blood from the newborn.

CLINICAL CONTRAINDICATIONS

Any method of blood drawing is contraindicated in the newborn with a known or suspected bleeding diathesis as establishing hemo-stasis may be difficult.

Venipuncture in the absence of bleeding diathesis is not contraindicated unless the skin is infected or if the vessel is potentially needed for central line or peripheral IV.

EQUIPMENT FOR VENIPUNCTURE

The equipment used includes personal protective equipment (PPE) such as gloves, pacifier and sucrose, povidone iodine to cleanse the skin, specimen tubes, 23-gauge butterfly needle, 3-mL syringe, 2 × 2 gauze, saline wipe to remove residual iodine, and tape to hold the gauze or adhesive bandage to cover the puncture site.

STEPS

- Wash hands and assemble equipment.
- Swaddle the infant with the extremity to be punctured exposed or have an additional assistant hold the infant.
- Don gloves and give the baby a pacifier with sucrose.
- Cleanse the site over the vein with povidone iodine and allow to dry.
- Insert a 23-gauge butterfly needle at a 45° angle into the vein.
- Once blood appears in the butterfly tubing, draw the desired volume into a 3-mL syringe.
- Remove the needle and apply pressure to the puncture site with 2 × 2 gauze until hemostasis is attained.
- Cleanse the excess iodine from the skin and, if necessary, apply gauze or an adhesive bandage over the site.

ASSESSMENT AND CARE POST-PROCEDURE

Evaluate for residual bleeding, hematoma, and peripheral circulation.

DOCUMENTATION

Record the site punctured, size of needle used, amount of blood drawn, tolerance of procedure, and residual bleeding, hematoma, or peripheral trauma.

BLOOD DRAW BY ARTERIAL STICK

DEFINITION

This practice refers to obtaining blood from a peripheral artery stick. The most common arteries used are the radial arteries and the posterior tibial arteries. Avoid the use of brachial arteries, which can result in brachial nerve damage; temporal arteries, which can result in temporal nerve damage; or femoral arteries, which can result in osteomyelitis of the hip joint.

CLINICAL INDICATIONS

Arterial puncture is indicated when drawing blood gases or large quantities of blood in a single sample for special tests such as those needed for genetic and metabolic disorders where microvolumes are insufficient for reliable results. Arterial puncture is also indicated for tests where tourniquet application may alter the reliability of results such as serum lactate and ammonia levels.

CLINICAL CONTRAINDICATIONS

Arterial stick should be reserved for special tests as listed. Arteries may only be used for one stick and often cannot be reused. If the artery is necessary for cannulation to establish a peripheral arterial line, then it should not be punctured for one-time labs.

EQUIPMENT

- Sterile PPE gloves
- Pacifier and sucrose, as appropriate
- Facility antiseptic, such as povidone iodine swab
- Sterile 2 × 2 gauze (two)
- Sterile saline wipe

- 23-gauge butterfly needle
- Syringe(s) needed to collect specimen(s)
- Specimen tubes
- Transilluminator light

STEPS

- Identify the infant, verify facility consent obtained if indicated, and inform the parents of the procedure necessity.
- Wash hands, don appropriate PPE, and give the infant a pacifier with sucrose. Swaddle the infant as needed or obtain assistance from another person to contain the infant.
- Perform a modified Allen test to confirm collateral circulation if either radial or posterior tibial arteries are to be used.
- As needed, use transilluminator light to identify the artery.
- Don sterile gloves if the facility requires.
- Cleanse the skin over the artery using facility-approved antiseptic (i.e., povidone iodine, chlorhexidine, or alcohol) and allow to air dry completely.
- Clean off residual antiseptic with sterile saline.
- Insert a 23-gauge butterfly needle, bevel up, at a 30° to 45° angle into the identified artery.
- Connect the syringe when blood flows into the butterfly tubing.
- Draw the desired specimen volume, applying steady slow pressure on the syringe plunger to avoid collapsing the artery.
- Remove the needle and quickly apply pressure over the puncture site using sterile 2 × 2 gauze.
- Maintain pressure until hemostasis is attained.
- Cleanse the residual blood and antiseptic with saline or water wipe and cover the site with gauze taped over the site with mild pressure.
- Monitor for bleeding.

ASSESSMENT AND CARE POST-PROCEDURE

Evaluate circulation distal to the puncture site, site for bleeding, and surrounding area for evidence of hematoma formation.

DOCUMENTATION

Document the Allen test result if indicated, tolerance of the procedure, pain score and pain management, aseptic technique, artery punctured, needle size, success in obtaining specimen, and subsequent bleeding or hematoma at site.

BLOOD DRAW FROM VENIPUNCTURE

DEFINITION

Blood draws in the newborn are performed to obtain serum or whole blood specimens for laboratory testing.

CLINICAL INDICATIONS

This procedure is most commonly used when obtaining over 1 mL of blood from the newborn.

CLINICAL CONTRAINDICATIONS

Any method of blood drawing is contraindicated in the newborn with a known or suspected bleeding diathesis as establishing hemostasis may be difficult.

Venipuncture in the absence of bleeding diathesis is not contraindicated unless the skin is infected or if the vessel is potentially needed for central line or peripheral IV.

EQUIPMENT FOR VENIPUNCTURE

- PPE including gloves
- Pacifier and sucrose
- Povidone iodine to cleanse skin

- Specimen tubes
- 23-gauge butterfly needle
- 3-mL syringe
- 2 × 2 sterile gauze
- Saline wipe to remove residual iodine
- Tape to hold gauze or adhesive bandage to cover the puncture site

STEPS

- Wash hands and assemble equipment.
- Swaddle the infant with the extremity to be punctured exposed or have an additional assistant hold the infant.
- Don gloves and give the baby a pacifier with sucrose.
- Cleanse the site over the vein with povidone iodine and allow to dry.
- Insert a 23-gauge butterfly needle at a 45° angle into the vein.
- Once blood appears in the butterfly tubing, draw the desired volume into a 3-mL syringe.
- Remove the needle and apply pressure to the puncture site with 2 × 2 gauze until hemostasis is attained.
- Cleanse the excess iodine from the skin and, if necessary, apply gauze or adhesive bandage over the site.

ASSESSMENT AND CARE POST-PROCEDURE

Evaluate for residual bleeding, hematoma, and peripheral circulation.

DOCUMENTATION

Record the puncture site, size of needle used, amount of blood drawn, tolerance of procedure, and residual bleeding, hematoma, or peripheral trauma.

BLOOD DRAW FROM A CENTRAL OR PERIPHERAL ARTERIAL CATHETER

DEFINITION

If the infant has a central or peripheral arterial line, blood can be drawn from the catheter without traumatizing the infant by a needle stick.

CLINICAL INDICATIONS

The goal is to obtain a blood specimen without the trauma associated with puncturing a peripheral vein, artery, or heel.

CLINICAL CONTRAINDICATIONS

There is seldom a contraindication to drawing blood from a previously established central or peripheral arterial line. Rapid aspiration or infusion through the catheter is contraindicated in the extremely low-birth-weight infant as changes in blood flow volume can result in intraventricular hemorrhage (IVH).

EQUIPMENT

■ PPE gloves

■ Appropriate-sized syringe to draw specimen

■ Appropriate specimen tubes

■ Syringe to clear line

■ Syringe with flush solution or saline

STEPS

■ Wash hands and don PPE gloves.

■ Clamp the line or close the stopcock, connect the syringe to the catheter or stopcock, interrupt infusion, unclamp the line or open the stopcock, and draw back 0.5 mL to clear the line, then clamp the catheter or close the stopcock. Disconnect and cap this syringe to keep it sterile.

■ Connect the specimen-collecting syringe, unclamp the line or open the stopcock, and draw the required specimen volume. Clamp the line or close the stopcock.

■ Connect the syringe used to clear the line, unclamp or open the stopcock, and return the blood drawn off to clear the line. Clamp the line or close the stopcock.

■ Connect the syringe with flush, unclamp or open the stopcock, and slowly flush the line to clear it of residual blood.

■ Resume infusion.

ASSESSMENT AND CARE POST-PROCEDURE

Verify that line is infusing with fluid without residual blood or air in line.

DOCUMENTATION

Document volume of specimen obtained, lab specimens sent, complications if any.

BLOOD DRAW BY HEEL STICK

DEFINITION

The goal is obtaining a whole blood specimen from a heel puncture.

CLINICAL INDICATIONS

Heel stick blood draw is indicated to obtain small quantities of blood as with capillary blood gas, whole blood glucose screen or Accu-Chek, newborn screening test (blood spot test), or one routine blood assay.

CLINICAL CONTRAINDICATIONS

Heel stick blood draw is contraindicated in the extremely immature newborn, if the perfusion is poor, if the heel has been traumatized, if adequate flow cannot be obtained after puncture, or if a large quantity of blood is needed for a lab test. Excessive squeezing of the heel results in trauma and can alter the integrity of the specimen for testing.

EQUIPMENT

- Personal protective equipment (PPE)
- Heel warmer
- Facility-approved antiseptic (i.e., povidone iodine or alcohol wipe)
- Newborn or premature size lancet
- Microtainer with scoop lid, newborn screen spot paper, or capillary tube
- Two 2 × 2 gauze
- Tape or adhesive bandage

STEPS

- Wash hands.
- Activate the heel warmer, wrap the heel warmer around the heel, and attach with adhesive.
- Don gloves and give the baby a pacifier with sucrose or put the baby to the mother's breast.
- Remove the heel warmer after the heel is warmed (usually 2–3 minutes).
- Cleanse the area of the heel to be punctured with iodine or alcohol swab and wipe off residue with clean gauze.
- Lance either the outer or inner lateral aspect of the heel with a lancet.

- Gently squeeze the foot to produce blood flow from the punctured site.
- Obtain a specimen.
- Cover the puncture site with clean gauze and apply pressure for hemostasis.
- Apply taped gauze or adhesive bandage over the puncture site.

ASSESSMENT AND CARE POST-PROCEDURE

Examine the punctured heel for trauma from squeezing and persistent bleeding from the puncture site.

DOCUMENTATION

Document the heel punctured and site of puncture, specimen obtained, infant tolerance, and visible trauma or residual bleeding from the site.

INTRAVASCULAR CANNULATION

INSERTION OF INTRAVENOUS CATHETER

Patricia Johnson

DEFINITION

Intravenous catheters involve insertion of a catheter into a peripheral vein for infusing intravenous fluids, medications, blood, or blood products.

CLINICAL INDICATIONS

These are placed when there is a need for intravenous access for medication, fluid, or blood product infusion.

CLINICAL CONTRAINDICATIONS

Contraindications include circulatory compromise of the surrounding tissue or infection of skin overlying the vein.

EQUIPMENT

- Flat surface with adequate heat source to prevent cold stress
- Swaddling blanket
- Gloves
- Pacifier
- Sucrose
- Facility-approved skin disinfectant (povidone iodine, alcohol)
- 22- to 27-gauge IV catheter
- T-connector
- 3-mL syringe with normal saline for infusion to flush catheter
- Single-use tourniquet or latex-free 1/4-inch cut and cleaned rubber band
- Transparent bio occlusive dressing
- Securing adhesive tape 1/2 to 1 inch
- Sterile 2 × 2 gauze
- Cotton balls, arm board as needed
- Transilluminator to visualize vein

STEPS

- Wash hands and don gloves.
- Confirm the infant's identity and need for IV access from the provider.
- Position the infant on a warm flat surface.
- Swaddle as necessary or obtain assistance to stabilize the infant during the procedure.
- Provide a pacifier with optional sucrose.
- Flush the T-connector with saline flush and keep connections sterile.
- Identify the vein with optional use of transilluminator: plantar surface of hand or foot, scalp, forearm, or leg. Veins on the hands

and feet are often easier to see and access. Avoid using antecubital and saphenous veins that may be needed for blood draws or percutaneous central line access if IV access is required longer than 1 week.

- ■ Apply a tourniquet proximal to the vein to dilate the vein.

- ■ Cleanse the skin over the vein.

- ■ Insert the catheter bevel up. Once blood flashes into the catheter reservoir, thread the plastic part of the catheter into the vein and retract the needle.

- ■ Remove the tourniquet.

- ■ Connect the T-connector and flush the catheter to verify patency.

- ■ If unable to flush or the tissue proximal to the catheter tip becomes distended with fluid, apply pressure above the catheter tip and pull the catheter out, applying pressure to the insertion site for hemostasis.

- ■ Attempt again with a new catheter in an alternative location. Each person should attempt insertion only twice, after which another clinician should make an attempt.

- ■ Once the catheter is inserted and flushes easily, secure with the transparent dressing and tape. Use the other securing or limb stabilizing devices to protect the IV from dislodging when the baby moves.

ASSESSMENT AND CARE POST-PROCEDURE

Verify the patency of the IV immediately after insertion, after securing, and before attaching infusion equipment. Monitor the integrity of the surrounding skin and insertion site frequently to avoid excessive extravasation of infusate into the surrounding tissue if accidentally dislodged. Monitor for signs of phlebitis or other evidence of infection.

DOCUMENTATION

Document the site of insertion, number of attempts, infant's tolerance, blood loss, and complications.

CHEST TUBE INSERTION

Katherine M. Newnam

DEFINITION

Placement of a tube is done to remove air from the plural space with negative pressure set-up using suction.

CLINICAL INDICATIONS

■ Tension pneumothorax with cardiorespiratory compromise

■ Pneumothorax compromising ventilation and oxygen delivery

■ Drainage of plural effusion

■ Obtain fluid for diagnostic purposes

CLINICAL CONTRAINDICATIONS

■ Skin integrity at site and coagulation status

■ Possible complications include: bleeding, infection, pain, and nerve injury. These occur in less than 2% of all neonates who undergo chest tube insertion.

EQUIPMENT

■ Cleaning solution (2% chlorhexidine, povidone-iodine)

■ Prepackaged chest tube tray:

  ▪ Sterile drape

  ▪ Suture

  ▪ Curved hemostats

  ▪ Scalpel

  ▪ Scissors

  ▪ Needle holder

■ Chest tube (10 French for < 2 kg or 12 French for > 2 kg)

- Sterile water (to clean off cleaning solution following procedure)
- Pain medications and/or sedation as indicated
- Sterile gloves
- Sterile gown
- Mask/hat
- Positioning aids (blanket rolls)
- Pleur-Evac or similar system

STEPS

- Locate and assemble supplies.
- Position the patient with positioning aids to elevate the affected chest (approximately 45°–60°).
- Locate the site (second to third intercostal space at the midclavicular line or midaxillary at the 4th–6th intercostal space).
- Administer pain medications/sedation as indicated.
- Wash hands, don sterile gloves, and organize supplies in a sterile fashion.
- Cleanse the area.
- Drape the patient.
- Administer 1% lidocaine to anesthetize the area.
- Make a small incision in the skin over the rib.
- Insert a closed curved hemostat into the incision and spread the tissues open to the depth of the rib.
- Then puncture the pleura with the hemostat (you may hear air escape).
- Insert the chest tube through the opening (with or without a trocar) and use the hemostat to guide the tube depth to about 2 to 4 cm based on the infant's size.
- Attach the chest tube to the closed suction system (Pleur-Evac).
- Suture the chest tube in place and dress the site as indicated.

ASSESSMENT AND CARE POST-PROCEDURE

■ Monitor vital signs and oxygen saturations.

■ Obtain follow-up chest x-ray.

■ Monitor for additional pain management and complications.

DOCUMENTATION

■ Date and time of the procedure

■ Location (site of entry)

■ Clinical indications

■ Equipment used (including size of the chest tube)

■ Vital signs prior to and following procedure

■ Pain control measures (medication/comfort care)

■ Number of attempts

■ Patient tolerance to procedure/problems encountered

■ Fluid/air removal

■ Blood loss

■ Chest AP results prior to and following procedure

■ Stabilization plan

NEEDLE ASPIRATION

Katherine M. Newnam

DEFINITION

The emergent percutaneous insertion of a needle for the removal of fluid, blood, or air from the plural space.

CLINICAL INDICATIONS

Clinical indications include symptoms of cardiorespiratory compromise or failure, as well as the size of the air leak (pneumothorax) and general condition.

CLINICAL CONTRAINDICATIONS

Other considerations are skin integrity at the site and coagulation status. Possible complications include: bleeding, infection, pain, and nerve injury. The risk factors for therapeutic needle thoracentesis are less than 1% of all neonates undergoing this procedure.

EQUIPMENT

- Needle (#23- #25-gauge butterfly needle or #22- #24-gauge angiocath)
- Cleaning solution (2% chlorhexidine, povidone-iodine)
- Sterile water (to clean off cleaning solution following procedure)
- T-connector
- Three-way stopcock
- 10- or 20-mL syringe
- Sedation as indicated
- Sterile gloves
- Sterile 2 × 2 gauze
- Sterile drape
- Positioning aids (blanket rolls)

STEPS

- Place the patient in a supine position with the positioning aid under the affected side.
- Maintain thermoregulation and monitor vital signs/oxygen saturation during the procedure.
- Assemble equipment (if using an angiocath, attach the T-connector to the end of the IV catheter and the three-way stopcock to the end of the T-connector. The aspiration syringe can be attached to the stopcock. If using the butterfly needle, attach the

stopcock to the end of the tubing and the syringe to the stopcock for aspiration).

■ Locate landmarks at the second intercostal space, midclavicular line.

■ Wash hands, don sterile gloves, and organize supplies in a sterile fashion.

■ Drape the patient.

■ Cleanse the area.

■ Insert the needle firmly into the identified space, advancing it until a "pop" is felt.

■ Use the syringe to aspirate air and/or fluid from the plural space.

■ Secure the needle in place with dressing and monitor for an accumulation of air leak.

ASSESSMENT AND CARE POST-PROCEDURE

■ Monitor vital signs and oxygen saturations.

■ Set up for chest tube insertion.

DOCUMENTATION

■ Date and time of the procedure

■ Indications

■ Equipment used

■ Vital signs prior to and following procedure

■ Pain control measures (medication/comfort care)

■ Number of attempts

■ Patient tolerance to procedure

■ Chest AP results prior to and following procedure

ENDOTRACHEAL INTUBATION

Katherine M. Newnam

DEFINITION

The placement of an orotracheal or nasotracheal tube into the trachea between the glottis and carina in order to provide artificial ventilation.

CLINICAL INDICATIONS

- To provide respiratory support through mechanical ventilation
- To obtain sputum sample for culture
- To clear the trachea of meconium
- To alleviate airway obstruction or subglottic stenosis
- To administer surfactant
- To inspect the lower airway

EQUIPMENT

- Sterile suction catheter (8 or 10 French to clear oral secretions)
- Suction canister and apparatus
- Endotracheal tube (see Table 14.1)
- Laryngoscope handle with appropriate-sized blade and light source (see Table 14.1)
- Bag and mask or T-piece for ventilation
- Oxygen source
- Stylet
- Gloves
- CO_2 detector
- Securing device (tape, neobar, etc.)
- Meconium aspirator (as condition warrants)
- Pulse oximeter with heart rate monitor
- Pre-procedural pain management if route available

TABLE 14.1 Endotracheal Tube Size and Placement		
Infant's Weight (kg)	**Tube Size (mm)**	**Insertion Depth (cm)**
< 1	2.5	< 7
1–2	3	7–8
2–3	3.5	8–9
> 3	3.5–4	> 9

Source: Data from the American Heart Association Emergency Cardiac Care Committee and Subcommittees (1992) and Kattwinkel (2011).

STEPS

■ Prepare and check the working order of all equipment (prior to infant delivery).

■ Place the infant supine in a "sniffing position."

■ Suction the oropharynx to clear secretions.

■ Provide artificial ventilations until the heart rate, oxygen saturation, and color are stable and monitor throughout the procedure.

■ Hold the laryngoscope with your left hand and gently insert the blade into the neonate's mouth.

■ Sweep the tongue to the side to visualize the field.

■ Lift the blade vertically to visualize the glottis by vertically lifting the epiglottis.

■ Gentle external pressure may be required over the thyroid cartilage to visualize vocal cords.

■ Pass the endotracheal tube along the right side of the mouth and through the cords as they open during inspiration.

■ Advance the tube into the trachea to the appropriate level (see Table 14.1).

■ Use a CO_2 detector to confirm placement and auscultate lung fields for breath sounds and symmetry.

■ Secure the endotracheal tube (ETT) with the securing device.

■ Obtain a chest x-ray to confirm the proper placement of the ETT and evaluate the lung fields.

ASSESSMENT AND CARE POST-PROCEDURE

Monitor for complications, including tracheal perforation, esophageal perforation, improper tube position, tube obstruction, or dislodgement. Provide continued respiratory support and monitoring. Use blood gas analysis serial x-rays as indicated.

DOCUMENTATION

The procedure notes should describe the rationale for the procedure, method, medications administered, equipment used, and infant tolerance of the procedure. Vital signs following the procedure should be documented with a plan for continued care.

REFERENCES

American Heart Association Emergency Cardiac Care Committee and Subcommittees. (1992, October 28). Guidelines for cardiopulmonary resuscitation and emergency cardiac care. Emergency Cardiac Care Committee and Subcommittees, American Heart Association. Part I. Introduction. *JAMA*, *268*(16), 2171–2183.

Kattwinkel, J. (2011). Neonatal resuscitation textbook (6th ed.). Elk Grove Village, IL: American Academy of Pediatrics and American Heart Association. Retrieved from http://shop.aap.org/Textbook-of-Neonatal-Resuscitation-6th-Edition

INSERTION OF PERCUTANEOUS INTRAVENOUS CENTRAL CATHETER

Elizabeth (Liz) Sharpe

DEFINITION

A peripherally inserted central catheter (PICC) is a long catheter inserted into a peripheral vein, then threaded to place the catheter tip at the superior vena cava (SVC) or inferior vena cava (IVC).

For catheters inserted into the veins of the upper extremity or scalp, the optimal catheter tip location for central placement is in the SVC (FDA, 1989; INS, 2011; Pettit & Wyckoff, 2007). For catheters inserted into the veins in the lower extremities, the optimal catheter tip location for central placement is in the IVC between the right atrium and diaphragm (Pettit & Wyckoff, 2007).

A midline catheter is a long catheter inserted into a peripheral vein, then threaded to

- Below the axilla if inserted in an upper extremity
- The external jugular vein if inserted in a scalp vein
- Below the groin if inserted in a lower extremity

CLINICAL INDICATIONS

The Centers for Disease Control and Prevention (CDC) recommend that patients who require in excess of 6 days of therapy should be considered for more than a peripheral intravenous device, that is, either a PICC or midline catheter. Early assessment for vascular access needs supports minimizing the number of attempts and trauma to the patient and increased availability of sites and success. Clinical indications for long-term venous access include:

- Hyperosmolar medications (> 600 mOsm/L)
- Parenteral nutrition
- Prolonged intravenous therapy
- Irritant or vesicant medications

CLINICAL CONTRAINDICATIONS

General contraindications include:

- Uncontrolled bacteremia or fungemia
- Family withholding consent
- Coagulopathy or thrombocytopenia
- Inability to identify an appropriate vein

Site selection considerations include:

■ Fracture and/or birth injury

■ Decreased venous return

■ Skin breakdown

■ Site or vessel needed for another purpose

Some examples of situations where the site may be needed for another purpose include when an infant is a candidate for a ventricular reservoir or ventriculo-peritoneal shunt and scalp vessels should be avoided. Similarly, for an extracorporeal membrane oxygenation (ECMO) candidate, the right upper extremity should be avoided. In infants with congenital heart defects, consider the site of intended future surgeries.

EQUIPMENT

■ Hat, mask

■ Sterile gown

■ Sterile gloves

■ Sterile tape measure

■ Sterile tourniquet

■ Sterile drapes for maximum sterile barrier precautions

■ Catheter

■ Introducer

■ Scissors and/or trim tool

■ Sterile forceps

■ Skin antiseptic (chlorhexidine gluconate or povidone iodine)

■ Sterile flush solution

■ Sterile 10-mL syringes (2)

■ Sterile extension tubing

■ Sterile gauze

■ Sterile water or saline

- Sterile skin-closure strips or adhesive padded foam
- Transparent dressing and stabilization device (if available)

PROCEDURE STEPS

Personnel inserting central venous catheters should receive specialized training upon their hire, annually thereafter, and when this task is added to their job responsibilities.

- Evaluate needs and duration of intended therapy.
- Discuss with the family and obtain informed consent.
- Perform physical assessment for vein selection.
- Determine the catheter insertion length by measuring the distance from the intended insertion site along the vein track to SVC for upper extremity or scalp vessels or to IVC for lower extremity vessels.
- Gather the central line kit, catheter, introducer, sterile gloves, maximum sterile barriers, and other needed supplies.
- Prepare the patient for the procedure, including pharmacologic and developmental comfort measures.
- Don hair covering and mask.
- Perform hand hygiene.
- Prepare a sterile field and assemble equipment.
- Prepare the catheter by flushing and trimming to the premeasured length.
- Position the patient as developmentally appropriate.
- Prepare the insertion site by disinfecting the skin with an antimicrobial agent. Allow the antiseptic to dry on the skin according to the manufacturer's directions. Chlorhexidine gluconate or povidone iodine may be used. Chlorhexidine may be used with caution in premature infants or infants younger than 2 months of age. These products may cause irritation or chemical burns.
- Utilize maximum sterile barrier precautions to isolate the extremity or insertion site.
- Apply a sterile tourniquet.

■ Insert the introducer bevel up at a 15° to 30° angle and observe for blood return. Remove the needle from over the sheath introducers.

■ Remove the tourniquet.

■ Place the catheter in an introducer lumen using nontoothed forceps and a thread catheter in small increments.

■ Remove the introducer per manufacturer's directions.

■ Apply gentle pressure to the site until bleeding stops.

■ Verify the inserted catheter length and any externally lying catheter.

■ If a catheter with stylet is used, remove the stylet slowly at this time.

■ Aspirate to confirm blood return and flush to confirm patency.

■ Attach Luer-lock extension tubing if not part of the catheter apparatus, with care to eliminate air entry into the tubing.

■ Secure the catheter temporarily with skin closure tapes while awaiting radiographic confirmation.

■ Confirm the catheter tip location in SVC or IVC.

■ Reposition the catheter if not in SVC or IVC.

■ Obtain radiographic reconfirmation of the catheter tip location.

■ Remove povidone iodine from the skin and allow to dry.

■ Secure the catheter to the skin and apply a sterile transparent occlusive dressing.

■ Document the procedure, including any repositioning, radiographic confirmation, premedication, catheter specifics including brand and lot number, trimmed length, inserted length, and patient tolerance.

ASSESSMENT AND CARE POST-PROCEDURE

■ Assess the condition of the insertion site hourly including an evaluation of dressing integrity, erythema, leakage, or exposed catheter.

■ Confirm that the catheter tip location (central or midline) correlates with the properties of the infusate (osmolarity, irritant, or vesicant).

- Limit dextrose concentration to no greater than D12.5% if the catheter tip location is not central in SVC or IVC.
- Change the dressing when it becomes loose, nonocclusive, moist, soiled, or according to manufacturer's directions.
- Maintain adequate minimum infusion rates to prevent occlusion.
- Flush with no smaller than a 5- or 10-mL syringe or per manufacturer's directions (INS, 2011).
- If heparin locking, flush with 1 mL normal saline and 1 mL 10 units/mL heparin every 6 hours (INS, 2011).

DOCUMENTATION

- Indication for the procedure
- Consent and parent education
- Correct patient identification
- Patient preparation including pain management strategies and response
- Site preparation including type of antiseptic
- Brand, type, gauge/size, lot number, and number of lumens of catheter
- Style, size of introducer
- Presence of stylet
- Description of procedure including visualization technology
- Insertion site
- Number of attempts
- Length of catheter and, if trimmed, original length and trimmed length
- Inserted length of catheter and externally lying catheter
- Securement method including stabilization and dressing type
- Complications encountered and any repositioning required

■ Initial and final radiographic confirmation of catheter tip location

■ Patient tolerance of procedure

■ Date, time, and name of clinician performing the procedure

In addition to patient-specific documentation in the health record, some institutions require completion of a standardized tool for adherence to recommended practices. Some of these components include: hand hygiene, maximum sterile barrier precautions, chlorhexidine for skin antisepsis, and continued daily evaluation of line necessity.

REFERENCES

Food and Drug Administration Task Force. (1989). Precautions necessary with central venous catheters. FDA Drug Bulletin, July (15).

Infusion Nurses Society (INS). (2011). Policies and procedures for infusion nursing (4th ed.). Norwood, MA: INS.

Pettit, J., & Wyckoff, M. (2007). *Peripherally inserted central catheters guidelines for practice* (2nd ed.). Glenview, IL: National Association of Neonatal Nurses.

INSERTION OF UMBILICAL CATHETER

Patricia Johnson

DEFINITION

Umbilical artery and umbilical vein catheters are often inserted into sick and premature newborns admitted to intensive care nurseries to facilitate vascular access for lab testing, continuous monitoring, and infusion of intravascular fluids.

CLINICAL INDICATIONS

■ **An umbilical artery catheter** is indicated in infants who require blood gas monitoring, central blood pressure monitoring, and possibly frequent blood sampling for laboratory specimens. It is generally accepted that if the infant requires mechanical ventilation and/or supplemental oxygen at greater than 0.4 FiO_2, umbilical artery catheters are indicated for blood gas monitoring.

■ **An umbilical vein catheter** is indicated for stable vascular access in infants who require uninterrupted glucose infusions, medication drip infusions, and hyperosmolar parenteral nutrition.

CLINICAL CONTRAINDICATIONS

■ **Umbilical artery catheter contraindications:** Contraindications for umbilical arterial catheter insertion include local vascular compromise, peritonitis, necrotizing enterocolitis, omphalitis, omphalocele, and acute abdomen etiology.

■ **Umbilical vein catheter contraindications:** Contraindications for umbilical venous catheter insertion include peritonitis, necrotizing enterocolitis, omphalitis, and omphalocele.

EQUIPMENT

■ Cardiorespiratory monitor

■ Radiant warmer

■ PPE including sterile gloves, sterile gown, mask, and hat for inserter

■ PPE for assistant including sterile gown, gloves, mask, and hat

■ Measuring tape

■ Facility antiseptic, povidone iodine

■ Sterile umbilical tape

■ Sterile curved hemostats (two), iris forceps, scissors, straight forceps, needle holder, pick ups

■ Sterile towels (two or three)

■ Sterile scalpel #11 or #15

- Umbilical catheters: 3.5 French for infants less than 1,200 g and 5 French for infants greater than 1,200 g with optional duel lumen catheter for insertion in umbilical venus catheter (UVC)
- Sterile three-way stopcocks for each catheter with neutral clave for second port of optional dual lumen catheter
- Three sterile 3-mL syringes, one sterile 5- to 6-mL syringe, one sterile heparinized blood gas syringe
- Two sterile needles
- Sterile saline
- 3.0 or 4.0 silk suture with noncutting needle
- Hydrocolloid
- Bio occlusive dressing
- Exam light
- Immobilizing device, diaper with tape for across legs, gauze with tape or safety pins or posy straps
- Transducer set up
- Sterile saline wipes
- Optional use of commercial umbilical catheter insertion tray

STEPS

- Wash hands and don PPE gloves.
- Identify the patient and confirm consents available as appropriate.
- Immobilize extremities to provide optimal exposure of umbilicus.
- Assist inserter with PPE gloves.
- Perform time-out procedure.
- Don sterile PPE gloves.
- Prepare a sterile field with an open commercial tray or sterile towel.
- Open selected catheters and drop on sterile field.

- Open stopcocks and drop on the sterile field.

- Open syringes and drop on the sterile field.

- Hold the saline vials for the inserter to aspirate saline in one 3-mL syringe and one 5- to 6-mL syringe.

- Hold the umbilical cord vertical with a straight hemostat to allow for adequate antiseptic application on and around the cord.

- After the inserter cuts the cord, remove the cord and discard or, if requested, put aside for the parent.

- After the catheters are inserted and sutured in place, confirm the insertion length.

- Obtain any specimens obtained, label, and send them to the laboratory.

- Perform a whole blood glucose screen.

- Call for an ordered x-ray to confirm position.

- Flush the catheters every 5 minutes with a small amount of saline to maintain patency until an x-ray is obtained and the catheter tip position is confirmed.

- Adjust the catheter out as needed and as directed by the inserter.

- Clean the excess antiseptic from the skin around the umbilicus.

- Apply hydrocolloid around the cord and secure the catheters with transparent adhesive dressing.

- Attach a pressure transducer to the arterial line.

- Attach the designated fluid to infuse in the catheter at a designated rate.

- Discard used supplies and equipment as appropriate.

ASSESSMENT AND CARE POST-PROCEDURE

Monitor circulation, maintain continuous infusion, and use appropriate care to maintain the sterility of the connections and prevent exposure to contaminated surfaces.

DOCUMENTATION

Document time-outs, consents, patient tolerance, complications, insertion length for both catheters, adjustment of catheter insertion length as appropriate, time started infusion fluid and rates, and specimens obtained and resulted.

URINARY CATHETER

Patricia Johnson

DEFINITION

Urinary catheters are tools used for straight bladder catheterization and Foley catheterization.

CLINICAL INDICATIONS

Urinary catheters are inserted into the bladder via the urethra to obtain urine one time to relieve urinary retention, evaluate the presence of urine, obtain a sterile urine specimen for culture, or inject contrast for an image study of the bladder and urination (cystogram). Indwelling catheters are used to monitor continuous urine output or when bladder function may be compromised by medications or soft tissue obstructing normal urination.

CLINICAL CONTRAINDICATIONS

Contraindications include perineal infection that may contaminate the urinary tract by introducing infection into the bladder. Risks of the procedure include the development of a catheter-associated urinary tract infection (CAUDI) or trauma to the urethra or bladder.

EQUIPMENT

■ Urinary catheter, silicone or polyurethane, should be soft and of the appropriate size (3.5–8 French). For infants less than 1,000 g, use a 3.5 French catheter; for infants who are 1,000 to 1,800 g, use a 5 French catheter; and for infants over 1,800 g, use an 8 French catheter. Catheters should be balloon free as balloons can result in pressure trauma to the fragile urethra.

■ Sterile specimen cup/receptacle for one-time catheterization

■ A sterile closed drainage system if using indwelling catheters

■ Sterile towel

■ Povidone-iodine swabs (aseptic swabs)

■ Water-soluble lubricant

■ Saline or water wipes

■ Sterile gloves

■ Pacifier

■ Sucrose

STEPS

■ Prepare equipment.

■ Wash hands.

■ Place the infant supine on a flat surface with adequate thermal maintenance.

■ Swaddle the upper body and/or obtain assistance of someone to contain the infant and provide a pacifier with optional sucrose.

■ Remove the diaper and place a pad or clean diaper under the buttocks.

■ Abduct the thighs in a frog position to fully expose the perineum.

■ Don sterile gloves.

■ Place the catheter tip in the sterile lubricant.

■ Place one sterile drape under the baby and one drape over the thighs and abdomen.

- Expose the urethra:
  - In the male newborn, if uncircumcised, retract the foreskin with the nondominant hand to reveal the meatus.
  - In the female newborn, spread the labia majora with the nondominant hand to reveal the urethral meatus superior to the vaginal opening.
- Cleanse the exposed urethral opening area with aseptic solution on a swab (i.e., povidone-iodine).
- Take the catheter in the dominant (sterile) hand and insert it into the urethra meatus, advancing until urine flow is evident in the tubing. If obstruction is encountered, do not attempt to force it through the obstruction. Alter the angle of insertion but then discontinue and alert the provider.
  - Insert the catheter a maximum of 2 in. (5 cm) in a male newborn who is less than 750 g and 2.3 in. (6 cm) in a male who weighs more than 750 g.
  - Insert the catheter a maximum of 1 in. (2.5 cm) in a female newborn who is less than 750 g and 2 in. (5 cm) in a female who weighs more than 750 g.
- Once the catheter in in place, obtain a sterile specimen or connect to the closed drainage system.
- If the catheter is intended to be indwelling, secure with bio-occlusive dressing.

ASSESSMENT AND CARE POST-PROCEDURE

Note the length of the catheter extending from the meatus. Assess the perineum for trauma, and the urine flow if using an indwelling catheter. Assess for evidence of blood or stool in the urine, or if urine is leaking around the catheter.

DOCUMENTATION

Document the length of the catheter used and how far it is inserted in centimeters, tolerance of the procedure, securing of indwelling catheter, amount of specimen collected and labeled, and lab assays requested.

RESUSCITATION AND STABILIZATION

Jana L. Pressler

DEFINITION OF RESUSCITATION

Resuscitation refers to emergency lifesaving procedures to bring someone who is unconscious or close to death back to a viable condition (Editors of Webster's New World College Dictionaries, 2014). Resuscitative efforts are completed to revive someone when his or her heart has stopped beating and/or he or she has stopped breathing (Hazinski, Samson, & Schexnayder, 2010). Permanent brain damage or death can occur within minutes of the heart stopping or breathing stopping, indicating that the individual is in need of immediate actions to restore his or her life.

Resuscitation is short for *cardiopulmonary resuscitation* (CPR) (Field et al., 2010). CPR is a combination of chest compressions and rescue breathing. Chest compressions keep oxygen-rich blood flowing until the victim's heartbeat can be adequately restored. Rescue breathing is a way of providing oxygen to a victim's lungs until breathing can be restored. Guidelines for CPR have been established by the International Liaison Committee on Resuscitation (ILCOR). The pediatric working group of the ILCOR Committee who discussed and reviewed neonatal resuscitation consisted of representatives from nine groups:

■ American Heart Association (AHA)

■ European Resuscitation Council (ERC)

■ Heart and Stroke Foundation of Canada (HSFC)

■ Australian Resuscitation Council (ARC)

■ New Zealand Resuscitation Council (NZRC)

■ Resuscitation Council of Southern Africa (RCSA)

■ Council of Latin America for Resuscitation (CLAR)

■ Steering Committee of the American Academy of Pediatrics (AAP)

■ World Health Organization (WHO)

According to ILCOR, CPR involves chest compressions at least 5 cm (2 in.) deep and at a rate of at least 100 per minute. A rescuer might provide artificial respirations (breaths) by exhaling into the victim's mouth or through use of a bag-valve mask applied to the nose and mouth that pushes air into a victim's lungs. The current AHA guidelines emphasize that the administration of high-quality chest compressions should take precedence over artificial respirations, especially for untrained rescuers administering CPR (Hupfl, Selig, &, Nagele, 2010).

Depending on their health status, neonates can require CPR at the time of delivery and/or any time throughout the first postnatal month. Approximately 5% to 10% of newborns require some degree of CPR at birth (e.g., stimulation to breathe), with approximately 1% to 10% of babies born in a hospital reportedly requiring assisted ventilation (Perlman et al., 2010). WHO has estimated that birth asphyxia accounts for 19% of the five million neonatal deaths occurring worldwide each year. WHO notes that neonatal outcomes might be improved through implementation of CPR training for more than one million infants annually (WHO, 1995).

Based on those statistics, it is critical that the knowledge and skills required to complete CPR techniques successfully be taught to all neonatal care providers. Although oftentimes newborns' needs for CPR are predictable, newborns' needs for CPR also occur without warning. Knowing this vital fact can alert caregivers of CPR's primary importance, especially in health care facilities that do not routinely provide neonatal intensive care; CPR already would be administered more frequently in these facilities.

CLINICAL INDICATIONS

CPR is an emergency procedure required to preserve intact brain function when a person's heart has stopped beating, and/or a person has stopped breathing. CPR is indicated for any unresponsive neonate who is not breathing, or is breathing only in agonal gasps (Handley et al., 2005). If a neonate has a pulse but is not breathing (respiratory arrest), artificial respirations are needed. However, due to the difficulty that untrained rescuers have in assessing the presence or absence of a pulse correctly, the AHA guidelines for CPR recommend that untrained rescuers not be instructed to check for a pulse, while trained rescuers have the option to check for a pulse (Hupfl et al., 2010).

Stabilization of a person's vital signs is required when a person's heart is not performing well enough to adequately circulate oxygenated blood and/or a person is not breathing adequately such that he or she is receiving sufficient oxygen and exhaling carbon dioxide. All neonates who need full resuscitation must subsequently be brought to a stabilized condition. A neonate might not require full resuscitation, yet still need to have his or her vital signs stabilized. Or a neonate might require resuscitation and need postresuscitation stabilization (for more details, see the section Definition of Stabilization).

CLINICAL CONTRAINDICATIONS

CPR is likely to be effective only if implemented *within 6 minutes after circulation stops* (Cummins, Eisenberg, Hallstrom, & Litwin, 1985). That timed effectiveness reflects the fact that permanent brain cell damage occurs after 6 minutes even if fresh blood infuses the cells. The brain cells have been shown to become dormant in as little as 4 to 6 minutes in an oxygen-deprived environment and cannot survive the reintroduction of oxygen in a traditional resuscitation. Additional research is needed to determine the role that CPR, electroshock, and new advanced gradual resuscitation techniques have on brain cell damage and the timing of brain cell damage (Athanasuleas, Buckberg, Allen, Beyersdorf, & Kirsh, 2006).

One exception to the 6-minute CPR timing rule is cardiac arrest that occurs in conjunction with exposure to very cold temperatures. Hypothermia appears to protect the brain by slowing down metabolic and physiologic processes, greatly decreasing tissues' need for oxygen (Advanced Life Support Task Force of the International Liaison Committee on Resuscitation, 2003).

Noninitiation of resuscitation

The delivery of extremely premature infants and infants with severe congenital anomalies raises questions about whether to, and to what extent, initiate resuscitation (Byrne, Tyebkhan, &, Laing,

1994; Danzl & Pozos, 1994; Eich, Bräuer, & Kettler, 2005). In 1999, noninitiation of resuscitation in the delivery room was deemed to be appropriate for newborns with (a) confirmed gestation less than 23 weeks, (b) birth weight less than 400 g, (c) anencephaly, (d) confirmed trisomy 13, or (e) confirmed trisomy 18 (*Class IIb*). The 1999 data suggested that resuscitation of those newly born infants was very unlikely to result in survival without severe disability, if survival at all (Davies & Reynolds, 1992; Landwirth, 1993).

Successful management of younger, smaller, and sicker newborns is advancing on an ongoing and steady basis. To complicate the decision of which neonates should receive attempts to resuscitate further, antenatal information might be incomplete and/or unreliable. In situations of uncertain prognosis, including uncertain gestational age, resuscitation options include a trial of resuscitation and then discontinuation after a thorough assessment of the infant. In cases not highly likely to result in survival or survival without severe disability, initiation of resuscitation at the time of delivery does not mandate continued resuscitation and stabilization.

Noninitiation of resuscitative support and subsequent withdrawal of resuscitative support are considered to be ethically equivalent. However, the subsequent withdrawal of resuscitative support allows care providers more time to assimilate complete clinical information and provide counseling to the infant's family.

Discontinuation of resuscitation

Resuscitation is not required if a legal guardian has given the physician an advance directive to write a "do not resuscitate" or "allow a natural death" order due to the fetus or neonate having a known fatal health condition. Ongoing evaluation and discussion with parents and the health care team should guide continuation versus withdrawal of support. The ILCOR recommend that local discussions take place to formulate guidelines consistent with local resources and outcome data.

ETHICS

National and local protocols should direct the procedures that are followed. It is imperative that resuscitation procedures, protocols, policies, and neonatal outcomes be reviewed regularly by the primary neonatal care providers with updates shared as needed pertaining to changes made in resuscitation, delivery room, and intensive care practices.

SETTING

A clean and warm environment is best for conducting any infant resuscitations. Specific risk factors can predict that certain infants will require resuscitation; however, not all infants' resuscitation needs are predictable. Thus, to be prepared and safe, it is important to maintain the cleanliness and warmth of all hospital settings in case an infant's needs warrant resuscitation.

EQUIPMENT

No equipment is needed to perform basic CPR of a neonate or infant. One-person or two-person CPR can be performed without equipment. However, supplemental oxygen, an oxygen mask, an oxygenation saturation monitor, an endotracheal tube, an intubation handle and blade, IV supplies, and medications can be useful in both expediting and facilitating neonatal resuscitation. Wherever deliveries occur, a complete inventory of resuscitation equipment and supplies should be maintained and accessible (Perlman et al., 2010).

Important note

Additionally, according to the 2010 guidelines for CPR and emergency cardiovascular care (Field et al., 2010), if a neonate experiences cardiac fibrillation, an automated external defibrillator (AED) device could be helpful in defibrillating the neonatal victim and restoring his or her heart to a normal sinus rhythm. Note that the ILCOR advisory statement does not currently support a recommendation either for or against the use of AEDs on children under 12 months of age because there is insufficient evidence supporting its effectiveness (Perlman et al., 2010).

A recognized problem with using an AED device on a child who is younger than 12 months of age is that infants can have a "normal" heart rate of up to 205 beats per minute (bpm) (Field et al., 2010). The AED device interprets a 205 bpm heart rate as "tachycardia," then automatically charges and shocks the infant victim. In reality, that infant's heart rate was within normal limits and the infant did not need to be shocked. Because of this interpretive dilemma by the AED, children who are younger than 12 months need to be shocked only using manual settings of the AED device by caregivers who have completed an approved competency course for using the AED device with infants.

The AHA has adopted these guidelines for use of the AED in infants but has made it very clear that a "more advanced defibrillator" is preferred for use in infants. In infants, the energy dosage across the external chest wall is 2 to 6 W-sec/kg body weight to reverse ventricular fibrillation (Hazinski, 2010). For the AED paddle positions in infants, the anterior paddle should be midline of the chest, slightly to the left. The posterior paddle should be on the posterior chest wall. Since the best decision of which AED device should be used for infants is left up to advanced care providers, courses presently addressing different AED devices and their appropriate use are included in ACLS, PALS, and health care provider CPR classes.

SUPPLIES

Personnel should wear gloves and other appropriate protective barriers when handling newly born infants during resuscitation. Standard precautions should be followed carefully, particularly in situations where blood and body fluids are likely to be present. All fluids from neonatal patients should be treated as potentially infectious (Perlman et al., 2010).

The ECC guidelines present a list of supplies and equipment useful for resuscitation (Perlman et al., 2010, p. I–347).

Neonatal resuscitation supplies and equipment

- ■ Suction equipment
  - ▓ Bulb syringe
  - ▓ Mechanical suction and tubing
  - ▓ Suction catheters, 5F or 6F, 8F, and 10F or 12F
  - ▓ 8F feeding tube and 10-mL syringe
  - ▓ Meconium aspiration device
- ■ Bag-and-mask equipment
  - ▓ Neonatal resuscitation bag with a pressure-release valve or pressure manometer (the bag must be capable of delivering 90%–100% oxygen)
  - ▓ Face masks, premature and newborn sizes (masks with cushioned rim are preferred)
  - ▓ Oxygen with flowmeter (flow rate up to 10 L/min) and tubing (including portable oxygen cylinders) (also, a pulse oximeter, probe, and infant cuff [Donn & Engmann, 2003])
- ■ Intubation equipment
  - ▓ Laryngoscope with straight blades, No. 0 (preterm) and No. 1 (term)
  - ▓ Extra bulbs and batteries for laryngoscope (two for Welch Allyn standard handle laryngoscope, might require AA, pen-lite AA, C, D, or one 2.5 V or 3.5 V nickel–cadmium battery for a fiber-optic halogen HPX handle)
  - ▓ Endotracheal tubes, 2.5, 3.0, 3.5, and 4.0 mm ID (inside diameter)
  - ▓ Stylet (optional)
  - ▓ Scissors
  - ▓ Tape or securing device for endotracheal tube
  - ▓ Alcohol sponges
  - ▓ CO_2 detector (optional)
  - ▓ Laryngeal mask airway (optional)

■ Medications

■ Epinephrine 1:10,000 (0.1 mg/mL)—3 mL or 10 mL ampules

■ Isotonic crystalloid (normal saline or Ringer's lactate) for volume expansion—100 to 250 mL

■ Sodium bicarbonate 4.2% (5 mEq/10 mL)—10 mL ampules

■ Naloxone hydrochloride 0.4 mg/mL—1 mL ampules; or 1.0 mg/mL—2 mL ampules

■ Normal saline, 30 mL

■ Dextrose 10%, 250 mL

■ Normal saline "fish" or "bullet" (optional)

■ Feeding tube, 5F (optional)

■ Umbilical vessel catheterization supplies

■ Sterile gloves

■ Scalpel or scissors

■ Povidone-iodine solution

■ Umbilical tape

■ Umbilical catheters, 3.5F, 5F

■ Three-way stopcock

■ Syringes, 1, 3, 5, 10, 20, and 50 mL

■ Needles, 25-, 21-, and 18-gauge or puncture device for needle-less system

■ Miscellaneous

■ Gloves and appropriate personal protection equipment

■ Radiant warmer or other heat source

■ Firm, padded resuscitation surface

■ Clock (timer optional)

■ Warmed linens

■ Stethoscope

■ Tape, 1/2 or 3/4 in.

■ Cardiac monitor and electrodes, and/or pulse oximeter with probe (optional in delivery room)

■ Oropharyngeal airways

STEPS TO RESUSCITATION

The International Guidelines 2000 recommendations for resuscitation (Perlman et al., 2010) form the basis of the procedures stated, followed by recommendations comprising the Neonatal Algorithm from the Neonatal Advanced Life Support (NALS) (Louis, Sundaranm, & Kumar, 2014). It is essential that the knowledge and skills required for resuscitation be taught to all providers of neonatal care. The Neonatal Resuscitation Program (NRP) developed by the AAP and the AHA offer the same curricula.

To be more versatile in meeting the needs of diverse environments, the essential components comprising the International Guidelines (Perlman et al., 2010) procedures are presented using four approaches. The caregiver needs to select one of these approaches that seems best for his or her setting, and then follow the steps described. Rather than from differences in interpretation of scientific evidence and outcomes, controversies about these approaches arise mostly from local and regional preferences or traditions, training networks, and differences in availability of equipment and medication. Each approach varies in the level of detail provided and the extent to which supplies, equipment, and medications are mentioned.

First resuscitation approach

The first approach separates neonatal resuscitation into *four categories of action*:

A. Basic steps, including rapid assessment plus initial steps in stabilization

B. Ventilation, including bag-mask or bag-tube ventilation

C. Chest compressions

D. Administration of medications and/or fluids

Note that intubation can be required during any of these A to D action steps. Also, all newborns require the rapid assessment described in the basic steps.

Resuscitation Category of Action I: Basic steps, including rapid assessment plus initial steps in stabilization. Newborns exhibiting a "normal" rapid assessment (which is similar to an Apgar [1953] assessment producing a score of 7 to 10, or excellent), will require only routine newborn care. If a newborn fits within this assessment category, he or she

■ Is free of meconium and/or meconium staining (sign of stress)

■ Is spontaneously crying and/or breathing (respiration)

■ Has good muscle tone (activity)

■ Has pink skin color (appearance)

■ Is of term gestation (age)

Routine stabilizing newborn care consists of supplying warmth, clearing the airway, and drying amniotic fluid off of the newborn. If any of the rapid assessment findings in the first 30 seconds warrant a caregiver's concern, the newborn might need to:

■ Have his or her airway cleared

■ Be stimulated to breathe

■ Be repositioned

■ Be given supplemental oxygen

Resuscitation Category of Action II: Ventilation, including bag-mask or bag-tube ventilation. If findings from the first 30 seconds postnatally indicated that the newborn was apneic—and/or his or her heart rate was less than 100 bpm—then positive-pressure ventilation using a self-inflating bag and mask should be applied during the next 30 seconds. If the newborn's heart rate does not increase to 100 bpm or higher within 1 minute, and the newborn's color is cyanotic, the newborn needs to be ventilated with a self-inflating bag attached to supplemental oxygen. During this time, the newborn's respirations, heart rate, and color need to be monitored continuously until the newborn's heart rate is over 100 bpm and his or her color is pink.

Chest compressions with ventilations need to be administered at a 3:1 ratio because ventilation is critical to reversal of newborn asphyxial arrest. Furthermore, higher ratios may decrease ventilation needs. If the neonate's arrest is known to be from cardiac etiology, a higher ratio (15:2) should be considered.

If epinephrine is indicated, a dose of 0.01 to 0.03 mg/kg should be administered IV as soon as possible. If the endotracheal route is needed for administering epinephrine because an IV is not in place, a larger dose (0.05–0.1 mg/kg) likely will be required (Hazinski, 2010; Louis et al., 2014).

Resuscitation Category of Action III: Chest compressions. If findings during the 90 seconds postnatally indicated that the newborn's heart rate was less than 60 bpm, chest compressions should be administered immediately. If the neonate's heart rate remains below 60 bpm after completing chest compressions for 1 minute, in addition to continuing chest compressions, the newborn might need endotracheal intubation plus supplemental oxygen.

Resuscitation Category of Action IV: Administration of medications and intravenous fluids. If the newborn has now been intubated, the fourth action is to administer

- Ventilations with a self-inflating bag attached to supplemental oxygen
- Epinephrine 0.01 mg/kg IV of a 1:10,000 solution, followed by
- IV fluids of 0.9% NaCl at 10 mL/kg

Second resuscitation approach

The second approach uses the AHA's algorithm/flow chart for newborn resuscitation based on *time elapsed following birth.* The techniques are described in the flow chart that follows (Perlman et al., 2010, p. 349). Steps are broken into four, 30-second intervals, as shown in the first column of Table 14.2.

Third resuscitation approach

The third approach is based on airway, breathing, and circulation or A-B-C. Because arrest is more likely to be of a respiratory etiology in newborns, resuscitation should be attempted with the proper A-B-C

TABLE 14.2 Newborn Resuscitation

Approximate Time	Birth	Response	Care
First 30 seconds [Step 1]	▪ Clear of meconium ▪ Crying or breathing ▪ Good muscle tone ▪ Pink color ▪ Term gestation	Yes------→	Routine care Provide warmth Clear airway Dry newborn's skin
	If no, then ↓		
	▪ Provide warmth ▪ Position, clear airway ▪ Dry, stimulate, reposition ▪ Give O$_2$ as necessary		
	Next ↓		
	▪ Evaluate respirations ▪ Evaluate heart rate and color	**Response**	**Care**
		Breathing------→ and HR > 100 plus color is pink	Supportive care

		Response	Care
Second 30 seconds [Step 2]	Apneic? ↓ or HR < 100?	Ventilate baby--------→ and HR > 100 plus color is pink	Ongoing care
	■ Provide positive-pressure ventilation[a]		
Third 30 seconds [Step 3]	HR < 60↓ ↑ HR > 60	**Response**	**Care**
	■ Provide positive-pressure ventilation[a] ■ Administer chest compressions		
Thereafter … [Step 4]	↕	**Response**	**Care**
	HR < 60?		Endotracheal intubation might be considered
	■ Administer epinephrine[a]		

[a] "Newborn" or "newly born" refers to an infant who is within *the first minutes to hours after birth* (Perlman et al., 2010). Traditionally, a "neonate" is defined as an infant during his or her first 28 days postnatally. Infancy begins at birth and extends through 12 months of age. Although the preceding guidelines and neonatal resuscitation steps focus on newborn infants, most resuscitative principles apply for the first 28 days through early infancy. HR, heart rate.

sequence and not the circulation first, then airway and breathing sequence, unless there is a known cardiac etiology (Hazinski, Chahine, Holcomb, & Morris, 1994). The A-B-C sequence is recommended because the etiology of neonatal arrests is nearly always asphyxia (Suominen, Rasanen, & Kivioja, 1998). Thus, resuscitation, if needed, should be addressed according to checking:

- For whether the airway (A) is clear
- For breathing (B), and then
- For circulation (C)

Note that if a neonate does require resuscitation, stabilizing steps can be completed once a neonate is fully resuscitated. If a neonate does not require full resuscitation, but only needs to have his or her health status stabilized, then only stabilization of the neonate needs to occur.

First, the caregiver needs to check whether or not the neonate's airway is clear. If it is not clear, the airway needs to be suctioned. *Second*, the caregiver needs to check for breathing. If breathing is not present, artificial respirations need to be administered. *Third*, to assess circulation in a neonate, the caregiver should assess for a pulse. Pulse in neonates is assessed at either the brachial or femoral artery using the caregiver's index and middle finger. If a neonate's pulse is not present at his or her brachial or femoral artery, then the caregiver needs to initiate chest compressions for the neonate.

AIRWAY

Suctioning the airway after birth is only for babies with obvious obstruction or who require positive-pressure ventilation.

- Suctioning during delivery has been shown to have no value.
- Despite the lack of evidence, continue current practice of endotracheal suctioning of nonvigorous babies with meconium-stained amniotic fluid.

When used by trained providers, a laryngeal mask can be used as an alternative method for establishing an airway, especially if the bag-mask ventilation is ineffective for the newborn or attempts at tracheal intubation have been unsuccessful (AHA-*Class Indeterminate*). Exhaled CO_2 detection can be useful in the secondary confirmation of tracheal tube intubation in newborns, particularly when clinical assessment is equivocal (AHA-*Class Indeterminate*).

BREATHING

When giving artificial respirations, make sure of the following:

■ Rate is at 40 to 60 breaths per minute

■ Neonate's chest rise is visible

■ Administer positive end-expiratory pressure (PEEP), if needed

CHEST COMPRESSIONS

The AHA guidelines for CPR and emergency cardiovascular care developed a protocol for neonatal resuscitation named NALS (Lamberg & Raghavendra Raghu, 2014; Louis et al., 2014). NALS advises how to give chest compressions to neonates. This includes:

■ If the pulse at the brachial or femoral artery is absent, begin compressions using the two-thumb method.

■ The two-thumb method of CPR has been shown to require less force to generate the same blood pressure as the two-finger technique (Manisterski et al., 2002). Thus, it is easier to correctly perform chest compressions with neonates using the two-thumb method.

■ The two-thumb method is described as less draining on a rescuer and the rescuer is able to deliver compressions of a higher quality over a longer time period than using the two-finger technique (Kattwinkel et al., 2010). Logic would suggest that the two-thumb method is best for single and multiple rescuers. Yet practical concerns have been raised in the single rescuer using the two-thumb chest compression method while simultaneously being capable of managing the airway adequately.

■ Therefore, in some circumstances of a single rescuer, the two-finger technique may be more appropriate.

The two thumb-encircling hands chest compression method is preferred for chest compressions in newborns and older infants when size allows (*Class IIb*). For chest compressions, a relative depth of compression (one third of the anterior–posterior diameter of the chest), rather than an absolute depth, is recommended. Infant chest compressions should be completed as follows:

- Use the thumb-encircling method.
- Place thumbs directly over the lower half of the sternum between the nipples.
- Press your thumbs down at least one third of the antero-posterior chest diameter ($\approx$ 5–7 mm).
- Chest compression depth should be at least one third the antero-posterior chest diameter.
- Allow complete chest recoil after each chest compression.
- A minimum of 100 compressions should be delivered per minute.
- The compression-to-ventilation ratio should be 3:1.
- If an advanced airway is present, chest compressions should be continued.
- Minimize interruptions in chest compressions to less than 10 seconds.
- Chest compressions should be sufficiently deep to generate a palpable pulse.

Fourth resuscitation approach

The fourth approach uses the Pediatric Working Group of the ILCOR's advisory statement that was published in 1999 (Kattwinkel et al., 1999). That statement listed the following principles of newborn resuscitation:

A. Caregivers capable of initiating resuscitation should attend every delivery. A minority (< 10%) of newborns require active resuscitative interventions to establish a vigorous cry or regular respirations, maintain a heart rate greater than 100 bpm, and achieve pink color and good tone.

B. When meconium is observed in the amniotic fluid, deliver the newborn's head, and suction meconium from the hypopharynx on delivery of the head. If the newborn has absent or depressed respirations, heart rate less than 100 bpm, or poor muscle tone, carry out direct tracheal suctioning to remove meconium from the airway.

C. Of primary concern is the establishment of adequate ventilation. Provide assisted ventilation with attention to oxygen delivery, inspiratory time, and effectiveness as judged by chest rise if stimulation does not achieve prompt onset of spontaneous respirations or if the heart rate is less than 100 bpm.

D. Provide chest compressions if the heart rate is absent or remains less than 60 bpm despite adequate assisted ventilation for

TABLE 14.3 NALS Algorithm
Time: 0–30 Seconds
1. Initial evaluation ■ Term gestation? ■ Breathing or crying? ■ Good muscle tone?
2. Routine care if initial evaluation findings are normal ■ Provide warmth ■ Clear airway if necessary ■ Dry newborn ■ Ongoing evaluation
3. Measures if initial evaluation findings are abnormal ■ Provide warmth ■ Clear airway if necessary ■ Dry, stimulate, and reposition
4. Secondary evaluation ■ Respirations ■ Heart rate ■ Color

(continued)

TABLE 14.3 NALS Algorithm (*continued*)
Time: 30–60 Seconds
5. If the heart rate is greater than 100 bpm, the baby is pink, and he or she has nonlabored breathing, proceed with routine care.
6. If the heart rate is greater than 100 bpm and the baby is cyanotic or has labored breathing, proceed with the steps that follow: ■ Clear the airway, if the infant has obvious airway obstruction (Suominen et al., 1998), and begin monitoring pulse oximetry oxygen saturation (SpO_2) ■ Consider giving supplementary oxygen ■ Consider continuous positive airway pressure (CPAP) ■ If the baby improves, institute postresuscitation care
7. If the heart rate is less than 100 bpm and the baby is gasping or apneic, proceed as follows: ■ Clear the airway if the infant has obvious airway obstruction, and begin SpO_2 monitoring ■ Provide positive-pressure ventilation ■ Consider supplementary oxygen ■ If the baby improves, institute postresuscitation care
Time: 60–90 Seconds
8. If the heart rate is less than 60 bpm, proceed with the following steps: ■ Begin chest compressions ■ Consider intubation; intubate if there is no visible chest rise
9. Reassess heart rate ■ If the heart rate is greater than 60 bpm, stop compressions and continue ventilations. ■ If the heart rate is less than 60 bpm, administer epinephrine and/or a volume expander.

NALS, Neonatal Advanced Life Support.

Source: Louis et al. (2014).

30 seconds. Coordinate chest compressions with ventilations at a ratio of 3:1 to achieve approximately 90 compressions and 30 breaths per minute.

TABLE 14.4 Extra Resuscitation Guidance

I. Drug therapy

- Epinephrine 0.01–0.03 mg/kg IV
- Crystalloid 10 mL/kg IV
- Naloxone is not recommended

II. Target preductal SpO$_2$

- 1 minute: 60%–65%
- 2 minutes: 65%–70%
- 3 minutes: 70%–75%
- 4 minutes: 75%–80%
- 5 minutes: 80%–85%
- 10 minutes: 85%–95%

III. Compressions

- Check pulse at brachial or femoral artery
- Compression landmarks: Lower half of sternum between the nipples
- Method: Thumb-encircling
- Depth: At least one third antero-posterior chest diameter
- Allow complete chest recoil after each compression
- Compression rate: At least 100 compressions per minute
- Compression-to-ventilation ratio of 3:1
- Continuous compressions if advanced airway is present
- Minimize interruptions in compressions to less than 10 seconds

IV. Airway

- Suctioning after birth is only to be completed for babies with obvious obstructions, or who require positive-pressure ventilation.
- Suctioning during delivery has been shown to have no value.
- Despite lack of evidence, continue current practice of endotracheal suctioning of nonvigorous babies who have meconium-stained amniotic fluid.

(continued)

TABLE 14.4 Extra Resuscitation Guidance (*continued*)
V. Ventilations
Rate of 40–60 breaths per minute ■ Watch for visible chest rise ■ If available, administer positive end-expiratory pressure (PEEP) ■ Special circumstances such as extremely low birth weight or congenital diaphragmatic hernia
VI. Factors that should prompt consideration of intubation
■ Nonvigorous meconium-stained newborn ■ Ineffective bag-mask ventilation ■ CPR is being performed
Special circumstances such as extremely low birth weight or congenital diaphragmatic hernia

Sources: Field et al. (2010); Kattwinkel et al. (2010); Louis et al. (2014); Orlowski (1986).

E. Administer epinephrine if the heart rate remains less than 60 bpm despite 30 seconds of effective assisted ventilation and chest compressions.

The foregoing ILCOR principled approach serves as a compressed and abbreviated form of the NALS algorithm (see Table 14.3) (Lamberg & Raghavendra Raghu, 2014). The NALS approach that follows combines time elapsed with nine specific resuscitation assessment and therapeutic activities. Extra resuscitation guidance from three AHA resources in the form of six separate recommendations on drug therapy, target preductal SpO_2, compressions, airway, ventilations, and factors that should prompt consideration of intubation are detailed in Table 14.4 (Field et al., 2010).

Next are additional guidelines for facilitating and supporting resuscitative efforts. These specific aids might help answer questions that arise during resuscitations.

Only a very small percentage of neonates will need chest compressions and medications (Hupfl et al., 2010). However, it might be useful to access some basic information on epinephrine, volume expansion, and vascular access. For example:

■ Epinephrine: Administer epinephrine if the heart rate remains less than 60 bpm after a minimum of 30 seconds of adequate ventilation and chest compressions (*Class I*). Epinephrine administration is especially indicated in the presence of asystole.

■ Fluid choice for acute volume expansion: Emergency volume expansion can be accomplished by an isotonic crystalloid solution—such as normal saline or Ringer's lactate (*Class IIb*).

■ Alternative routes for vascular access: Intraosseous access can be used as an alternative route for medications/volume expansion if umbilical or other venous access is not readily available (*Class IIb*).

ASSESSMENT AND CARE POST-PROCEDURE

■ Because there are considerable assessments and reassessments completed during resuscitation, coordination between and among resuscitation care providers is critical.

■ At least one care provider should oversee the overall resuscitative event.

■ Another care provider should keep a written record of events that have taken place and the neonate's response.

■ Additional help should be requested when needed. Referral or tertiary centers should be called for advice and/or assistance with transport.

■ Termination of resuscitation is difficult and should follow local protocols and medical direction.

DOCUMENTATION

■ Procedure notes should be written for all procedures completed.

■ All lab results should be listed and/or noted as pending.

■ All working diagnoses should be noted.

■ All plans for additional diagnostics and therapeutic interventions should be noted.

■ Informed consent(s) should be included, if any consents were needed as part of the resuscitation.

■ Parent(s) should have seen/touched the neonate before or following the resuscitation.

- Staff consultations should be written and included in the medical record.

- Any pertinent information regarding heritable and familial conditions should be noted.

- Notification of any referring physicians and the mother's obstetrician should be noted.

- The family's religious preference, particularly Jehovah's Witness, should be noted.

DEFINITION OF STABILIZATION

Stabilization refers to a state where a person's vital signs are within normal limits (Athanasuleas et al., 2006). In order to transition a neonate to a steadfast and stable state—such that his or her heart rate and breathing are within normal limits—interventions that require a variety of supplies and equipment might be needed. Because there are so many different interventions required for stabilizing a particular condition or set of conditions, only a general discussion of stabilization is presented here.

STABILIZATION OR CONTINUING CARE AFTER RESUSCITATION

As part of stabilization, ongoing and/or supportive care, monitoring, and appropriate diagnostic evaluation are necessary after resuscitation (Perlman et al., 2010). Once adequate ventilation and circulation are established, the neonate should be maintained within, or transferred to, an environment where close monitoring and ongoing care can be provided.

In terms of vital signs, postresuscitation monitoring should include monitoring of the heart rate, respiratory rate, arterial oxygen saturation, administered oxygen concentration, and blood gas analysis at regular intervals and as indicated. Blood pressure should be assessed and documented. Blood glucose also should be assessed during stabilization after resuscitation.

In terms of laboratory tests, ongoing blood glucose screening and calcium levels should be obtained. A chest radiograph may help identify the underlying causes of the arrest or detect respiratory complications.

In terms of treatments, additional care might include treatment of hypotension with volume expanders or pressors, treatment of possible infections, and initiation of appropriate fluid therapy. Documentation of assessments and additional interventions should be recorded.

Further information about specific stabilizing caregiving is accessible from the S.T.A.B.L.E. Program resource (Karlsen, 2013). The S.T.A.B.L.E. Program for neonatal caregivers was developed to meet the educational needs of health care providers who deliver stabilization care to neonates. S.T.A.B.L.E. education is very helpful in reducing infant morbidity and mortality. It is useful in postresuscitations, pretransports, and at other times when a neonate's condition is unstable in one or more body systems. S.T.A.B.L.E. is the most widely used neonatal education program to focus exclusively on stabilization care of sick infants. Based on a mnemonic, S.T.A.B.L.E. stands for the *six assessment and care modules* in the program: Sugar and safe care, temperature, airway, blood pressure, lab work, and emotional support. A seventh module, *quality improvement*, stresses the professional responsibility of improving and evaluating care provided to sick infants.

S.T.A.B.L.E. (Karlsen, 2013) endorses recommendations pertinent to six areas.

1. *Sugar and safe care* that reviews the importance of establishing IV access. Neonates are at risk for developing hypoglycemia. IV fluid administration must be monitored to determine hydration and glucose status. Safe patient care that eliminates and prevents errors is a top priority.

2. *Temperature* reviews special thermal needs of infants, including avoiding hyperthermia (*Class III*) and selective cerebral hypothermia as a protection against brain injury in the asphyxiated infant (*Class Indeterminate*).

3. *Airway* reviews evaluation of respiratory distress, basic chest x-ray evaluation, useful initial ventilator settings, and respiratory treatments. For babies born at term, room air should be given 100% oxygen during positive-pressure ventilation (Suominen et al., 1998).

Lower inspired oxygen concentrations may be useful in some settings; data are insufficient to justify a change from the recommendation that 100% oxygen be used if assisted ventilation is required. Any supplementary oxygen administered should be regulated by blending oxygen and air, using oximetry measured from the right upper extremity to guide titration of the blend delivered (Suominen et al., 1998). If supplemental oxygen is unavailable and positive-pressure ventilation is required, use room air (*Class Indeterminate*).

4. *Blood pressure* reviews risk for hypovolemic, cardiogenic, and septic shock in infants, and how to assess and treat shock.

5. *Lab work* focuses on neonatal infection, the complete blood count, and initial antibiotic treatment for suspected infection.

6. *Emotional support* reviews the crisis surrounding the birth of a sick neonate and how to support the infant's family.

REFERENCES

Advanced Life Support Task Force of the International Liaison Committee on Resuscitation. (2003). ILCOR advisory statement. Therapeutic hypothermia after cardiac arrest. *Circulation*, *108*, 118–121. doi:10.1161/01.CIR.0000079019.02601.90

Apgar, V. (1953). A proposal for a new method of evaluation of the newborn infant. *Current Researches in Anesthesia & Analgesia*, *32*(4), 260–267. doi:10.1213/00000539-195301000-00041

Athanasuleas, C. L., Buckberg, G. D., Allen, B. S., Beyersdorf, F., & Kirsh, M. M. (2006). Sudden cardiac death: Directing the scope of resuscitation towards the heart and brain. *Resuscitation*, *70*(1), 44–51. doi:10.1016/j.resuscitation.2005.11.017

Byrne, P. J., Tyebkhan, J. M., & Laing, L. M. (1994). Ethical decision-making and neonatal resuscitation. *Seminars in Perinatology*, *18*, 36–41.

Cummins, R. O., Eisenberg, M. S., Hallstrom, A. P., & Litwin, P. E. (1985). Survival of out-of-hospital cardiac arrest with early initiation of cardiopulmonary resuscitation. *American Journal of Emergency Medicine*, *3*(2), 114–119. doi:10.1016/0735-6757(85)90032-4

Danzl, D. F., & Pozos, R. S. (1994). Accidental hypothermia. *New England Journal of Medicine*, *331*(26), 1756–1760. doi:10.1056/NEJM199412293312607

Davies, J. M., & Reynolds, B. M. (1992). The ethics of cardiopulmonary resuscitation. I: Background to decision making. *Archives of Disease in Childhood, 67,* 1498–1501.

Donn, S. M., & Engmann, C. (2003). Neonatal resuscitation: Special procedures. In S. M. Donn (Ed.), *Michigan manual of neonatal intensive care* (3rd ed., pp. 33–41). Philadelphia, PA: Hanley & Belfus.

Editors of Webster's New World College Dictionaries. (2014). *Webster's new world college dictionary* (5th ed., pp. 1240, 1411). New York, NY: Macmillan.

Eich, C., Bräuer, A., & Kettler, D. (2005). Recovery of a hypothermic drowned child after resuscitation with cardiopulmonary bypass followed by prolonged extracorporeal membrane oxygenation. *Resuscitation, 67*(1), 145–148. doi:10.1016/j.resuscitation.2005.05.002

Field, J. M., Hazinski, M. F., Sayre, M. R., Chameides, L., Schexnayder, S. M., Hemphill, R., ... Vanden Hoek, T. L. (2010). Part 1: Executive summary: 2010 American Heart Association guidelines for cardiopulmonary resuscitation and emergency cardiovascular care. *Circulation, 122*(18, Suppl. 3), S640–S656. doi:10.1161/CIRCULATIONAHA.110.970889

Handley, A. J., Koster, R., Monsieurs, K., Perkins, G. D., Davies, S., Bossaert, L., & European Resuscitation Council. (2005). European Resuscitation Council guidelines for resuscitation 2005. Section 2. Adult basic life support and use of automated external defibrillators. *Resuscitation, 67*(Suppl. 1), S7–S23.

Hazinski, M. F. (Ed.). (2010). *Highlights of the 2010 American Heart Association guidelines for CPR and ECC–Pediatric advanced life support* (pp. 20–24). Retrieved from http://www.heart.org/idc/groups/heart-public/@wcm/@ecc/documents/downloadable/ucm_317350.pdf

Hazinski, M. F., Chahine, A. A., Holcomb, G. W., & Morris, J. A. (1994). Outcome of cardiovascular collapse in pediatric blunt trauma. *Annals of Emergency Medicine, 23,* 1229–1235.

Hazinski, M. F., Samson, R., & Schexnayder, S. (Eds.). (2010). *Handbook of emergency cardiovascular care for healthcare providers.* Dallas, TX: American Heart Association.

Hupfl, M., Selig, H. F., & Nagele, P. (2010). Chest compression-only CPR: A meta-analysis. *Lancet, 376*(9752), 1552–1557. doi:10.1016/S0140-6736(10)61454-7

Karlsen, K. (2013). *The S.T.A.B.L.E. program, learner/provider manual: Post-resuscitation/pre-transport stabilization care of sick infants—Guidelines for neonatal healthcare providers* (6th ed.). Salt Lake City, UT: S.T.A.B.L.E.

Kattwinkel, J., Niermeyer, S., Nadkarni, V., Tibballs, J., Phillips, B., Zideman, D., ... Osmond, M. (1999). ILCOR advisory statement: Resuscitation of the newly born infant. An advisory statement from the Pediatric Working Group of the International Liaison Committee on Resuscitation. *Circulation, 99,* 1927–1938. doi:10.1161/01.CIR.99.14.1927

Kattwinkel, J., Perlman, J. M., Aziz, K., Colby, C., Fairchild, K., Gallagher, J., ... Zaichkin, J. (2010). Part 15: Neonatal resuscitation. 2010 American Heart Association guidelines for cardiopulmonary resuscitation and emergency cardiovascular care. *Circulation, 122,* S909–S919. doi:10 .1161/CIRCULATIONAHA.110.971.119

Lamberg, J. J., & Raghavendra Raghu, M. (2014, March 21). *NALS-neonatal resuscitation.* Retrieved from http://emedicine.medscape.com/article/2172079-overview

Landwirth, J. (1993). Ethical issues in pediatric and neonatal resuscitation. *Annals of Emergency Medicine, 22,* 502–507.

Louis, D., Sundaranm, V., & Kumar, P. (2014). Pulse oximeter sensor application during neonatal resuscitation: A randomized controlled trial. *Pediatrics, 133*(3), 476–482. doi:10.1542/peds.2013-2175

Manisterski, Y., Vaknin, Z., Ben-Abraham, R., Efrati, O., Lotan, D., Berkovitch, M., ... Paret, G. (2002). Endotracheal epinephrine: A call for larger doses. *Anesthesia & Analgesia, 95*(4), 1037–1041.

Orlowski, J. P. (1986). Optimum position for external cardiac compression in infants and young children. *Annals of Emergency Medicine, 15,* 667–673.

Perlman, J. M., Wyllie, J., Kattwinkel, J., Atkins, D. L., Chameides, L., Goldsmith, J. P., ... Neonatal Resuscitation Chapter Collaboration. (2010). Part 11: Neonatal resuscitation. 2010 international consensus on cardiopulmonary resuscitation and emergency cardiovascular care science with treatment recommendations. *Circulation, 122*(Suppl. 2), S516–S538. doi:10.1161/CIRCULATIONAHA.110.971127

Suominen, P., Rasanen, J., & Kivioja, A. (1998). Efficacy of cardiopulmonary resuscitation in pulseless paediatric trauma patients. *Resuscitation, 36,* 9–13.

World Health Organization. (1995). *The world health report 1995: Bridging the gaps.* Report of the Director-General. Geneva, Switzerland: World Health Organization.

WHOLE BODY COOLING

Georgia R. Ditzenberger and Susan T. Blackburn

OBJECTIVE

The objective is to provide whole body cooling to eligible neonates with hypoxic-ischemic encephalopathy.

GENERAL INFORMATION

- Whole body cooling therapy will be provided to newborns meeting eligibility criteria. The neonatologist or pediatric neurologist will evaluate the newborn and determine whether the newborn meets the criteria for whole body cooling.

- The newborn will undergo whole body cooling therapy to achieve and maintain an esophageal temperature of 33.5°C.

- Cooling therapy is a 72-hour period of maintaining the esophageal body temperature at 33.5°C.

- On completion of 72 hours of body cooling, the newborn will be rewarmed over a 6-hour period.

  - A physician or neonatal nurse practitioner (NNP) must complete the whole body cooling order set in the electronic chart to initiate this protocol.

  - A physician or NNP must complete the rewarming order set in the electronic chart to initiate rewarming the newborn.

- Risks to newborn:

  - Blood pressure changes: either hypo- or hypertension

  - Respiratory pattern changes; may require ventilator support

  - Abnormal clot formation

  - Skin breakdown

  - Metabolic acidosis

IMPLEMENTATION

- ◼ Equipment and supplies:
  - ▣ Radiant warmer
  - ▣ Electric cooling unit with a probe adapter cable and one set of connecting hoses
  - ▣ One newborn-sized (22 in. × 33 in.) cooling blanket
  - ▣ Two single-patient-use esophageal probes (one for esophageal temperature and one for skin temperature monitoring)
  - ▣ Distilled/sterile water
  - ▣ Tape to secure esophageal probe
- ◼ Electric cooling unit set up; follow manufacturer's guidelines:
  - ▣ Fill the water reservoir; monitor the water level while unit is in use and add water as needed.
  - ▣ Connect the hoses.
  - ▣ Be sure the power switch is OFF prior to inserting the power plug into a grounded receptacle.
  - ▣ Once the unit is plugged into a grounded receptacle, turn the unit on.
  - ▣ Press and hold the test lights button:
    - • Observe that all lights function properly
    - • Confirm the audible alarm sounds are functioning
  - ▣ Place a blanket on the radiant warmer.
  - ▣ The blanket should be flat and the two hose clamps OPEN to allow the blanket to fill.
  - ▣ Water will begin to circulate into the blanket.
    - • Check for leaks
    - • Do not use pins or sharp objects on the blanket
  - ▣ After the blanket has filled, check the level of water in the reservoir; refill as needed to keep the green line on the float visible.
  - ▣ Do not overfill the reservoir.

■ Precool the blanket before the newborn is placed on the blanket:

　■ Operate the electric cooling unit in the Manual Control Mode.

　■ Change the temperature scale by pressing the Celsius/Fahrenheit button to display "Celsius."

　■ Set the temperature desired to 33.5°C.

　■ The unit will cool as required to bring the blanket temperature to the set point.

■ Temperature probes:

　■ Esophageal probe insertion:

　　• Soften the esophageal probe prior to insertion by placing it in warm water for a few minutes.

　　• Do *not* use lubricants.

　　• Nasal placement of the probe is preferred.

　　• Position the esophageal temperature probe in the lower third of the esophagus.

　　• Measure the distance from the nares to the ear to the sternum minus 2 cm.

　　• Mark the probe with an indelible pen before inserting.

　　• Secure the probe by taping it to the newborn's nose.

　　• Probe position may be confirmed with the next routine chest radiographic examination.

　　• Connect the esophageal probe to the probe adapter cable and plug into the probe jack on the electric cooling unit skin probe.

　　• Position over the abdomen; affix to skin with a radiant warmer temperature probe reflective patch.

　　• Skin temperature probe and cable are compatible with the cardiorespiratory monitor and are connected directly into the monitor's temperature module.

■ Cooling the newborn:

   ▨ Place the newborn directly on the cooling blanket on the radiant warmer in the supine position:

   • The newborn's entire head and body should be resting on the cooling blanket.

   • There should be nothing between the newborn and the cooling blanket (no receiving blankets, cloth diapers, gel pads, etc.).

   ▨ The radiant warmer must be OFF.

   ▨ Any other exogenous heat source must be OFF.

   ▨ Change the electric cooling unit to Automatic Control Mode:

   • Make sure the SET POINT is 33.5°.

   • The unit will cool as required to bring the newborn's esophageal temperature to the SET POINT.

■ Maintain the SET POINT at 33.5°:

   ▨ This is the desired esophageal temperature for the next 72 hours.

   ▨ Once the newborn's esophageal temperature reaches the set point of 33.5°, a single blanket layer, such as a thin receiving blanket, may be used between the newborn and the cooling blanket to minimize soiling the cooling blanket.

   ▨ Patient temperature display will flash until the newborn's temperature is within 1°C of the SET POINT.

   ▨ Expect some fluctuation around the SET POINT; it should not be more than ±1°C.

■ Monitor temperatures:

   ▨ Record the esophageal, skin, axillary, and blanket water temperatures in the electronic patient record.

   ▨ Temperatures should be recorded:

   • Every 15 minutes for 2 hours

   • Then, every hour for 4 hours

   • Then every 2 hours until completion of the 72 hours of cooling

■ Assess skin integrity, perfusion, vital signs, and potential complications every hour.

REWARMING THE NEWBORN

■ Verify the rewarming order set is in the electronic patient chart:

　▨ The newborn is rewarmed gradually, increasing the esophageal temperature at a rate of 0.5°C per hour over a 6-hour period.

　　• Every hour, increase the electric cooling unit SET POINT by 0.5°C.

　　• During rewarming, temperatures should be recorded every hour until the skin temperature is stable at 36.5°C.

　▨ At the end of the 6-hour rewarming period, turn on the radiant warmer skin control 0.5°C higher than the newborn's current skin temperature.

　▨ Continue to increase the radiant warmer skin control by 0.5°C every hour until the newborn's axillary temperature is 36.5°C.

　　• Avoid rewarming any faster than 6 hours

　　• Avoid axillary temperatures greater than 37°C

　▨ Remove the cooling blanket from beneath the newborn.

　▨ Remove the esophageal probe and discard.

ADDITIONAL CHAPTER RESOURCES

American Heart Association Emergency Cardiac Care Committee and Subcommittees. (1992). Guidelines for cardiopulmonary resuscitation and emergency cardiac care. *Journal of the American Medical Association, 268*(16), 2171–2183.

Arterial Puncture for Blood Gas Analysis, Neonatal. (2014). *Lippincott's nursing procedures and skills.* Retrieved from http://procedures.lww.com/lnp/view .do?pId=1460395

Barrington, K. J. (1999). Umbilical artery catheters in the newborn: Effects of heparin. *Cochrane Database of Systematic Reviews, 1999*(1), CD000507.

Bindler, R. C., & Ball, J. W. (2011). *Clinical skills manual for pediatric nursing: Caring for children* (5th ed.). Upper Saddle River, NJ: Prentice Hall.

Capillary Blood Sampling, Neonatal. (2014). *Lippincott's nursing procedures and skills.* Retrieved from http://procedures.lww.com/lnp/view.do?pId= 1460423

Centers for Disease Control and Prevention. (2011). *Guidelines for the prevention of intravascular catheter-related infections [Online].* Retrieved from http://www .cdc.gov/hicpac/pdf/guidelines/bsi-guidelines-2011.pdf

Cloherty, J. P., Eichenwald, E. C., Hansen, A. R., & Stark., A. R. (2012). *Manual of neonatal care* (7th ed.). Philadelphia, PA: Lippincott Williams & Wilkins.

College of Respiratory Therapists of Ontario. (2009). *Chest needle & chest tube insertion—Clinical best practice guideline.* Retrieved from http://www.crto.on.ca/ pdf/PPG/Chest_Tube_CBPG.pdf

Gardner, S. L., Carter, B. S., Enzman-Hines, M. I., & Hernandez., J. A. (2011). *Merenstein and Gardner's handbook of neonatal intensive care* (7th ed.). St. Louis, MO: Mosby.

Gomella, T. L., & Cunningham, M. (2013). *Neonatology* (7th ed.). New York, NY: Lange Medical Books/McGraw-Hill.

Gorski, L. (2011). Infusion nursing standards of practice. *Journal of Infusion Nursing, 34*(1S), S1–S110.

Gunn, A. J., Battin, M. R., Gluckman, P. D., Gunn, T. R., & Bennet, L. (2005). Therapeutic hypothermia: From lab to NICU. *Neonatal Intensive Care, 19,* 35–40.

Hatfield, L. A., Chang, K., Bittle, M., Deluca, J., & Polomano, R. C. (2011). The analgesic properties of intraoral sucrose: An integrative review. *Advances in Neonatal Care, 11,* 83–92. doi:10.1097/ANC.0b013e318210d043

Hazinski, M. F., Samson, R., & Schexnayder, S. (Eds.). (2010). *Handbook of emergency cardiovascular care for healthcare providers.* Dallas, TX: American Heart Association.

Ikuta, L. M., & Beauman, S. S. (Eds.). (2011). *Policies, procedures, and competencies for neonatal nursing care.* Glenview, IL: National Association of Neonatal Nurses.

Indwelling Urinary Catheter (Foley) Insertion, Neonatal Female. (2014). *Lippincott's nursing procedures and skills.* Retrieved from http://procedures.lww .com/lnp/view.do?pId=1459600

Kenner, C., & Lott, J. (2014). *Comprehensive neonatal nursing care* (5th ed.). New York, NY: Springer Publishing Company.

Kenner, C., & McGrath, J. M. (2010). *Developmental care of newborns and infants: A guide for health professionals* (2nd ed.). Glenview, IL: National Association of Neonatal Nurses.

MacDonald, M., & Ramesethu, J. (Eds.). (2012). *Atlas of procedures in neonatology* (5th ed.). Philadelphia, PA: Lippincott Williams & Wilkins.

Marschall, J., Mermel, L. A., Fakih, M., Hadaway, L., Kallen, A., O'Grady, N. P., ... Yokoe, D. S. (2014). SHEA/IDSA practice recommendation: Strategies to prevent central line–associated bloodstream infections in acute care hospitals: 2014 update. *Infection Control and Hospital Epidemiology, 35,* 753–771. Retrieved from http://www.jstor.org/stable/10.1086/676533

O'Grady, N., Alexander, M., Burns, L., Dellinger, E., Garland, J., Heard, S., ... Saint, S. (2011). Guidelines for the prevention of intravascular catheter-related infections. *American Journal of Infection Control, 4,* S1–S34.

Phillips, G. W., & Zideman, D. A. (1986). Relation of infant heart to sternum: Its significance in cardiopulmonary resuscitation. *Lancet, 1*(8488), 1024–1025.

Shankaran, S., Laptook, A. R., Ehrenkranz, R. A., Tyson, J. E., McDonald, S. A., & Donavan, E. F. (2005). Whole-body hypothermia for neonates with hypoxic-ischemic encephalopathy. *New England Journal of Medicine, 353*(15), 1574–1584.

Sharpe, E. (2007). Tiny patients, tiny dressings. *Advances in Neonatal Care, 7*(3), 150–162.

Standard 33. (2011). Site selection. Infusion nursing standards of practice. *Journal of Infusion Nursing, 34,* S40–S43.

Standard 41. (2011). Umbilical catheters. Infusion nursing standards of practice. *Journal of Infusion Nursing, 34,* S52–S53.

Standard 45. (2011). Flushing and locking. Infusion nursing standards of practice. *Journal of Infusion Nursing, 34,* S59–S63.

Standard 57. (2011). Phlebotomy. Infusion nursing standards of practice. *Journal of Infusion Nursing, 34,* S77–S80.

The Joint Commission. (2015). *National patient safety goals for critical access hospitals effective January 1, 2015.* Oakbrook Terrace, IL: The Joint Commission.

Tyson, J. E., Younes, N., Verter, J., & Wright, L. L. (1996). Viability, morbidity, and resource use among newborns of 501- to 800-g birth weight: National Institute of Child Health and Human Development Neonatal Research Network. *Journal of the American Medical Association, 276,* 1645–1651.

Umbilical Catheter Blood Withdrawal. (2014). *Lippincott's nursing procedures and skills*. Retrieved from http://procedures.lww.com/lnp/view.do?pId=1460032

Umbilical Catheter Insertion, Assisting, Neonate. (2014). *Lippincott's nursing procedures and skills*. Retrieved from http://procedures.lww.com/lnp/view.do?pId=1460033

Venipuncture, Neonatal. (2014). *Lippincott's nursing procedures and skills*. Retrieved from http://procedures.lww.com/lnp/view.do?pId=1460676

Verger, J. T., & Lebet, R. M. (Eds.). (2008). *AACN procedure manual for pediatric acute and critical care*. St. Louis, MO: Saunders.

Verklan, M. T., & Walden, M. (2015). *Core curriculum for neonatal intensive care nursing* (5th ed.). St. Louis, MO: Elsevier Saunders.

Verklan, M. T., & Walden, M. (Eds.). (2015). *Core curriculum for neonatal intensive care nursing* (5th ed.). Philadelphia, PA: Saunders.

Walden, M., & Gibbins, S. (Eds.). (2012). *Newborn pain assessment and management: Guidelines for practice* (3rd ed.). Glenview, IL: National Association of Neonatal Nurses.

World Health Organization. (2009). *WHO guidelines on hand hygiene in health care: First global patient safety challenge, clean care is safer care*. Retrieved from http://whqlibdoc.who.int/publications/2009/9789241597906_eng.pdf

Woten, M., & Walsh, K. (n.d.). Cinahl information systems. In D. Pravikoff (Ed.), *Arterial blood gases: Performing arterial puncture in the neonate*. Retrieved from http://web.b.ebscohost.com/nrc/detail?sid=c1de5bf6-fa4c-46bd-bc5f-d1560a1991a8%40sessionmgr112&vid=3&hid=115&bdata=JnNpdGU9bnJjLWxpdmU%3d#db=nrc&AN=T70785

Diagnostic Tests

Samual L. Mooneyham

OVERVIEW

Care of the neonate typically involves numerous diagnostic procedures and tests to identify dysfunction related to birth, prematurity, illness, or congenital malformations. This chapter highlights the commonly used methods for developing a medical or surgical diagnosis in the newborn and infant.

DIAGNOSTIC IMAGING IN INFANTS

Diagnostic imaging in newborns and infants is unique. Significant differences exist, not just in size, but also in the origin and imaging appearance of disease entities, anatomic proportions, exposure factors, radiation protection, and methods of immobilization (Hilton & Edwards, 2006; Huda et al., 2001; Swischuk, 1997, 2003).

CONDITIONS REQUIRING DIAGNOSTIC IMAGING

Pathologic conditions commonly encountered in adults often are not found in infants, and many abnormal conditions are exclusive to the newborn period. Examples of these pathologic conditions are the congenital abnormalities of the newborn, such as atresias of the gastrointestinal (GI) tract, severe congenital heart defects (CHD), surgical causes of respiratory distress, spina bifida, and bilateral choanal atresia. These lesions, which are lethal if left untreated, often are symptomatic in the first days after birth. Medical problems related to premature and postmature birth, intrauterine growth disturbances, nonlethal developmental defects, genetic abnormalities, and perinatal asphyxia are of greatest concern in the newborn period. In addition, malignant tumors, such as neuroblastoma and Wilms' tumor, may appear in the newborn period and up to approximately 4 years of age. Certain infections, such as cytomegalovirus (CMV), toxoplasmosis, and syphilis, have a distinct radiographic and ultrasonographic presentation if exposure occurred in utero rather than in the neonatal period (Hilton & Edwards, 2006; Martin, Fanaroff, & Walsh, 2011; Swischuk, 1997, 2003).

ANATOMIC PROPORTIONS

The anatomic proportions of infants are very different from those of adults, and the younger the infant, the more marked the differences. A thorough knowledge of these proportions is essential for correct patient positioning to limit field exposure and for accurate interpretation of diagnostic imaging (Dowd & Tilson, 1999; Hilton & Edwards, 2006). It is important that only the area in question, but the whole of the area in question, appear in the imaging field.

As shown in Figure 15.1, the newborn's head is large in proportion to the body, and the cranial vault is large in proportion to the area of the face. The neck is short, and the diaphragm is high. The kidneys are low, about midway between the diaphragm and symphysis pubis. The abdomen is large because of the relative size of the liver and stomach. The pelvic cavity is very small, and the bladder extends above the symphysis pubis. The chest, pelvis, and limbs are small in proportion to the abdomen (Hilton & Edwards, 2006; Swischuk, 1997, 2003). In an anteroposterior (AP) projection, the neonate's lungs appear wider than they are long and much higher up in the thoracic cavity than is normally expected (Hilton & Edwards, 2006; Swischuk, 1997, 2003). The diaphragm is located just below the level of the nipples. On a lateral projection, the posterior aspect of the lungs may extend to twice the depth of the anterior part (Swischuk, 1997, 2003).

The newborn's abdomen bulges laterally wider than the pelvis, and the bulge contains abdominal organs displaced by the large liver and stomach. Care must be taken to include this area of the

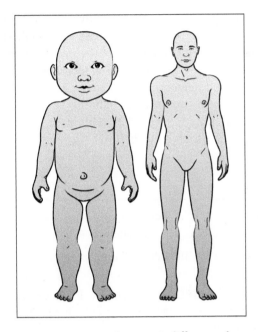

FIGURE 15.1. Proportional anatomic differences between a neonate and an adult.

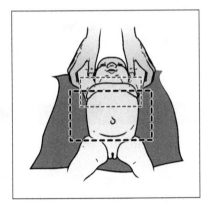

FIGURE 15.2. Neonatal radiographs should be limited to only the area of interest. Total body radiographs should be avoided. The top box (light dashed lines) defines the area of interest for an AP chest radiograph. The bottom box (heavy dashed lines) defines the area of interest for an AP abdominal film. The gonad shield has been omitted for illustrative purposes.

abdomen in the imaging field (Hilton & Edwards, 2006; Swischuk, 1997, 2003). Irradiation should encompass the smallest possible body area consistent with production of the necessary information (Dowd & Tilson, 1999). Often the field is too large, particularly in premature infants and newborns. Arms and legs should not appear on the abdominal film, nor should half the skull and abdomen appear on a chest film (Figure 15.2) (Hilton & Edwards, 2006; Martin et al., 2011; Swischuk, 1997, 2003).

REFERENCES

Dowd, S. B., & Tilson, E. R. (1999). *Practical radiation protection and applied radiobiology* (2nd ed.). Philadelphia, PA: Saunders.

Hilton, S., & Edwards, D. K. III. (2006). *Practical pediatric radiology.* (3rd ed.). Philadephia, PA: Saunders Elsevier.

Huda, W., Chamberlain, C. C., Rosenbaum, A. E., & Garrisi, W. (2001). Radiation doses to infants and adults undergoing head CT examinations. *Medical Physics, 28*(3), 393-399.

Martin, R., Fanaroff, A., & Walsh, M. (2011). *Neonatal-perinatal medicine.* (9th ed.). St. Louis, MO: Elsevier Mosby.

Swischuk, L. E. (1997). *Differential diagnosis in pediatric radiology* (3rd ed.). Baltimore, MD: Lippincott Williams & Wilkins.

Swischuk, L. E. (2003). *Imaging of the newborn, infant, and young child* (5th ed.). Baltimore, MD: Lippincott Williams & Wilkins.

TYPES OF DIAGNOSTIC IMAGING

The four major diagnostic imaging methods are x-ray (roentgenologic) imaging, radionuclide imaging, ultrasonographic imaging, and magnetic resonance imaging (MRI) (Bushong, 1999, 2000, 2003, 2013; Juhl, 1998; Treves, 2014). This chapter discusses each of these imaging modalities in relation to the biophysical principles responsible for producing the image, the potential risks of the procedure, and the nursing care of the newborn or infant undergoing such an examination. Table 15.1 summarizes the types of diagnostic imaging commonly used for neonates.

TABLE 15.1 Diagnostic Imaging Methods Commonly Used for Neonates

Technique	Indications and Advantages	Limitations	Potential Risks	Comments	Cost
Roentgenologic Techniques					
Radiographic imaging	Most frequently used initial diagnostic screening mode	Detects only four different levels of photon absorption (air, fat, water, and mineral); two-dimensional (2D) projection of three-dimensional (3D) structures	Ionizing radiation; thermal stress of cool film plate	Proper positioning of infant is essential; child must be monitored during procedure	$
Xeroradiographic imaging	Used to evaluate soft tissue structures	Tissue structures defined by relative amounts of air, fat, water, and minerals; seldom used since advent of newer diagnostic imaging methods	Higher level of ionizing radiation than with routine radiographs	Proper positioning of infant is essential; child must be monitored during procedure	$$

(continued)

TABLE 15.1 Diagnostic Imaging Methods Commonly Used for Neonates *(continued)*

Technique	Indications and Advantages	Limitations	Potential Risks	Comments	Cost
Roentgenologic Techniques					
Fluoroscopic imaging	Used to evaluate motion or function of cardiovascular, gastrointestinal, and genitourinary systems; may be used to guide therapeutic or diagnostic procedures	Images rely on greater radiation and/or movement of contrast material; improper diagnostic sequencing may delay informational yield; contrast material may have physiologic consequences	Much higher level of ionizing radiation than with routine radiographs; thermal stress of cool radiology environment	Proper positioning of infant is essential; child must be monitored during procedure	$$–$$$$
CT	Used to provide detailed, superior characterization of various soft tissue densities that cannot be detected by conventional radiographs	Motion artifact may cause blurring of scans; radiation dose depends on scan time; contrast material may have physiologic consequences	Ionizing radiation; thermal stress of cool environment	Proper positioning of infant is essential; child must be monitored during procedure	$$$

				$
Ultrasound imaging	Does not use ionizing radiation, but rather uses sound waves to depict anatomic and functional motion of tissue; sound waves can be directed in a beam in a variety of planes; portable; different graphic displays are available	Ultrasound technique is operator dependent; does not provide as much information on organ function such as urography; reveals less anatomic detail than CT; scan is adversely affected by the presence of bone and air	Thermal stress may occur with application of cool scanning gel to infant's skin; there are no known deleterious effects from clinical use of ultrasound imaging	Proper positioning of infant is essential; child must be monitored during procedure
Radionucleotide imaging	Used to trace anatomic proportions and a wide range of physiologic functions in virtually	Diagnostic yield depends on uptake of radionucleotide by different organs; radionucleotides are	Thermal stress during nucleotide scanning	Proper positioning of the infant is essential; maximum
				$$

(continued)

TABLE 15.1 Diagnostic Imaging Methods Commonly Used for Neonates (continued)

Technique	Indications and Advantages	Limitations	Potential Risks	Comments	Cost
Roentgenologic Techniques					
	every organ in the body; amount of ionizing radiation emitted by injected agent is significantly less than the amount required for corresponding radiograph	rarely organ specific; limited anatomic resolution		radiation exposure is not always the organ of interest; child must be monitored during procedure	
PET and SPECT	Both techniques have greater sensitivity and qualifications of the distribution and density of radioactivity to depict the "metabolic" function	PET scanning requires access to a cyclotron to produce the positrons used in scans	Thermal stress during nucleotide scanning	Proper positioning of infant is essential; child must be monitored during procedure	$$$$$$

of tissue; 3D imaging is possible with computer reconstruction; dose of nucleotide is the same; artifactual lesions can be eliminated; amount of ionizing radiation emitted by injected agents (carbon 11, oxygen 15, nitrogen 13) is significantly less than the amount required for corresponding radiograph			

(continued)

TABLE 15.1 Diagnostic Imaging Methods Commonly Used for Neonates (continued)					
Technique	Indications and Advantages	Limitations	Potential Risks	Comments	Cost
Roentgenologic Techniques					
MRI	Uses magnetic fields and radio waves to produce images; the region of the body scanned can be controlled electronically, and hardware does not limit scanning sites; scans are free of high-intensity artifacts; newer scanning techniques can quantify many pathologic conditions	Availability and cost; limited use in unstable infants on life support; monitoring equipment must be free from interference with magnetic field	Does not use ionizing radiation to produce images; limited access to infant during procedure	Proper positioning is essential; must be monitored during procedure	$$$$$

PET, primary evaluation team; SPECT, single photon emission computed tomography.

X-RAY IMAGING (ROENTGENOLOGY)

The principles of conventional radiography have not changed since the discovery of x-rays in the late 1800s. However, the equipment and techniques have become far more sophisticated; current radiographic methods include tomography, fluoroscopy, computed tomography (CT), and digital radiography.

ROENTGENOLOGIC BIOPHYSICAL PRINCIPLES

When an x-ray beam is directed toward a part of the body, differential absorption of the x-ray photons by different types of body tissue occurs. A beam of x-ray photons is variously attenuated as it passes through the body tissues, producing a shadow image that is recorded on photographic film; the absorbed x-ray photons interact with the tissue, causing ionization in the body (Alpen, 1998; Bushong, 2013; Dowd & Tilson, 1999; Juhl, 1998). Bone and metal fragments absorb x-ray photons and therefore appear white on the radiographic film, whereas air-containing structures, such as lungs and gas-filled bowel, absorb few x-ray photons and appear black. Soft tissues and blood vessels appear as intermediate shades of gray.

A radiograph gives a two-dimensional projection of three-dimensional structures. This simple imaging technique can distinguish only among air, fat, and tissues with densities approximately equal to those of water or metals, but it continues to be enormously valuable and is still the diagnostic imaging method most often used in neonatal care.

XERORADIOGRAPHY

Xeroradiography is a radiographic imaging technique used to evaluate soft tissue. With this technique, the electrical charge of a photoconductive plate is altered in proportion to the intensity of the transmitted radiation image (Alpen, 1998; Bushong, 2013; Dowd & Tilson, 1999; Juhl, 1998). With soft tissue structures that differ only slightly in density, this method provides much better contrast than conventional radiography. It also provides an "edge effect" at the margins of discontinuous structures and therefore is indicated for the detection of nonmetallic foreign bodies and for evaluation of complex upper airway abnormalities in the neonate (Hilton & Edwards, 2006; Juhl, 1998; Swischuk, 2003). The radiation exposure involved is 6 to 12 times greater than that with conventional radiographs (Alpen, 1998; Hilton & Edwards, 2006; Juhl, 1998; Swischuk, 2003).

CONVENTIONAL X-RAY TOMOGRAPHY

Tomography is a radiologic method of imaging a "slice" of tissue at a specific level. Coordinated movement of the x-ray tube and film cassette gives a defined image in the two planes of interest, whereas the structures in front of or behind this plane are blurred out (Alpen, 1998; Bushong, 2000; Juhl, 1998). Tomography is useful in many circumstances, but its usefulness has been overshadowed by the development of CT.

COMPUTED TOMOGRAPHY

CT scanning obtains cross-sectional images rather than the shadow images of conventional radiography. Conventional radiography is based on variable attenuation of the x-ray beam as it passes through tissue. Conventional radiographs cannot produce a detailed characterization of various soft tissue densities. Bone is the densest, absorbs the largest amount of x-rays, and appears white; air is the least dense and appears black; soft tissues are displayed as intermediate shades of gray. CT detects changes in density in very small areas of tissue and allows identification of various components of soft tissue, such as subarachnoid space, white matter, gray matter, and ventricles (Alpen, 1998; Bushong, 2000, 2013; Juhl, 1998). CT demonstrates tissue structure with precise clarity, showing superior anatomic detail compared with conventional radiographic imaging (Alpen, 1998; Bushong, 2013; Juhl, 1998). CT permits two-dimensional visualization of entire anatomic sections of tissue, which aids the determination of the extent of the disease or malformation. Anatomic and physiologic information can be visualized despite overlying gas and bone. Contrast enhancement can measure blood flow and help define pathologic abnormalities (Bushong, 2000; Swischuk, 1997, 2003). Bolus injection of contrast material allows excellent visualization of vascular structures.

As good as CT is as an imaging modality, it is still not a radiologic microscope; CT does have its drawbacks. It also uses ionizing radiation, and because the computers require a cool room for proper equipment performance, the neonate's environment is altered significantly, a circumstance that must be considered.

RADIOGRAPHIC CONTRAST AGENTS

Plain radiography can differentiate only four kinds of body tissue: tissue containing gas (lung and bowel), fatty tissue and tissue containing calcium (bone or pathologic calcifications), and tissues of water density (solid organs, muscle, and blood). To demonstrate blood vessels that are in solid organs or surrounded by muscle or to demonstrate other hollow structures, artificial radiographic contrast agents must be introduced. The contrast medium may be negative or positive and may be injected, swallowed, or administered as an enema (Hilton & Edwards, 2006; Swischuk, 1997, 2003).

Negative contrast media absorb less radiation than adjacent soft tissues and therefore cast a darker radiographic image. Gases such as air, oxygen, and carbon dioxide can be used as negative contrast media. Because negative media provide a limited amount of contrast for conventional radiography, they are seldom used (Martin et al., 2011; Swischuk, 1997, 2003).

Positive contrast media use elements with a high atomic number, which absorb much more radiation than surrounding soft tissues and therefore cast a lighter image. Barium and iodine are the two elements currently used. Barium sulfate, a relatively stable, nontoxic compound, is the major contrast agent used for outlining the walls of the GI tract.

Iodine-containing salts that are excreted by the kidneys are used for a wide variety of urographic and angiographic studies. The kidneys also excrete the newer nonionic, iodine-containing media. Because of their lower osmolality, these agents are less painful than iodine-containing salts when injected into arteries, and they are rapidly replacing the older contrast agents (Box 15.1) (Hilton & Edwards, 2006; Martin et al., 2011; Swischuk, 1997, 2003).

Box 15.1   Radiopharmaceuticals Used in Neonatal Diagnostic Imaging

- Technetium 99m sulfur or tin colloid: used for imaging liver, spleen, bone marrow, ventilation, and gastrointestinal bleeding
- Albumin microspheres: used for imaging lung perfusion Pyrophosphate, diphosphate: used for imaging skeletal and myocardial infarcts
- Pertechnetate: used for imaging thyroid, brain, and gastrointestinal tract
- Diethylenetriaminepentaacetic acid (DTPA) glucoheptonate: used for imaging kidney and brain
- Hepatoiminodiacetic acid (HIDA): used for imaging biliary system
- Iodine 131: used for imaging thyroid and fibrinogen and for clot localization
- Xenon 131, krypton 81 m: used for imaging lung ventilation
- Thallium 201: used for imaging myocardial perfusion and for testicular localization

FACTORS AFFECTING RADIOGRAPHIC QUALITY

Several factors determine the technical quality of a radiograph, including film exposure, phase of respiration, motion, tube angulation, and infant positioning. If one of these factors is unsatisfactory, the film may be misinterpreted. When nurses have an understanding of these factors, the technical quality of radiographs is improved.

Film exposure

If the film is underexposed, the dorsal disk spaces are lost, and the lungs and other structures have a homogeneous, "whitewashed" appearance. If the film is overexposed, the pulmonary vascular markings are progressively lost until the lungs have a black, "burned out" appearance (Hilton & Edwards, 2006; Swischuk, 1997, 2003).

Phase of respiration

The phase of respiration at the time the film is obtained affects the appearance of the radiograph considerably (Figure 15.3). On an expiratory film, the heart may appear grossly enlarged, the lung fields may appear opaque (which may simulate diffuse atelectasis), and the diaphragm is located above the seventh rib (Hilton & Edwards, 2006; Swischuk, 1997, 2003). On an inspiratory film, the diaphragm is at the eighth rib, the cardiothymic diameter is normal, and the pulmonary vascularity is prominent. The right hemidiaphragm is slightly higher than the left. If the right hemidiaphragm is at or above the level of the seventh rib, the film was obtained in the expiratory phase or the infant has hypoaerated (Hilton & Edwards, 2006; Swischuk, 1997, 2003).

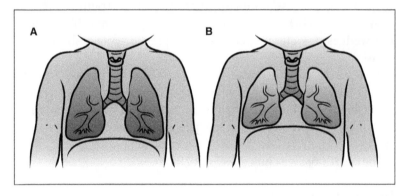

FIGURE 15.3. Differences in appearance between inspiration (A) and expiration (B) in a neonatal chest radiograph. On full inspiration, the diaphragm is located at the eighth rib, and the lungs appear larger and darker. During expiration, the diaphragm is at or above the seventh rib, and the lung fields appear smaller and lighter. The heart size may also appear larger on expiratory films.

Motion

If the infant moves just as the radiograph is made, the resulting film is blurred. Motion causes blurring of the hemidiaphragms, the cardiovascular silhouette, and all fine pulmonary detail (Hilton &

Edwards, 2006; Swischuk, 1997, 2003). Movement blur on diagnostic images can be prevented by fast imaging and adequate immobilization.

Speed

A short exposure time is essential for obtaining clear images. This can be achieved by limiting the duration of exposure to the energy source and by increasing the use of computed imaging.

Immobilization

The nursing staff is primarily responsible for ensuring adequate immobilization during diagnostic imaging. Inadequate immobilization is an important cause of poor quality in neonatal images. Proper immobilization techniques improve image quality, shorten the examination time, and eliminate the need for repeat studies (Hilton & Edwards, 2006; Swischuk, 1997, 2003). Proper immobilization may be less traumatic than manual restraint alone. An immobilization board may be required, or tape, foam rubber blocks and wedges, towels, diapers, or clear plastic acetate sheets may be used.

Physical risks to neonates are associated with immobilization. Infants lie still only when they are very ill. Otherwise, they greatly resent being forcibly restrained, especially in an unusual position. A number of immobilization devices are available, but the best means is a pair of adequately protected adult hands (Hilton & Edwards, 2006; Swischuk, 1997, 2003).

Tube angulation

Another factor is angulation of the x-ray tube, along with improper field limitation. Often on neonatal films, the infant's chest appears mildly lordotic, with the medial clavicular ends projected on or above the dorsal vertebrae. This results in a rather peculiar chest configuration. The preossified anterior arcs of the upper ribs are positioned superior to the posterior arcs (Figure 15.4). The lordotic projection tends to increase the apparent transverse cardiac diameter, making it difficult to determine the size of the heart. Lordotic projections result when the x-ray tube is angled cephalad, when the x-ray beam is centered over the abdomen, or when an irritable infant has arched the back at the time of the film exposure (Hilton & Edwards, 2006; Swischuk, 1997, 2003). If the x-ray tube is angled caudad or the x-ray beam is centered over the head, the anterior rib arcs are angulated sharply downward in relation to the posterior arcs (Hilton & Edwards, 2006; Swischuk, 1997, 2003).

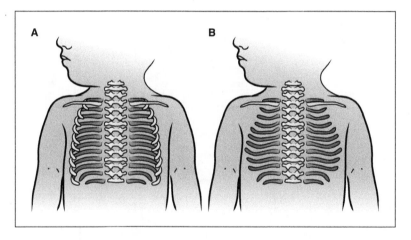

FIGURE 15.4. Skeletal position in a normally positioned radiograph (A) and in a film obtained with cephalad positioning of the x-ray (B).

Infant positioning

If the infant is rotated, a false impression of a mediastinal shift may be created (Figure 15.5) (Hilton & Edwards, 2006; Swischuk, 1997, 2003). The direction and degree of rotation can be estimated by comparing the lengths of the posterior arcs of the ribs from the costovertebral junction to the lateral pleural line at a given level. The infant is rotated toward the side with the greatest posterior arc length (Hilton & Edwards, 2006; Swischuk, 1997, 2003). Another measurement for determining the degree of rotation is the distance from the medial aspect of the clavicles to the center of the vertebral body at the same level. If the infant is properly positioned, the medial aspects of the clavicles should be equidistant from the center of the vertebral body (Hilton & Edwards, 2006; Swischuk, 2003). The distance is greater on the side toward which the infant is rotated. On a lateral view, rotation can be readily determined by observing the amount of offset between the anterior tips of the right and left sets of ribs.

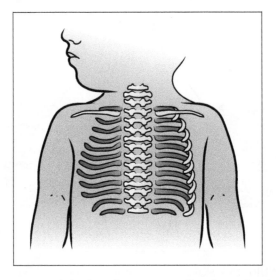

FIGURE 15.5. Skeletal configuration in a film obtained with the infant rotated to the right.

Before any chest film is interpreted, these factors must be systematically evaluated. Through experience this evaluation becomes automatic, and the film can be scanned rapidly.

RADIOLOGIC PROJECTIONS

Radiologic projections are the geometric views of the radiograph, and they vary among institutions and radiologists. They can be customized to the specific infant or clinical condition. For example, the skull may require a simple AP film to make the diagnosis of a fracture, whereas a complete skull series may be necessary for evaluation of congenital malformations. In the neck and upper airway, a lateral film in inspiration with the infant's head extended may be sufficient for the evaluation of stridor, or a xeroradiograph of the soft tissue structures of the neck may be required. Because the radiation dose is much greater with a xeroradiograph than with a plain lateral neck film, the indications for this examination should be clear (Swischuk, 1997).

For evaluation of the spine, the AP projection is most commonly used. Oblique views of the spine usually are difficult to obtain in infants because it is difficult to position and immobilize babies. Also, the diagnostic information gained does not outweigh the risk of the greater radiation exposure required to obtain such views. For evaluation of congenital hip dysplasia, an AP view of the entire pelvis and both hips is required. Gonadal exposure should be minimized with proper shielding during radiographic examination of the hips. Assessment of skeletal maturation in the infant requires an AP film of the left hemiskeleton, and a long bone series requires a film of the upper and lower extremities (Hilton & Edwards, 2006; Swischuk, 1997, 2003).

Chest radiographs are the most frequently performed diagnostic imaging procedure in the neonatal intensive care unit (NICU). In most cases, an AP projection from a supine position is satisfactory for evaluating the infant's chest, heart, lung fields, endotracheal tube, line placement, and pneumothorax (air leak complications related to mechanical ventilation). The cross-table view allows verification of pleural chest tube being placed anteriorly or posteriorly. Lateral decubitus is used to evaluate small pneumothorax and small pleural fluid collection; these can be hard to see on an AP view. Upper right shows abdominal perforation, which shows free air under the diaphragm (rarely used). Lateral projections of the chest often are poorly positioned, have diminished technical quality, and require greater radiation exposure of the infant. For the experienced radiographer, an AP film in the supine position is sufficient in most cases. In rare cases, a lateral chest film with esophageal barium contrast may be requested for evaluation of the left atrium of the heart (Gomella, Cunningham, & Eyal, 2013; Hilton & Edwards, 2006; Swischuk, 1997, 2003; Verklan & Walden, 2015).

Abdominal x-ray films also are frequently obtained in the NICU. The most commonly used radiographic projections are the AP, cross-table lateral, and left lateral decubitus views (Hilton & Edward, 2006; Swischuk, 2003). Because the infant's abdomen is relatively cylindric, a lateral view provides more information than it does in an older child or adult. AP views define the gas pattern, intestinal displacement, some masses, ascites, and placement of lines such as umbilical catheters or intestinal tubes, whereas the cross-table lateral view is recommended in the diagnosis of abdominal perforation, and left lateral decubitus view is for diagnosis intestinal perforation, free intra-abdominal air (Gomella et al., 2013; Hilton & Edwards, 2006; Swischuk, 2003).

A FEW GENERAL PRINCIPLES

1. Exposure time should be kept short to prevent movement blur and limit the radiation dose.

2. Radiographic technicians should be knowledgeable about factors and variables that affect exposure so repeat films occasioned by poor technique can be avoided.

3. A repeated infant x-ray is the major cause of the largest dose of unnecessary radiation (Hilton & Edwards, 2006; Swischuk, 1997, 2003); every possible precaution should be taken to ensure that the first attempt produces a film of diagnostic quality.

4. Before a repeat is done, the film should be shown to the radiologist or neonatologist who requested it; although the quality may not be ideal, it may provide sufficient information.

Radiation exposure can also be reduced by using other diagnostic imaging modalities, when possible, that do not use ionizing radiation to create an image (e.g., ultrasonography, MRI) (Swischuk, 1997, 2003). If radiologic imaging is the best diagnostic approach for the infant's condition, it may be important to "customize" the examinations, to limit the area examined, and to reduce the number of follow-up films.

Plain films should be obtained first. Then, if indicated, a dye contrast study (e.g., excretory urograph) should be performed, because the contrast material is rapidly eliminated from the body. Last, barium contrast studies should be obtained (Hilton & Edwards, 2006; Swischuk, 1997, 2003). Barium contrast studies are performed after the others because (a) barium interferes with any nuclear scintigraphic scans, body computed tomograms, and ultrasonographic scans, and (b) barium is slowly eliminated from the GI tract, which delays further diagnostic evaluation. Additional radiation exposure is possible if the barium must be completely eliminated before the next imaging procedure (Hilton & Edwards, 2006; Swischuk, 1997, 2003).

Adequate patient preparation is another means of reducing radiation exposure (Hilton & Edwards, 2006; Swischuk, 1997, 2003). If GI and genitourinary (GU) imaging are both to be performed, the GU examination should be scheduled first. Although each institution has its own policies, in preparation for a GU examination such as excretory urography, the infant should be kept on nothing by mouth (NPO) status for no longer than 3 hours; this can be accomplished by withholding the early morning feeding and scheduling the examination for 8 a.m. No preparation is necessary for excretory urography in infants with abdominal masses, trauma, or GU emergencies. If the infant has impaired renal function, the radiologist and the neonatologist should discuss the condition thoroughly so that the risks of this procedure are minimized. For an infant who has been feeding, the baby is prepared for a GI contrast study by keeping the child on NPO status for no longer than 3 hours before the examination. Generally, if a contrast study of the entire GI tract has been requested, the lower GI series is performed before the upper GI series (Hilton & Edwards, 2006; Swischuk, 1997, 2003). This allows time for elimination of the barium in the colon and prevents the barium from interfering with the diagnostic quality of the upper GI study. Colon preparation usually is unnecessary in the neonate and should be avoided in infants with an acute abdominal condition and in those suspected of having Hirschsprung disease (Swischuk, 1997, 2003).

COLLABORATIVE CARE

Radiation protection

Any radiation is considered harmful to the infant, and all efforts must be made to reduce radiation exposure without forgoing diagnostic information. Radiation exposure can have both genetic and somatic effects (Bushong, 2013; Dowd & Tilson, 1999; NCRP, 1993a, 1993b, 1993c). Reduction of radiation exposure should be the goal for sites that are sensitive genetically (gonads) and somatically (eyes, bone marrow). Methods of reducing radiation exposure include performing examinations only when they are clinically indicated, selecting the appropriate imaging modality, using the lowest radiation dose that achieves an image of diagnostic quality, avoiding repeat examinations, reducing the number of films obtained, using appropriate projections with tight field limitation, ensuring proper positioning and immobilization, and shielding the gonads (Alpen, 1998; Dowd & Tilson, 1999; Hilton & Edwards, 2006; NCRP, 1993a, 1993b, 1993c).

If the gonads are not within the area of interest, gonadal exposure depends on the adequacy of field limitation. The maximum gonadal dose occurs when the gonads are unshielded and exposed to the primary x-ray beam. This dose declines rapidly as the distance from the gonads to the primary beam increases. Gonadal exposure in an AP film that includes the gonads can be reduced by 95% with proper contact shielding (Dowd & Tilson, 1999). The gonads should be shielded whenever they are within 5 cm of the primary x-ray beam.

Contact gonadal shields are easy to make from 0.5-mm thick lead rubber sheets, and they should be sized for gender and age (Figure 15.6) (Swischuk, 1997, 2003). In males, proper positioning of the shield avoids obscuration of any bony detail of the pelvis if the upper edge of the shield is placed just below the pubis and if the testicles have descended into the scrotum. In females, the position of the ovaries varies with bladder distention. Because of their anatomic location, the ovaries cannot be shielded without obscuring lower abdominal and pelvic structures. The lower margin of the gonad shield should be placed at the level of the pubis, and the upper margin should cover at least the lower margin of the sacroiliac joints (Hilton & Edwards, 2006; Swischuk, 1997, 2003).

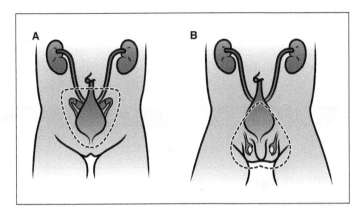

FIGURE 15.6. Anatomic placement of gonad shield for female infants (A) and for male infants (B).

Radiation safety

The three ways to reduce radiation exposure of personnel are (a) shorten the duration of radiation exposure, (b) increase the distance from the radiation source, and (c) provide radiation shielding between the nurse and the radiation source (Alpen, 1998; Bushong, 2013; Dowd & Tilson, 1999; NCRP, 1993a, 1993b, 1993c). Portable radiologic examinations are the most common form of diagnostic imaging routinely performed in the NICU. During these procedures, there is a tendency for all the nurses to leave the room when an exposure is being produced; consequently, other infants may be left unattended for that short period. Because of this practice, parents have expressed fear about their infants facing environmental radiation hazards.

It appears that if certain basic radiation precautions are observed, nurses and other NICU personnel need not leave the room during x-ray exposures. However, staff members should stay 30 cm (1 foot) or farther from the infant being radiographed. Care must be taken to ensure that if a horizontal beam film is obtained (e.g., in a cross-table lateral projection), no one is in the direct x-ray beam; this is because the radiation dose in the primary beam is considerably higher than in the scattered portion. When a horizontal beam is used, it should not be directed at any other patient or person.

Any employee within 30 cm (1 foot) of the incubator or one who is holding the infant for the exposure should wear a lead apron and gloves. Table 15.2 summarizes the process of systematic interpretation of radiographic images in the neonate.

TABLE 15.2 Radiographic Interpretation	
Technical Evaluation	**Characteristics**
Film density and contrast	The intravertebral disk spaces should be visible through the cardiothymic silhouette. Underexposed films appear whitish with progressive loss of spaces; overexposed films have a "burned out" appearance with loss of pulmonary vascular markings.
Phase of respiration	The respiratory phase affects the appearance of the lung fields. During expiration, the cardiothymic silhouette appears larger, and the lung fields appear more opaque; the hemidiaphragms usually are at the level of the seventh rib. During inspiration, the cardiothymic silhouette is normal, pulmonary vascularity is seen, and the lung fields are clear. Adequate inspiration puts the right hemidiaphragm at the level of the posterior eighth rib; the right hemidiaphragm usually is slightly higher than the left during basal breathing.
Motion	Radiology personnel must check for motion at the time the film is taken. Motion is detected by blurring of the hemidiaphragms and cardiothymic silhouette. Motion obscures all fine pulmonary vascular detail, which makes the films unsatisfactory for evaluation of the lung fields.
Tube angulation and patient positioning	Anteroposterior (AP) films of the newborn appear lordotic, with the medial ends of the clavicles projecting on or above the second dorsal vertebra.

(continued)

TABLE 15.2 Radiographic Interpretation (*continued*)	
Technical Evaluation	**Characteristics**
	If the tube has been angled cephalad, the lordosis is exaggerated, with the anterior arcs of the ribs positioned superior to the posterior arcs. The cardiothymic silhouette appears larger because the view is through the transverse diameter of the heart. This occurs if the infant arches during the procedure or if the beam has been centered over the abdomen. Caudad angulation of the beam over the head results in distortion of the chest, with the anterior ribs arcs angled sharply downward in relation to the posterior arcs.
Rotation of the patient	Assessment of rotation is critical in determining whether mediastinal shift is present. Lateral rotation may lead to the false impression of a mediastinal shift. The trachea shifts toward the side of the rotation, and the contours of the heart are altered. The direction and degree of rotation are estimated by comparing the lengths of the posterior arcs of the ribs on both sides. The side with the longest posterior arc is the side to which the patient is rotated. Rotation also results in unequal lengths of the clavicles when they are measured from the medial aspects to the center of the vertebral body at the same level. The patient is rotated to the side with the longer clavicle.
Heart size and pulmonary vascularity	These features are difficult to determine in the newborn in the first 24 hours of life because of the dynamic cardiovascular alterations that occur during this period. Changes in the transitional circulation are associated with an increase in pulmonary blood flow and in blood return to the left atrium, a decrease in blood return and lower

(*continued*)

TABLE 15.2 Radiographic Interpretation (*continued*)	
Technical Evaluation	**Characteristics**
	pressure in the right atrium, and changes in systemic and pulmonary arterial pressures. The newborn's heart size is relatively larger in the first 48–72 hours because of those rapid changes. Heart size can be accurately assessed only during basal breathing, because the size is significantly altered during phases of the cardiac cycle and during hyperexpansion of the lung. After the first 24 hours, a cardiothoracic ratio above 0.6 is the upper limit of normal. Fetal lung fluid is reabsorbed, and the air spaces are filled with air on inspiration. The resorption of lung fluid enhances the appearance of the pulmonary lymphatics, resulting in an apparent increase in vascularity at birth. Transient tachypnea of the newborn is characterized by perihilar streaky infiltrates with increased pulmonary vascularity and good lung inflation.
Cardiothymic silhouette	The cardiac configuration is difficult to determine in the newborn largely because of the variation in size and shape of the thymus. The aortic knob and main pulmonary artery are obscured by the thymus, which frequently has a wavy border. A tuck may be seen in the left lobe of the thymus at the lateral margin of the right ventricle, a feature called a *sail sign*. The apex of the heart has a more cephalad position and assumes a more caudal position over time. The elevation of the apex is due to the relative right ventricular hypertrophy of the fetus. After birth, as the left ventricle becomes more prominent, the cardiac apex descends. The thymus involutes rapidly under the stress of delivery and over the next 2 weeks of life may enlarge slightly.

(*continued*)

TABLE 15.2 Radiographic Interpretation (*continued*)	
Technical Evaluation	**Characteristics**
Aeration of the lungs	Satisfactory inspiration positions the hemidiaphragms at the posterior arcs of the eighth rib. Expansion and radiolucency of the right and left sides are equal. If the sides are not comparable, a right and left lateral decubitus film should be obtained to evaluate for fluid levels or air. The lungs may bulge slightly through the ribs. On lateral projection, the hemidiaphragms should be smoothly domed. The AP and transverse diameters of the chest vary with age and disease. In a normal newborn, the AP and transverse diameters are equal. Over time, the transverse diameter increases, giving the chest cavity an oblong appearance. Air-trapping diseases produce a more rounded configuration, whereas hypoaeration results in a more flattened AP diameter. With hypoaeration, the right hemidiaphragm is located at the seventh rib, the posterior arcs have a more downward slope, and the transverse diameter of the chest is reduced. Laterally, hypoaeration results in increased doming of the diaphragm. With hyperaeration, the hemidiaphragm is located below the level of the ninth rib, the diaphragm is flattened, and the posterior rib arcs are horizontal. Hyperaeration also results in greater bulging of the lungs through the intercostal spaces and an increased diameter of the upper thorax.
Pulmonary infiltrates	Films should be evaluated for areas of increased pulmonary lucency or density. The characteristics and distribution of densities may lead to a diagnosis. Infiltrates should be described with regard to their distribution (unilateral, bilateral) and nature (alveolar, reticulated, diffuse, nondiffuse, patchy, streaky).

(*continued*)

TABLE 15.2 Radiographic Interpretation (*continued*)	
Technical Evaluation	**Characteristics**
Mediastinal shift	The examiner evaluates for mediastinal shift by determining if the trachea, heart, and mediastinum are in normal position. In general, the shift occurs toward the side with the diminished lung volume or away from the hemithorax with the increased lung volume. Rotation of the patient must first be excluded.
Liver size	The edges of the liver should be clearly defined, and the size of the organ should correlate well with the size determined by palpation, especially when the intestines are filled with air. If insufficient gas is present in the abdomen, the size of the liver cannot be determined. Atelectasis obscures the upper margin of the liver. Radiographically, the size of the liver is not altered by the phase of respiration, as it is during palpation. Liver size may vary with progression of right-sided heart failure. The position of the liver may be altered by congenital malformations such as situs inversus.
Abdominal gas pattern	Swallowing air produces gas in the stomach. The gas pattern must be interpreted in light of the infant's history. In the newborn, stomach air is present, with progression of air through the small bowel at 3 hours of life and rectal air by 6 hours. With bowel obstruction, gaseous distention progresses until at some point the bowel is blocked; beyond that point there is a paucity of air or a gasless bowel. Lack of haustra in the colon makes it possible to distinguish the small and large bowels on the radiograph. A gasless abdomen may be seen with prolonged gastrointestinal decompression, severe dehydration, acidosis, oversedation, brain injury, diaphragmatic hernia, midgut volvulus, and esophageal atresia.

(*continued*)

TABLE 15.2 Radiographic Interpretation (*continued*)	
Technical Evaluation	**Characteristics**
	Marked aerophagia may be due to mechanical ventilation, tracheoesophageal fistula, necrotizing enterocolitis, and mesenteric vascular occlusion. Free peritoneal air rises to the highest level and outlines superior structures; therefore, it is best demonstrated on a left lateral decubitus film.
Catheter and tube positions	All catheter and tube positions should be evaluated and reported each time a radiograph is made. The position of these devices may provide clues to the underlying disease, and malpositioning of tubes and catheters may be life threatening. The trachea is positioned to the right in the midmediastinum, anterior, and slightly to the right of the esophagus. The carina is located at T_4. In the right aortic arch, the trachea is found slightly to the left of the vertebral column. Endotracheal tubes optimally are placed in the midtrachea. If the tip is too low (below T_4) or too high (above the thoracic inlet), ventilation is suboptimal. Inadvertent esophageal intubation has occurred when the tip of the tube is below T_4 but is still in the midline or when the trachea can be visualized apart from the tube. Nasogastric (NG) tube placement should be reported. NG tubes may be too short (seen in the distal esophagus) or too long (seen in the duodenum or jejunum), or they may be coiled in the esophagus (tracheoesophageal atresia). The location of vascular catheters must be evaluated. Central catheters should be placed with the tip in the superior part of the inferior cava. Umbilical artery catheters ideally should be located in the high (T_6–T_9) or low (L3–L5) position, away from major arterial branches. Umbilical venous catheters should be positioned with the tip in the inferior vena cava and not in a hepatic branch.

(*continued*)

TABLE 15.2 Radiographic Interpretation (*continued*)	
Technical Evaluation	**Characteristics**
Bony structures	The skeleton should be evaluated, especially the general configuration of the thoracic cage. Normally, over time, the cephalic portion of the thoracic cage becomes rounded and the transverse diameter increases. Hyperaeration exaggerates cephalic rounding, and the horizontal position of the rib arcs. Hypoaeration reduces the diameter of the upper thorax and increases the inferior slope of the rib arcs (bell-shaped thorax). The radiograph must be evaluated for fractures, dislocations, hypodensities, or other lucencies. Persistent elevation of the scapula and an ipsilateral elevated diaphragm (which occur secondary to phrenic nerve injury) may accompany Erb's palsy. Scans should be done for vertebral, rib, and other bony anomalies. Rib aplasia is associated with hemivertebrae, and complete or partial aplasia of the clavicles may be a manifestation of chromosomal abnormality. The proximal humeri can yield information related to congenital infections such as in rubella, syphilis, and cytomegalovirus infection. The bone density should be evaluated in relation to film penetration.

REFERENCES

Alpen, E. L. (1998). *Radiation biophysics* (2nd ed.). San Diego, CA: Academic Press.

Bushong, S. C. (1999). *Diagnostic ultrasound: Essentials of medical imaging series.* New York, NY: McGraw-Hill.

Bushong, S. C. (2000). *Computed tomography: Essentials of medical imaging series.* New York, NY: McGraw-Hill.

Bushong, S. C. (2003). *Magnetic resonance imaging: Physical and biological principles* (3rd ed.). St. Louis, MO: Mosby.

Bushong, S. C. (2013). *Radiologic science for technologists: Physics, biology, and protection* (10th ed.). St. Louis, MO: Elsevier Mosby.

Dowd, S. B., & Tilson, E. R. (1999). *Practical radiation protection and applied radiobiology* (2nd ed.). Philadelphia, PA: Saunders.

Gomella, T. L., Cunningham, M. D., & Eyal, F. G. (2013). *Neonatology: Management, procedures, on-call problems, diseases, and drugs.* (7th ed.). New York, NY: McGraw-Hill.

Hilton, S., & Edwards, D. K. III. (2006). *Practical pediatric radiology* (3rd ed.). Philadephia, PA: Saunders Elsevier.

Juhl, J. H., Crummy, A. B., & Kuhlman, J. E. (1998). *Paul and Juhl's essentials of radiologic imaging* (7th ed.). Philadelphia, PA: Lippincott Williams & Wilkins.

Martin, R., Fanaroff, A., & Walsh, M. (2011). *Neonatal-perinatal medicine* (9th ed.). St. Louis, MO: Elsevier Mosby.

National Council on Radiation Protection and Measurements. (1993a). *Risk-estimates for radiation protections* (NCRP Report No. 15). Bethesda, MD: Author.

National Council of Radiation Protection and Measurements. (1993b). *Research needs for radiation protection* (NCRP Report No. 117). Bethesda, MD: Author.

National Council on Radiation Protection and Measurements. (1993c). *A practical guide to the determination of human exposure to radiofrequency fields.* (NCRP Report No. 119). Bethesda, MD: Author.

Swischuk, L. E. (1997). *Differential diagnosis in pediatric radiology* (3rd ed.). Baltimore, MD: Lippincott Williams & Wilkins.

Swischuk, L. E. (2003). *Imaging of the newborn, infant, and young child* (5th ed.). Baltimore, MD: Lippincott Williams & Wilkins.

Treves, S. T. (2014). *Pediatric nuclear medicine and molecular imaging* (4th ed.). New York, NY: Springer Publishing Company.

Verklan, M., & Walden, M. (2015). *Core curriculum for neonatal intensive care nursing* (5th ed.). St. Louis, MO: Elsevier Mosby.

ULTRASONIC IMAGING

With neonates, ultrasonography frequently is used in the evaluation and treatment of internal anatomic structures. Ultrasonography has the following advantages as a diagnostic tool (Bushong, 1999, 2013; Martin et al., 2011; Swischuk, 1997, 2003).

■ It emits no ionizing radiation and has now known deleterious somatic or genetic effects; therefore, follow-up may be repeated at will.

■ Ultrasound waves can be directed as a beam.

■ Sound waves obey laws of reflection and refraction.

■ Ultrasound waves are reflected by objects of small size.

■ Ultrasonography can be used in a variety of transverse, longitudinal, sagittal, or oblique planes.

■ Ultrasonography is considerably less costly than either CT or MRI.

■ Ultrasound equipment is easily portable.

■ The examination is relatively painless and well tolerated.

■ Sedation is rarely required.

■ Ultrasonography relies on acoustic impedance of tissue to demonstrate anatomy.

■ Ultrasonography is diagnostically accurate.

The following are the principal disadvantages of ultrasonography (Bushong, 1999, 2013):

■ It is operator dependent.

■ It does not provide as much information on organ function as urography.

■ It has limited value as a screening procedure for "acute abdominal distress"; rather, the examination should focus on a particular area of interest.

■ CT is superior in demonstrating the extent of disease, because ultrasonography demonstrates a smaller area of interest and less anatomic detail.

■ Bone, excessive fat, and gas artifacts adversely affect ultrasonography.

Because of these drawbacks, certain parts of the body, such as the brain, must be imaged through an ultrasound "window," such as the anterior fontanel. In addition, because sound waves are poorly propagated through a gaseous medium, the transducer must have airless contact with the surface being examined, and parts of the body that contain large amounts of air are difficult to examine.

Ultrasonography also is useful as a diagnostic imaging method because it is reflected at tissue interfaces. A principle called "sonic momentum" describes the velocity of sound transmitted through tissue.

The major patterns of ultrasound reflection are anechoic, echoic, and mixed. An anechoic structure, which is described as sonar lucent, is a structure in which the acoustic medium is homogeneous and the sound waves are unimpeded. An anechoic structure may be fluid filled (bladder), cystic (hydronephrosis), or solid (lymphoma), as long as the tissue is homogeneous. Cystic structures usually have sharp echogenic margins anteriorly and posteriorly. Echoic structures are inhomogeneous and reflect sound waves. These tissues generally are solid and have a variety of densities (typical Wilms' tumor) or may be cystic (hemorrhagic Wilms' tumor). A mixed pattern of reflections has the combined qualities of anechoic and echoic tissues. In addition, ribs and calculi may cause imaging artifacts on an ultrasonographic image. These dense structures prevent further penetration of the ultrasound beam and cause a band-like region of decreased sound transmission beyond that point, called acoustic shadowing (Bushong, 1999).

When the tissue interface is moving (e.g., the movement of red blood cells in a vessel), the reflected ultrasound wave has a shifted frequency directly proportional to the velocity of the reflecting blood cells, in accordance with a principle called the Doppler effect. If the movement of the blood cells is toward the transducer, the frequency of the reflected wave is higher than the transmitted frequency. Conversely, movement of blood away from the transducer results in a lower frequency of the reflected wave (Bushong, 1999, 2013). The difference between the transmitted frequency and the reflected frequency is called the Doppler shift. It is the principle of sound frequency shifts that allows the application of the mathematic relationship between the velocity of the target and the Doppler frequency to calculate flow. This is used most commonly in the echocardiographic evaluation of the heart and in cerebral blood flow determinations (Bushong, 1999, 2013).

BIOLOGIC EFFECTS OF ULTRASONOGRAPHY

Ultrasonic imaging was introduced into obstetric practice in 1966. Since that time, despite the widespread use of this imaging modality and the use of multiple scans during an individual pregnancy, there have been no reports of manifested injury or late effects in human beings (or fetuses) exposed to diagnostic levels of medical ultrasound (Bushong, 1999).

Indications for ultrasonography in neonatal intensive care commonly include evaluation of brain parenchyma and ventricular size, myocardial function and structure, cholelithiasis, choledochal cysts, intestinal duplication, renal neoplasms, urinary tract dilation and duplication, pelvic masses, and skeletal anomalies of the spine and hips (Martin et al., 2011).

COLLABORATIVE CARE

The care of a neonate undergoing a diagnostic ultrasound examination ensures that any disruption of the infant's microenvironment is minimal. The infant's temperature can be maintained more easily if the ultrasound examination can be performed by using the transducer in the incubator.

MAGNETIC RESONANCE IMAGING

The theoretic basis for MRI is a development of research conducted since the 1940s for studying atomic nuclear structure, which resulted in the awarding of the Nobel Prize for physics in 1952 to Edward Purcell and Felix Block. In addition to the advances in atomic nuclear research, other developments were necessary, such as superconductivity and advances in computer programming, before this concept could be applied to diagnostic imaging. As an imaging modality, MRI has several advantages over CT and ultrasound (Bushong, 2003, 2013; Huda et al., 2001; Lansberg et al., 2001; Peled & Yeashurun, 2001; Schierlitz et al., 2001):

1. Like ultrasonography, MRI does not use ionizing radiation to produce the image, but rather uses magnetic fields and radio waves.

2. The magnetic resonance image depends on three separate molecular parameters that are sensitive to changes in structure and bioactivity rather than on x-ray photon interaction with tissue electrons as in CT.

3. The region of the body imaged with MRI is not limited by the gantry geometry, as it is with CT, but can be controlled electronically, allowing imaging in transverse planes and in true sagittal, coronal, and oblique planes.

4. Magnetic resonance images are free of the high-intensity artifacts produced in CT scans by sharp, dense bone, or metallic surgical clips.

The principal disadvantages of MRI are its high cost and limited availability. Its use for clinically unstable infants on life support also is restricted, because the strong magnetic field can interfere with monitoring devices, and access to the infant is limited during the procedure (Lansberg et al., 2001; Schierlitz et al., 2001; Swischuk, 1997, 2003; Peled & Yeashurun, 2001). Despite the disadvantages of MRI, its clinical applications are rapidly expanding.

BIOPHYSICAL PRINCIPLES

All particles in an atom have either a positive or a negative charge, or a "spin," like a tiny spinning top. The total spin of the protons and neutrons on the nucleus is the sum of the individual spins. Moving charges create magnetic fields, thus the nucleus of an atom develops north and south magnetic dipoles (Bushong, 2003, 2013; Dowd & Tilson, 1999; Juhl, 1998). In MRI, the strong magnetic field is imposed to align the molecular magnetic dipoles, and radio frequency pulses then are applied. The known specific frequency of these radio waves displaces the net magnetic moment by an amount determined by the strength and duration of the pulse. The frequency is directly proportional to the strength of the magnetic field and is known as the resonant frequency. After the pulse, the protons emit radio frequencies as they return to their original orientation. Therefore, the frequency of signals emitted by the protons after the application with radio frequency waves reflects their position in the tissue. Although in theory any stable nuclei can be used, hydrogen is the most abundant and has the strongest resonance (Bushong, 2003, 2013; Juhl, 1998).

When protons are placed in a magnetic field, proton alignment does not occur instantaneously, but rather increases exponentially with a time constant characterized by T1, or spin–lattice relaxation time, which reflects the interaction of the hydrogen nucleus with its molecular environment (Bushong, 2003, 2013; Juhl, 1998). T1 characterizes the return of the net magnetization from its displaced position to its normal vertical position resulting from spin–lattice interactions. To form an image, the radio frequency pulses must be applied repetitively. After each radio frequency pulse, the net magnetic force of the sample is reduced; therefore, too rapid a radio frequency repetition depletes the magnetization of the tissue, and an image cannot be produced. Hence, radio frequency pulses are sequenced with a certain time interval to allow the magnetic force to be reestablished. The longer the time interval, the greater the magnetic force, and the longer the imaging time required (Bushong, 2003, 2013; Juhl, 1998).

After exposure to the radio frequency pulse has occurred, the signal emitted from the sample of protons decays exponentially with a time constant referred to as T2, or spin–spin relaxation time. T2 reflects the magnetic interactions between protons. It characterizes the exponential loss of signal caused by dephasing or desynchronization of magnetic force, which results from spin–spin interactions (Bushong, 2003, 2013; Dort et al., 2001; Juhl, 1998). The interval between the application of a radio frequency pulse and the emitted signal depends on the alignment and synchronization of magnetic dipoles. A strong magnetic force results in a long interval for the emitted signal after the pulse; this explains the contrast between tissues with different values of T2 changes. T1 is not equal to T2, because each nucleus is not located within identical magnetic fields. Each hydrogen nucleus is subject to different local magnetic fields because of the presence or absence of other hydrogen nuclei (Bushong, 2003, 2013; Dort et al., 2001).

The third variable that affects image resolution with MRI is spin density. *Spin density* refers to the strength of the signal received from the nuclei before any of the decay processes have taken place (Bushong, 2003, 2013; Dort et al., 2001; Juhl, 1998). This strength is proportional to the number of nuclei within the detection volume of the scanner. Spin density is an indication of hydrogen concentration in the tissue.

A magnetic resonance image results from the mixture of these three properties (T1, T2, and spin density) unique to each tissue. The values of T1 and T2 for various tissues have been defined. A wide range of values exists among various types of tissue, and considerable differences have been documented between pathologic and normal tissue (Dort et al., 2001; Juhl, 1998). Each number defined for the relaxation times (T1 and T2) for various tissues depends on the primary external magnetic field and thus may vary from scanner to scanner. The visual projection of the magnetic resonance image is similar to that obtained in CT. By controlling the gradient field of radio frequency pulses, a series of projections at uniform angles through the tissue can be collected. The computer can then reconstruct the image and can emphasize the individual T1, T2, or spin density parameters to further define detail (Bushong, 2003, 2013; Dort et al., 2001; Juhl, 1998).

The spatial resolution of an MRI scan compares favorably to that obtained with CT. If the object scanned is of high tissue contrast, a lesion as small as 1 mm can be defined. As more data are collected on this imaging modality, even greater spatial resolution and enhanced three-dimensional images are being obtained. As stronger magnetic fields are used, the emitted signals become stronger, and greater resolution may be possible using even higher radio frequency pulses (Bushong, 2003, 2013; Dort et al., 2001).

MRI is better able than CT to detect differences between low-contrast structures. The difference in T1 and T2 MRI between biologic tissues frequently is 10% or more. For example, on CT scans, the x-ray photon attenuation coefficient between gray and white matter is approximately 0.5%, whereas the differences in T1, T2, and spin density between gray and white matter are great, allowing for more accurate definition of these two tissues (Bushong, 2003, 2013; Dort et al., 2001). Thus, MRI has become the diagnostic imaging mode of choice for certain neurologic conditions such as multiple sclerosis, cerebral infarctions, and periventricular leukomalacia. MRI may be useful in the early diagnosis of periventricular leukomalacia, before the characteristic cystic lesions have developed (Huppi et al., 2001; Krishnamoorthy et al., 2000; Peterson et al., 2000; Sie, Barkhof, Lafeber, Valk, & van der Knaap, 2000; Tierney, Varga, Hosey, Grafman, & Braun, 2001).

SAFETY OF MRI

MRI scanning uses three kinds of fields associated with the imaging process: (a) a static, moderately strong magnetic field; (b) a switched, weaker magnetic field gradient; and (c) radio frequency waves. The energies associated with the imaging process are approximately 10 to 8 eV/quantum, which are too weak to cause ionization or breakage of chemical bonds (Bushong, 2003, 2013; Dowd & Tilson, 1999). Energies associated with body temperature elevations are 100,000 to 1 million times greater, so these temperature effects are far more disruptive to chemical bonds than the energy associated with MRI (Bushong, 2003, 2013).

The hazards of MRI relate primarily to any ferromagnetic objects (e.g., tools, oxygen cylinders, watches, bank cards, pens, and paper clips) that are accelerated toward the center of the magnetic field. The magnetic propulsion of these objects can result in projectile damage; therefore, any patient with a pacemaker or an extensive metal prosthesis should be excluded from this imaging technique. In addition, MRI has not been fully tested with pregnant women.

REFERENCES

Alpen, E. L. (1998). *Radiation biophysics* (2nd ed.). San Diego, CA: Academic Press.

Bushong, S. C. (1999). *Diagnostic ultrasound: Essentials of medical imaging series.* New York, NY: McGraw-Hill.

Bushong, S. C. (2003). *Magnetic resonance imaging: Physical and biological principles* (3rd ed.). St. Louis, MO: Mosby.

Bushong, S. C. (2013). *Radiologic science for technologists: Physics, biology, and protection* (10th ed.). St. Louis, MO: Elsevier Mosby.

Dort, J. C., Sadler, D., Hu, W., Wallace, C., La Forge, P., & Sevick, R. (2001). Screening for cerebellopontine angle tumours: Conventional MRI vs T2 fast spin echo MRI. *Canadian Journal Neurological Sciences, 28*(1), 47–50.

Dowd, S. B., & Tilson, E. R. (1999). *Practical radiation protection and applied radiobiology* (2nd ed.). Philadelphia, PA: Saunders.

Huda, W., Chamberlain, C. C., Rosenbaum, A. E., & Garrisi, W. (2001). Radiation doses to infants and adults undergoing head CT examinations. *Medical Physics, 28*(3), 393–399.

Huppi, P. S., Murphy, B., Maier, S. E., Zientara, G. P., Inder, T. E., Barnes, P. D., & Volpe, J. J. (2001). Microstructural brain development after perinatal cerebral white matter injury assessed by diffusion tensor magnetic resonance imaging. *Pediatrics, 107*(3), 455–460.

Juhl, J. H., Crummy, A. B., & Kuhlman, J. E. (1998). *Paul and Juhl's essentials of radiologic imaging* (7th ed.). Philadelphia, PA: Lippincott Williams & Wilkins.

Krishnamoorthy, K. S., Soman, T. B., Takeoka, M., & Schaefer, P. W. (2000). Diffusion-weighted imaging in neonatal cerebral infarction: Clinical utility and follow-up. *Journal of Child Neurology, 15*(9), 592–602.

Lansberg, M. G., O'Brien, M. W., Tong, D. C., Moseley, M. E., & Albers, G. W. (2001). Evolution of cerebral infarct volume assessed by diffusion-weighted magnetic resonance imaging. *Archives of Neurology, 58*(4), 613-617.

Martin, R., Fanaroff, A., & Walsh, M. (2011). *Neonatal-perinatal medicine.* (9th ed.). St. Louis, MO: Elsevier Mosby.

Peled, S., & Yeshurun, Y. (2001). Superresolution in MRI: Application to human white matter fiber tract visualization by diffusion tensor imaging. *Magnetic Resonance in Medicine, 45*(1), 29–35.

Peterson, B. S., Vohr, B., Staib, L. H., Cannistraci, C. J., Dolberg, A., Schneider, K. C., ... Ment, L. R. (2000). Regional brain volume abnormalities and long-term cognitive outcome in preterm infants. *Journal of the American Medical Association, 284*(15), 1939–1947.

Schierlitz, L., Dumanli, H., Robinson, J. N., Burrows, P. E., Schreyer, A. G., Kikinis, R., & Tempany, C. M. (2001). Three-dimensional magnetic resonance imaging of fetal brains. *Lancet, 357*(9263), 1177–1178.

Sie, L. T., Barkhof, F., Lafeber, H. N., Valk, J., & van der Knaap, M. S. (2000). Value of fluid-attenuated inversion recovery sequences in early MRI of the brain in neonates with a perinatal hypoxic-ischemic encephalopathy. *European Radiology, 10*(10), 1594–1601.

Swischuk, L. E. (1997). *Differential diagnosis in pediatric radiology* (3rd ed.). Baltimore, MD: Lippincott Williams & Wilkins.

Swischuk, L. E. (2003). *Imaging of the newborn, infant, and young child* (5th ed.). Baltimore, MD: Lippincott Williams & Wilkins.

Tierney, M. C., Varga, M., Hosey, L., Grafman, J., & Braun, A. (2001). PET evaluation of bilingual language compensation following early childhood brain damage. *Neuropsychologia, 39*(2), 114–121.

CARDIAC PROCEDURES

ELECTROCARDIOGRAPHY

Electrocardiography is a noninvasive diagnostic tool used with neonates. It is most useful in the diagnosis and management of cardiac arrhythmias or in conjunction with other diagnostic measures to evaluate cardiac function, specifically the circulatory demands placed on individual heart chambers. In the neonatal period, however, electrocardiography is less helpful in evaluating cardiac anomalies associated with significant ventricular enlargement (Flanagan, Yeager, & Weindling, 2005).

ECHOCARDIOGRAPHY

Echocardiography, another noninvasive diagnostic procedure, commonly is used in the evaluation of the structure and function of the heart. This information can be important not only in the preoperative assessment of cardiac defects, but also in the postoperative evaluation of procedures. High-frequency sound waves send vibrations to the structures in the heart, which reflect energy, which is transmitted into a visual image. Echocardiography may be used prenatally as early as 11 weeks gestation when used transvaginally or 18 weeks gestation when used transabdominally (Erenberg, 2011).

Single-dimension echocardiography allows the evaluation of anatomic structures, including valves, chambers, and vessels. Two-dimensional echocardiography provides more in-depth information about relationships between the heart and the great vessels (Flanagan et al., 2005).

Doppler echocardiography is used in various forms in the evaluation of characteristics of blood flow through the heart, valves, and great vessels. It can measure not only cardiac output, but also flow velocity changes, as demonstrated in stenotic lesions. Regurgitation through insufficiently functioning valves can also be identified. Doppler studies can be used to show regurgitation through insufficiently functioning valves or to identify shunting, as through a patent ductus arteriosus (Zahka, 2011).

CARDIAC CATHETERIZATION

With the advent of more sophisticated echocardiography, especially Doppler echocardiography, cardiac catheterization is used increasingly as a therapeutic modality. The use of radiopaque dye allows clarification of congenital heart disease and helps to provide data that cannot be obtained from echocardiography.

Immobilization and constant monitoring of the neonate are required during cardiac catheterization. The infant must be restrained to maintain supine positioning. Electrocardiographic electrodes must also be placed to provide constant monitoring of vital signs. Sedation may be considered to maintain proper positioning during the procedure.

A local anesthetic is administered at the insertion site. A radiopaque catheter is inserted into an arm or leg vessel by percutaneous puncture or cut-down. Under fluoroscopy, the catheter is visualized and passed into the heart. Contrast medium is injected through the catheter to allow visualization of the various cardiac structures. Selected chambers and vessels of the heart can be evaluated for size and function. Intracardiac pressures and oxygen saturations can also be measured during this procedure. The use of balloons during catheterization can facilitate procedures such as septostomy, angioplasty, and valvuloplasty (Erenberg, 2011; Flanagan et al., 2005).

After the necessary information has been obtained, the catheter is carefully removed. If a cut-down was performed, the vessel is ligated and the skin is sutured. Pressure should be applied over a percutaneous puncture site to enhance clot formation. For continued bleeding problems, pressure dressings may be applied to the insertion site; these must be checked frequently for active bleeding. After cardiac catheterization, the vital signs should be measured frequently and compared with precatheterization baseline values. Evaluation of localized bleeding or of signs of hypotension resulting in changes in heart rate and blood pressure is essential. Assessment of the insertion site and affected extremity for bleeding, color, peripheral pulses, temperature, and capillary refill should continue for at least 24 hours after the procedure. In addition, the nurse must monitor for complications of catheterization, including hypovolemia (as a result of bleeding or fluid loss during the procedure), infection, thrombosis, or tissue necrosis.

REFERENCES

Erenberg, F. (2011). Fetal cardiac physiology and fetal cardiovascular assessment. In R. Martin, A. Fanaroff, & M. Walsh (Eds.), *Neonatal-perinatal medicine* (9th ed.). St. Louis, MO: Elsevier Mosby.

Flanagan, M. F., Yeager, S. B., & Weindling, S. N., (2005). Cardiac disease. In M. G. MacDonald, M. D. Mullett, & M. K. Seshia (Eds.), *Avery's neonatology pathophysiology & management of the newborn* (6th ed.). Philadephia, PA: Lippincott Williams & Wilkins.

Zahka, K. G. (2011). Approach to the neonate with cardiovascular disease. In R. Martin, A. Fanaroff, & M. Walsh (Eds.), *Neonatal-perinatal medicine* (9th ed.). St. Louis, MO: Elsevier Mosby.

GENETIC TESTING

CHROMOSOME ANALYSIS

High-resolution karyotyping and banding

Analysis of chromosome composition can assist in identification of various genetic disorders. A blood specimen is obtained from the infant and used to harvest an actual set of chromosomes. During active cell division, usually during metaphase, the chromosomes are photographed and then arranged in pairs by number. The chromosomes are also separated into regions, bands, and subbands. The end result, a karyotype with banding, is evaluated for the appropriate number of pairs, chromosome size, and structure. Specific genetic disorders can be associated with abnormal numbers of chromosomes (e.g., trisomy 21) or an abnormal chromosome structure, as in cri du chat syndrome, which reflects loss of part of the short arm of chromosome 5 (Kuller & Cefalo, 1996). Abnormal genes on the chromosomes can also cause genetic disorders, such as Duchenne muscular dystrophy, an X-linked recessive disorder.

High-resolution karyotype is widely used for infants with multiple congenital anomalies. This test consists of analysis of chromosomes from white blood cells. The cells are cultured and stimulated to divide, and then cell division is halted with a mitotic inhibitor in the prometaphase stage. In this stage, the chromosomes are at their longest length, and the stained band observed can reach 800 to 900. This test can take up to 2 weeks (Gomella et al., 2013).

Fluorescence in situ hybridization

Chromosomes can be further analyzed using fluorescence in situ hybridization (FISH) to detect syndromes that are not visible to the naked eye. The FISH process allows fluorescent-coated DNA probes to detect submicroscopic chromosomal deletions. It can be used with interphase and metaphase cells. This test is faster than high-resolution karyotyping (but still could take up to several weeks to complete). This test can provide a quick diagnosis for infants with trisomy 13, 18, 21, or Turner syndrome (Bajaj & Gross, 2011; Gomella et al., 2013; Martin et al., 2011; McLean, 2005).

Bone marrow cells may be analyzed for chromosomes if a more rapid evaluation is required. Skin fibroblast analysis is required when an infant has been transfused, making lymphocyte analysis inaccurate. In cases such as stillbirth, tissue biopsy specimens can be used for chromosome testing because viable lymphocytes are absent (Hamilton & Wynshaw-Boris, 2009).

Sweat chloride test

The sweat chloride test is used to evaluate for and confirm the diagnosis of cystic fibrosis. During the procedure the skin is stimulated with pilocarpine and a small electrical current for 5 minutes. The sweat is collected on a 2 × 2-in. gauze pad or filter paper for 30 minutes. Over this 30-minute period, 75 mg of sweat must be produced to ensure an appropriate sweat rate (National Committee for Clinical Laboratory Standards, 1994). A sweat chloride level below 40 mEq/L is normal. Levels between 60 and 165 mEq/L are considered diagnostic for cystic fibrosis (Wilford & Taussig, 1998). Sweat tests can be inaccurate if an inadequate amount of sweat is produced; if the sweat evaporates; or if the patient has edema.

Comparative genomic hybridization or chromosomal microarray analysis

The comparative genomic hybridization (CGH) and chromosomal microarray analysis (CMA) detects chromosomal deletions or duplication; this cytogenetic technique is relatively new. CGH/CMA compares reference standard DNA to the patient's DNA through a florescent technique. This test compares hundreds of regions across the entire genome to assess for the number of differences. It commonly assesses for microdeletion and microduplication, subtelomeric, and pericentromeric regions (Gomella et al., 2013).

NEWBORN SCREENING

Every infant born in a hospital in the United States undergoes newborn screening. Newborn screening is done before leaving the hospital, usually about day 1 or 2. Some states require follow up at about 2 weeks. All states are required to screen for 26 health conditions according to the March of Dimes (MOD) (2012). In addition, the MOD recommends that each state screen for 31. Some states are known to screen for 50 and more. For more information on newborn screens, please see http://www.marchofdimesusa.org/baby/bringinghome_newbornscreening.html (Newborn Screening, 2012).

REFERENCES

Bajaj, K., & Gross, S. (2011). Genetic aspects of perinatal disease and prenatal diagnosis. In R. Martin, A. Fanaroff, & M. Walsh (Eds.), *Neonatal–perinatal medicine* (9th ed.). St. Louis, MO: Elsevier Mosby.

Gomella, T. L., Cunningham, M. D., & Eyal, F. G. (2013). *Neonatology: Management, procedures, on-call problems, diseases, and drugs* (7th ed.). New York, NY: McGraw-Hill.

Hamilton, B. A., & Wynshaw-Boris, A., (2009). Basic genetics and patterns of inheritance. In R. K. Creasy, R. Resnik, J. D. Iam, C. J. Lockwood, & T. Moore (Eds.), *Creasy and Resnik's maternal-fetal medicine: Principles and practice.* (6th ed.). Philadelphia, PA: Saunders Elsevier.

Kuller, J. A., & Cefalo, R. C. (1996). *Prenatal diagnosis and reproductive genetics.* St. Louis, MO: Mosby.

March of Dimes (MOD). (2012). Bringing baby home. Retrieved from http://www.marchofdimesusa.org/baby/bringinghome_newbornscreening.html

Martin, R., Fanaroff, A., & Walsh, M. (2011). *Neonatal-perinatal medicine.* (9th ed.). St. Louis, MO: Elsevier Mosby.

McLean, S.D. (2005). Congenital anomalies. In M. G. MacDonald, M. D. Mullett, & M. K. Seshia (Eds.), *Avery's neonatology pathophysiology & management of the newborn* (6th ed.). Philadephia, PA: Lippincott Williams & Wilkins.

National Committee for Clinical Laboratory Standards. (1994). *Sweat testing: Sample collection and quantitative analysis: Approved guideline.* Wayne, PA: Author.

Newborn Screening. (2012, March). Retrieved from http://www.marchofdimesusa.org/baby/bringinghome_newbornscreening.html

Wilford, B. S., & Taussig, L. M. (1998). Cystic fibrosis: General overview. In L. M. Taussig & L. I. Landau (Eds.), *Pediatric respiratory medicine.* St. Louis, MO: Mosby.

GI PROCEDURES

BARIUM ENEMA

A barium enema is used in the evaluation of the structure and function of the large intestine. The diagnosis of disorders such as Hirschsprung disease and meconium plug syndrome can easily be supported by the use of this procedure.

For the enema procedure, either air or a contrast solution (e.g., barium sulfate) is instilled and a series of films are taken under fluoroscopy. The infant must be well restrained, starting in the supine position. As the contrast solution is instilled, its flow through the bowel is observed as the infant's position is changed. A series of abdominal x-ray films should be taken once the bowel has been filled with contrast solution. Follow-up films may also be necessary to document evacuation of the contrast solution from the bowel. Evaluation of the bowel is essential after this procedure to prevent constipation or obstruction. Assessment of bowel elimination is an important nursing concern after barium enema.

UPPER GI SERIES WITH SMALL BOWEL FOLLOW-THROUGH

As with the barium enema, barium sulfate or some other water-soluble contrast solution is used for the upper GI series with small bowel follow-through. However, the contrast solution is swallowed so that the upper GI tract can be examined. The three main areas examined are (a) the esophagus (for size, patency, reflux, and presence of a fistula or swallowing abnormality), (b) the stomach (for anatomic abnormalities, patency, and motility), and (c) the small intestine (for strictures, patency, and function).

Follow-up x-ray films may be desirable to evaluate both the emptying ability of the stomach and intestinal motility as the contrast material moves through the small bowel. Again, care of the infant includes assessment of temperature and cardiac and respiratory status throughout the procedure. The nurse should be alert for reflux or vomiting, which can be accompanied by aspiration. Evacuation of contrast material from the bowel remains a concern after upper GI series with small bowel follow-through and should be monitored by the nurse. It is also possible for fluid to be pulled out of the vascular compartment and into the bowel, resulting in hypotension. It is imperative that the health care team assess the infant for signs of these complications.

RECTAL SUCTION BIOPSY

Rectal biopsy is a procedure commonly used to help determine the presence or absence of ganglion cells in the bowel (the latter condition is seen in Hirschsprung disease). Before a rectal biopsy, it is essential to obtain bleeding times, prothrombin time, partial thromboplastin time, and platelet counts, as well as a spun hematocrit, to ensure that the infant is in no danger of excessive bleeding.

The infant is positioned supine with the legs held toward the abdomen. Small specimens of rectal tissue from the mucosal and submucosal levels are excised with a suction blade apparatus inserted through the anus into the bowel. The section of the pathology department that deals with the composition of ganglion cells evaluates the specimens.

Care of the infant after rectal suction biopsy should focus on assessments for bleeding or intestinal perforation. These assessments should include evaluation of vital signs for increased heart rate or decreased blood pressure, fever, persistent guaiac-positive stools, or frank rectal bleeding.

LIVER BIOPSY

Open or closed liver biopsy may be required for neonates. Open liver biopsy is a surgical procedure that requires general anesthesia, whereas a closed liver biopsy may be done using local anesthesia. As with the rectal biopsy, coagulation studies are essential, including bleeding time, platelet count, and spun hematocrit. Preoperative care may include sedation of the infant, requiring frequent monitoring of vital signs. Throughout the procedure, assessment of vital signs is essential for identifying changes in hemodynamics or respiratory status. After the procedure, assessment of vital signs for signs and symptoms of hemorrhage is essential. Indications of hemorrhage include decreases in the hemoglobin and hematocrit, which makes laboratory monitoring an important element of postbiopsy care. The biopsy site must be evaluated for signs of active bleeding, ecchymosis, swelling, or infection.

GENITOURINARY PROCEDURES

CYSTOSCOPY

Cystoscopy permits direct visualization of the urinary structures, including the bladder, urethra, and urethral orifices, allowing diagnosis of abnormalities in the structure of the bladder and urinary tract.

Cystoscopy is performed using general anesthesia. Preparation of the urethral opening with an antiseptic solution is followed by sterile draping. The lubricated cystoscope is inserted through the urethra, and the urinary structures are examined.

As with any patient who has had anesthesia, post-procedural care includes vital sign assessment. However, particular attention should be paid to assessing for adequate urinary output, the presence of hematuria, and signs of infection (Pagana & Pagana, 2013).

EXCRETORY UROGRAPHY AND INTRAVENOUS PYELOGRAPHY

Excretory urography and intravenous pyelography complement cystoscopic evaluation because they allow the examiner not only to evaluate structures but also to focus on the function of those structures. The intravenous route injects small amounts of contrast media, and as the contrast material is excreted through the urinary system, a sequence of x-ray films is taken. The configuration of organs and the rate of excretion of the contrast media are reflected in these films.

Excretory urography and intravenous pyelography are relatively safe for use in neonates and should cause no postprocedural complications.

VOIDING CYSTOURETHROGRAM

The purpose of a voiding cystourethrogram is to visualize the lower urinary tract after instillation of contrast media through urethral catheterization. The infant's bladder is emptied after catheterization and then filled with the contrast media. Serial films under fluoroscopy in a variety of positions are taken during voiding. After voiding, additional films are obtained. Pathologic results of a voiding cystourethrogram demonstrate residual urine in the bladder, such as with a neurogenic bladder, posterior valve obstructions, or vesicourethral reflux.

As with cystoscopy, the infant should be evaluated for hematuria; the baby also should be checked for signs of infection (fever, cloudy or sedimented urine, foul-smelling urine) in the event of contaminated catheterization.

ELECTROENCEPHALOGRAPHY

An electroencephalographic examination records the electrical activity of the brain. Numerous electrodes are placed at precise locations on the infant's head to record electrical impulses from various parts of the brain. This procedure can be important for diagnosing lesions or tumors, for identifying nonfunctional areas of the brain, or for pinpointing the focus of seizure activity.

The infant may require sedation during this procedure to prevent crying or movement. As much equipment as is safely possible should be removed to reduce electrical interference. Also, calming procedures, such as reducing light stimulation or warming the environment, may help quiet the infant during electroencephalography. The infant should be closely observed throughout the procedure for any signs of seizure activity.

RESPIRATORY PROCEDURES

PULSE OXIMETRY

Pulse oximetry is a widely used, noninvasive method of monitoring arterial blood oxygenation saturations (SaO_2). The SaO_2 is the ratio of oxygenated hemoglobin to total hemoglobin. A single probe, attached to an infant's extremity or digit, uses light emitted at different wavelengths, which is absorbed differently by saturated and unsaturated hemoglobin. The change in the light during arterial pulses is used to calculate the oxygen saturation. Pulse oximetry saturations reflect a more accurate measure of actual hemoglobin saturation. Saturations obtained by blood gas sample are calculated using a hemoglobin of 15 g% (Goetzman & Wennberg, 1999).

Proper placement of the probe should be assessed regularly, because movement, environmental light, edema, and diminished perfusion can reduce the accuracy of readings. The probe should be rotated every few hours to prevent skin breakdown at the site.

BRONCHOSCOPY

Bronchoscopy of the newborn is performed to visualize the upper and lower airways and to collect diagnostic specimens. The procedure can be done in the NICU using a flexible bronchoscope, or it can be performed under general anesthesia in the operating room using either a flexible or rigid bronchoscope. The flexible bronchoscope is preferable for examining the lower airways of an intubated patient or for examination of a patient with mandibular hypoplasia. A rigid bronchoscope is more advantageous in situations requiring removal of foreign bodies and for evaluation of patients with H-type tracheoesophageal fistula (TEF), laryngotracheoesophageal clefts, and bilateral abductor paralysis of the vocal cords (Wood, 1998). Examination of structures by direct visualization provides the opportunity to identify congenital anomalies, obstructions, masses, or mucous plugs and to evaluate stridor or respiratory dysfunction.

Bronchoscopy done at the bedside requires the nurse to assist with positioning, sedation, and monitoring of vital signs. Whether the infant undergoes flexible or rigid bronchoscopy, respiratory and cardiovascular monitoring should be continued in the immediate postprocedural period. Possible complications related to these procedures include bronchospasm, laryngeal spasms, laryngeal edema, or pneumothorax or bradycardia resulting in hypoxia.

SUMMARY

Marked technical advances over the past two decades have produced a variety of imaging methods for the diagnosis, treatment, and evaluation of neonates. Sizable expenditures have been directed toward improving image presentation and quality on the assumption that a trained clinical eye can make diagnostic use of the data provided. Investigations are useful only insofar as they reduce the diagnostic uncertainty. The final product of any radiologic imaging procedure is not a set of photographic pictures, but a diagnostic opinion that should be beneficial to management of the infant. Before initiating any imaging method, physicians should consider whether further information is really needed, and they should select the imaging technique that will give the required information with sufficient reliability and with minimal risk to the patient. The value of any diagnostic imaging examination must be balanced against the potential hazards. In addition to care of the newborn during and after a procedure, nursing care of newborns and infants undergoing diagnostic procedures requires a knowledge of the expected outcomes and methods so that the best result possible is obtained. Nurses also must be knowledgeable about normal values for the laboratory tests commonly used in the care of newborns and infants.

REFERENCES

Goetzman, B. W., & Wennberg, R. P. (1999). *Neonatal intensive care handbook* (3rd ed.). St. Louis, MO: Mosby.

Pagana, K. D., & Pagana, T. J. (2013). *Mosby's diagnostic and laboratory test reference* (11th ed.). St. Louis, MO: Elsevier Mosby.

Wood, R. E. (1998). Diagnostic and therapeutic procedures in pediatric pulmonary patients. In L. M. Taussig & L. I. Landau (Eds.), *Pediatric respiratory medicine*. St. Louis, MO: Mosby.

EXPANDED NEWBORN SCREENING: CRITICAL CONGENITAL HEART DISEASE

Wakako Eklund

The aim of performing an expanded newborn screening prior to discharge from the hospital is to identify certain treatable diseases during the early days of the newborn's life to make early interventions possible. These are generally healthy newborns and not typically NICU patients. This section is included here as there may be reasons neonatal nurses will encounter these newborns. The implementation of the expanded newborn screening has decreased mortality and morbidity related to various rare diseases, such as genetic or metabolic diseases (Centers for Disease Control and Prevention [CDC], 2008).

In the United States, screening for critical congenital heart disease (CCHD) with pulse oximetry has been recommended as a part of the expanded newborn screening, in addition to the blood sampling for multiple metabolic or genetic diseases and hearing screening for early recognition of congenital hearing deficit (Kemper et al., 2011). Efforts to implement uniform recommendation for CCHD screening are gaining momentum and pilot studies, multicenter studies, or regional implementations have been reported worldwide (Al Mazrouei, Moore, Ahmed, Mikula, & Martin, 2013; de-Wahl Granelli et al., 2014; Hom & Martin, 2014; Riede et al., 2010; Zhao et al., 2014).

The extent of the implementation or general understanding of the CCHD screening among health care providers may widely. The education related to CCHD screening aimed at early detection is an essential piece of the knowledge base for the nursing and other health professionals who care for the newborn population, as this screening has the potential to improve the outcome of CCHD patients by recognizing the disease earlier (Thangaratinam, Brown, Zamora, Khan, & Ewer, 2012).

BACKGROUND OF THE CCHD SCREENING IN THE UNITED STATES

In September 2010, the U.S. Health and Human Services Secretary's Advisory Committee on Heritable Disorders in Newborn and Children (SACHDNC) recommended that CCHD screening be added to the Recommended Uniform Screening Panel (RUSP) (Kemper et al., 2011; Mahle, Martin, Beekman, & Morrows, 2012; U.S. Department of Health and Human Services, 2013). This recommendation was made based on the previous studies that were conducted in Europe and in the United States (de-Wahl Granelli et al., 2009; Riede et al., 2010; Thangaratinam et al., 2012). Subsequently, the SACHDNC collaborated with the American College of Cardiology, the American Academy of Pediatrics, and the American Heart Association to develop strategies for successful implementation of CCHD screening in the United States (Kemper et al., 2011).

INCIDENCE

According to the CDC (2014a), congenital heart defects (CHDs) are the most commonly occurring birth defects; however, many of the babies born with these defects are living longer when appropriate interventions are provided. CHDs occur in seven to nine per 1,000 live births in the United States (Botto, Correa, & Erickson, 2001; Reller, Strickland, Riehle-Colarusso, Mahle, & Correa, 2008). This accounts for 1% of annual births, or approximately 40,000 births a year (Hoffman & Kaplan, 2002; Reller et al., 2008). Out of the entire universe of CHD cases, CCHD cases account for one sixth to one fourth, or 1 to 3 per 1,000 live births annually (Harris, Francannet, Pradat, & Robert, 2003; Hoffman & Kaplan, 2002; Oster et al., 2013; Pradat, Francannet, Harris, & Robert, 2003; Wren, Reinhardt, & Khawaja, 2008).

SIGNIFICANCE

If untreated, these infants' conditions would become life threatening and potentially lethal upon closure of the ductus arteriosus or other causes related to the physiological changes in the postnatal period

(Kemper et al., 2011). Earlier identification and initiation of treatment allows the infants to avoid the consequences of hypoperfusion, such as potential organ damage (Mahle et al., 2009). The delayed diagnosis leads to severe hemodynamic collapse and shock, leaving the infants in poorer preintervention condition. This unfortunately leads to poorer postintervention outcomes (Brown et al., 2006).

ASSESSMENT

Prenatal ultrasounds have limitation in identifying CCHD early. The most important clinical information that should be remembered by every nurse is that infants with CCHD may appear healthy, as a subtle decrease in saturation rate is often not detectable and no other symptoms may exist. Bedside nurses must be aware that, based on the type of structural defects, the newborn's presentation and resultant morbidity and mortality may differ. Some newborns with certain critical defects may present with a significant murmur or cyanosis, which leads to further evaluation including an echocardiograph by a specialist and likely an early diagnosis. Unfortunately, not all the cardiac defects present with recognizable murmur, vital sign changes, cyanosis, or other symptoms, and the newborns often appear healthy. This occurs more often when they have ductal dependent CHD during the period while the ductus is patent.

In the United States or worldwide, where routine discharges from the hospital after birth occur as early as 24 hours after birth, physiologic changes related to the defects do not present until after the hospital discharge. The benefit of recognizing the potential problem postnatally, and prior to discharge, is emphasized in regions where family of ill infants reside at a distance away from regional referral centers, or when a prenatal ultrasound was not always performed as a part of routine prenatal care.

Why is pulse oximetry important for CCHD?

The CCHD screening is performed with the use of a pulse-oximetry device familiar to most of the healthcare providers today. This device is painless to the babies and simple for anyone to learn to use. Pulse oximetry is recommended for CCHD screening to detect possible decrease in oxygen saturation. Many cases of CCHD, though not all, are accompanied by hypoxemia that is not visually detectable, but is detectable by pulse oximetry, during the early days of life (Mahle et al., 2009). If there is poor perfusion or vasoconstriction, caused by hypothermia or hypotension, an accurate saturation cannot be obtained, potentially leading to false positive CCHD screening results.

CCHD DEFINED: TARGETED DEFECTS

In the United States, for purposes of CCHD screening, CCHD is defined as a CHD that requires surgical or catheter intervention within the first year of life (Mahle et al., 2009).

The primary screening targets include the following CHDs (CDC, 2014b; Kemper et al., 2011; Mahle et al., 2009; 2012).

- Hypoplastic left heart syndrome
- Pulmonary atresia
- Tetralogy of fallot
- Total anomalous pulmonary venous return
- Transposition of the great arteries
- Tricuspid atresia
- Truncus arteriosus

Some defects are not included in this list, such as a coarctation of the aorta (CoA). CoA is the most frequently missed defect reported, and the diagnosis most likely to be missed even with the CCHD screening (Liberman et al., 2014; Mouledoux & Walsh, 2013; Peterson et al., 2014a). The CCHD screening may not have included CoA as one of the targeted diagnoses due to this reason; thus, clinicians must remain aware of the difficulty of identifying CoA by continuing with a thorough physical examination. The critical need to assess the pulses in the lower extremities of each newborn prior to discharge and at postdischarge check-ups cannot be overemphasized. Newborns with delayed CoA diagnosis have presented with symptoms such as tachypnea, cyanosis, murmur, poor feeding, respiratory distress, or circulatory collapse in need of rigorous resuscitation, or even death. According to Mouldoux and Walsh, the age of diagnosis for the missed CoA in state of Tennessee in 2011 ranged from 7 days to 30 days of life (Mouledoux & Walsh, 2013).

Bedside nurses who educate the parents at the time of discharge must inform the parents that the fact of passing CCHD screening does not rule out the presence of potential CCHD. The parents must be informed of danger signs and symptoms and the need to seek immediate care for further evaluation.

The potential impact of the CCHD screening

Peterson et al. (2014a) reported that nearly 30% of the babies with CCHD were not diagnosed until they were older than 3 days of age.

This would be a primary benefit of the CCHD screening, which is universally performed regardless of where the births occur, at 24 to 48 hours age before the newborns are discharged from the hospital. The finding that babies with other defects were more likely to be diagnosed early, and that those who appear healthy are missed more frequently, also suggests the value of screening every infant, whether or not the baby is symptomatic.

RECOMMENDED REGIONAL POLICY FOR THE CCHD SCREENING

Based on the Health and Human Services Department's Recommendations, in the United States, many states have enacted legislation to make CCHD screening a mandatory aspect of newborn screening or implementing programs in accordance with the national recommendation (as many as 40, as of late 2014).

NECESSARY EQUIPMENT AND THE SAMPLE PROTOCOL

Equipment needed

A Federal Drug Administration (FDA)-approved pulse oximeter (approved for newborn use) that is motion-tolerant.

Manufacturer-recommended probes that are disposable or reusable.

Protocol

Follow the manufacturer's recommendation to apply the probe by ensuring that the emitter and the detector portion of the probe are positioned appropriately.

The infant should not be cold or crying at the time of screening. (Nursing consideration: Educate the family in regards to the importance of CCHD screening and invite the family to assist to soothe the infant.)

Screen every infant shortly before discharge if less than 24 hours old or between 24 and 48 hours. Screening before 24 hours is associated with higher false positives (Thangaratinam et al., 2012).

Screening procedure

- Screen one foot, either the right or left
- 97% to 100% of infants pass the screening
- Passing does not definitively exclude the potential presence of CHDs.
- If any clinical findings suggest the possibility of CHDs, even with the passing reading, obtain further consultation for evaluation of CHDs.
- Lower than 90%: Immediately seek primary provider or specialist for further evaluation. (This process is determined by region; please investigate what is recommended in your region by your health authority.)
- 90% to 96%: Screen the right hand.
- Pass: If ≥ 95% in the right hand and foot and there is ≤ 3% difference between the right hand and the foot.
- Fail: If the right hand or foot reading is less than 90%, seek the primary provider or a specialist for further evaluation immediately.
- Rescreen in 1 hour: If 90% to 94% in the right hand and foot or greater than 3% difference is noted between the right hand reading and the foot.

- Pass: If ≥ 95% in the right hand or foot and ≤ 3% different is found between the right hand and foot.

- Fail: If less than the right hand or foot reading is still 90%. Seek the primary care provider or a specialist for further evaluation immediately. (Please investigate what is recommended in your region by your health authority.)

- 90% to 94% in the right hand, or there is greater than 3% difference between the right hand and foot.

- Rescreen in 1 hour.

- Pass: If ≥ 95% in the right hand or foot and there is ≤ 3% difference between the right hand and the foot.

- Fail: If less than 90% is found in the right hand or foot.

- Fail: If 90% to 94% in the right hand and foot or greater than 35% difference is found between the right hand and the foot and there is no clear cause of hypoxemia.

- In either of the latter two cases, please seek the primary care provider or a specialist for further evaluation.

- Do not rescreen.

SPECIAL CONSIDERATIONS

The current national recommendations for the CCHD screening do not include NICU patients. There is no specific guideline available at this time for the NICU population, and there is a potential for an increase in false negatives (Iyengar, Kumar, & Kumar, 2014; Manja, Mathew, Carrion, & Lakshminrusimha, 2015). It is prudent to observe the pulse oximeter reading on inpatients at 24 to 48 hours when stable, or once prior to discharge from the hospital. In any case, the CCHD screening is not intended to minimize or replace a careful physical examination by trained professionals and a thorough history taking to identify risk factors, such as family history of previous CHD or maternal risk factors associated with CHD (such as infant of a diabetic mother).

CONCLUSION

The presentation of a CCHD may be subtle or asymptomatic. The use of pulse oximetry is intended to increase the rate of early detection of CCHDs, which can allow the early initiation of treatment. It is very important that every birthing facility and hospital where births occur institute provisions to address these efforts toward early detection of CCHDs. The staff must be educated to perform the CCHD screening and to use the algorithm accurately.

REFERENCES

Al Mazrouei, S. K., Moore, J., Ahmed, F., Mikula, E. B., & Martin, G. R. (2013). Regional implementation of newborn screening for critical congenital heart disease screening in Abu Dhabi [Review]. *Pediatric Cardiology, 34*(6), 1299–1306. doi:10.1007/s00246-013-0692-0696

Botto, L. D., Correa, A., & Erickson, J. D. (2001). Racial and temporal variations in the prevalence of heart defects. *Pediatrics, 107*(3), E32.

Brown, K. L., Ridout, D. A., Hoskote, A., Verhulst, L., Ricci, M., & Bull, C. (2006). Delayed diagnosis of congenital heart disease worsens preoperative condition and outcome of surgery in neonates. *Heart, 92*(9), 1298–1302. doi:10.1136/hrt.2005.078097

Centers for Disease Control & Prevention (CDC). (2008). Impact of expanded newborn screening—United States, 2006. *Morbidity & Mortality Weekly Reports, 57*(37), 1012–1015.

CDC. (2014a). *Congenital heart defects (CHDs): Data and statistics.* Retrieved from http://www.cdc.gov/ncbddd/heartdefects/data.html

CDC. (2014b). *Congenital heart defects (CHDs): Information for healthcare providers.* Retrieved from http://www.cdc.gov/ncbddd/heartdefects/hcp.html

de-Wahl Granelli, A., Meberg, A., Ojala, T., Steensberg, J., Oskarsson, G., & Mellander, M. (2014). Nordic pulse oximetry screening—Implementation status and proposal for uniform guidelines. *Acta Paediatrica.* doi:10.1111/apa.12758

Harris, J. A., Francannet, C., Pradat, P., & Robert, E. (2003). The epidemiology of cardiovascular defects, part 2: A study based on data from three large registries of congenital malformations. *Pediatric Cardiology, 24*(3), 222–235. doi:10.1007/s00246-002-9402-9405

Hoffman, J. I., & Kaplan, S. (2002). The incidence of congenital heart disease. *Journal of the American College of Cardiology, 39*(12), 1890–1900.

Hom, L. A., & Martin, G. R. (2014). U.S. international efforts on critical congenital heart disease screening: Can we have a uniform recommendation for Europe? *Early Human Development, 90*(Suppl. 2), S11–S14. doi:10.1016/S0378-3782(14)50004-50007

Iyengar, H., Kumar, P., & Kumar, P. (2014). Pulse-oximetry screening to detect critical congenital heart disease in the neonatal intensive care unit. *Pediatric Cardiology, 35*(3), 406–410. doi:10.1007/s00246-013-0793-2

Kemper, A. R., Mahle, W. T., Martin, G. R., Cooley, W. C., Kumar, P., Morrow, W. R., ... Howell, R. R. (2011). Strategies for implementing screening for critical congenital heart disease. *Pediatrics, 128*(5), e1259–e1267. doi:10.1542/peds.2011-1317

Liberman, R. F., Getz, K. D., Lin, A. E., Higgins, C. A., Sekhavat, S., Markenson, G. R., & Anderka, M. (2014). Delayed diagnosis of critical congenital heart defects: Trends and associated factors. *Pediatrics, 134*(2), e373–e381. doi:10.1542/peds.2013-3949

Mahle, W. T., Martin, G. R., Beekman, R. H., 3rd, & Morrow, W. R. (2012). Endorsement of health and human services recommendation for pulse oximetry screening for critical congenital heart disease. *Pediatrics, 129*(1), 190–192. doi:10.1542/peds.2011-3211

Mahle, W. T., Newburger, J. W., Matherne, G. P., Smith, F. C., Hoke, T. R., Koppel, R., ... Grosse, S. D. (2009). Role of pulse oximetry in examining newborns for congenital heart disease: A scientific statement from the American Heart Association and American Academy of Pediatrics [Consensus Development Conference]. *Circulation, 120*(5), 447–458. doi:10.1161/CIRCULATIONAHA.109.192576

Manja, V., Mathew, B., Carrion, V., & Lakshminrusimha, S. (2015). Critical congenital heart disease screening by pulse oximetry in a neonatal intensive care unit. *Journal of Perinatology, 35*(1), 67–71. doi:10.1038/jp.2014.135

Mouledoux, J. H., & Walsh, W. F. (2013). Evaluating the diagnostic gap: Statewide incidence of undiagnosed critical congenital heart disease before newborn screening with pulse oximetry. *Pediatric Cardiology, 34*(7), 1680–1686. doi:10.1007/s00246-013-0697-1

Oster, M. E., Lee, K. A., Honein, M. A., Riehle-Colarusso, T., Shin, M., & Correa, A. (2013). Temporal trends in survival among infants with critical congenital heart defects. *Pediatrics, 131*(5), e1502–e1508. doi:10.1542/peds.2012-3435

Peterson, C., Ailes, E., Riehle-Colarusso, T., Oster, M. E., Olney, R. S., Cassell, C. H., … Gilboa, S. M. (2014a). Late detection of critical congenital heart disease among US infants: Estimation of the potential impact of proposed universal screening using pulse oximetry. *JAMA Pediatrics, 168*(4), 361–370. doi:10.1001/jamapediatrics.2013.4779

Pradat, P., Francannet, C., Harris, J. A., & Robert, E. (2003). The epidemiology of cardiovascular defects, part I: A study based on data from three large registries of congenital malformations. *Pediatric Cardiology, 24*(3), 195–221. doi:10.1007/s00246-002-9401-9406

Reller, M. D., Strickland, M. J., Riehle-Colarusso, T., Mahle, W. T., & Correa, A. (2008). Prevalence of congenital heart defects in metropolitan Atlanta, 1998–2005. *Journal of Pediatrics, 153*(6), 807–813. doi:10.1016/j.jpeds.2008.05.059

Riede, F. T., Worner, C., Dahnert, I., Mockel, A., Kostelka, M., & Schneider, P. (2010). Effectiveness of neonatal pulse oximetry screening for detection of critical congenital heart disease in daily clinical routine—Results from a prospective multicenter study. *European Journal of Pediatrics, 169*(8), 975–981. doi:10.1007/s00431-010-1160-1164

Thangaratinam, S., Brown, K., Zamora, J., Khan, K. S., & Ewer, A. K. (2012). Pulse oximetry screening for critical congenital heart defects in asymptomatic newborn babies: A systematic review and meta-analysis. *Lancet, 379*(9835), 2459–2464. doi:10.1016/S0140-6736(12)60107-X

U.S. Department of Health and Human Services. (2013). *Discretionary Advisory Committee on heritable disorders in newborn and children: Recommended uniform screening panel*. Retrieved from http://www.hrsa.gov/advisorycommittees/mchbadvisory/heritabledisorders/recommendedpanel

Wren, C., Reinhardt, Z., & Khawaja, K. (2008). Twenty-year trends in diagnosis of life-threatening neonatal cardiovascular malformations [Research Support, Non-U.S. Gov't]. *Archives of Diseases in Childhood—Fetal and Neonatal Edition, 93*(1), F33–F35. doi:10.1136/adc.2007.119032

Zhao, Q. M., Ma, X. J., Ge, X. L., Liu, F., Yan, W. L., Wu, L., … Neonatal Congenital Heart Disease Screening Group. (2014). Pulse oximetry with clinical assessment to screen for congenital heart disease in neonates in China: A prospective study. *Lancet, 384*(9945), 747–754. doi:10.1016/S0140-6736(14)60198-7

ADDITIONAL CHAPTER REFERENCES

Abramoff, M. D., Van Gils, A. P., Jansen, G. H., & Mourits, M. P. (2000). MRI dynamic color mapping: A new quantitative technique for imaging soft tissue motion in the orbit. *Investigative Ophthalmology Visual Science, 41*(11), 3256–3260.

Aoyagi, T., & Miyasaka, K. (2002). The theory and applications of pulse spectrophotometry. *Anesthesia & Analgesia, 94*(Suppl. 1), S93–S95.

Nolte, U. G., Finsterbusch, J., & Frahm, J. (2000). Rapid isotropic diffusion mapping without susceptibility artifacts: Whole brain studies using diffusion-weighted single-shot STEAM MR imaging. *Magnetic Resonance in Medicine, 44*(5), 731–736.

Peterson, C., Grosse, S. D., Glidewell, J., Garg, L. F., Van Naarden Braun, K., Knapp, M. M., ... Cassell, C. H. (2014b). A public health economic assessment of hospitals' cost to screen newborns for critical congenital heart disease. *Public Health Reports, 129*(1), 86–93.

Peterson, C., Grosse, S. D., Oster, M. E., Olney, R. S., & Cassell, C. H. (2013). Cost-effectiveness of routine screening for critical congenital heart disease in U.S. newborns. *Pediatrics, 132*(3), e595–e603. doi:10.1542/peds.2013-0332

Sinson, G., Bagley, L. J., Cecil, K. M., Torchia, M., McGowan, J. C., Lenkinski, R. E., & Grossman, R. I. (2001). Magnetization transfer imaging and proton MR spectroscopy in the evaluation of axonal injury: Correlation with clinical outcome after traumatic brain injury. *American Journal of Neuroradiology, 22*(1), 143–151.

Weissleder, R., & Mahmood, U. (2001). Molecular imaging. *Radiology, 219*(2), 316–333.

Wiesmann, M., & Seidel, G. (2000). Ultrasound perfusion imaging of the human brain. *Stroke, 31*(10), 2421–2425.

Yorgin, P. D., & Rhee, K. H. (1998). Gas exchange and acid-base physiology. In L. M. Taussig & L. I. Landau (Eds.), *Pediatric respiratory medicine.* St. Louis, MO: Mosby.

Common Laboratory Values

Samual L. Mooneyham

A wide variety of laboratory tests can be used in both the diagnosis and care of the newborn. The values given in this chapter represent the broader normal ranges, but values in a specific chapter may vary slightly, depending on the range the author considers to be within normal limits. Every attempt has been made to provide consistent diagnostic and laboratory values. However, many hospitals have compiled their own list of acceptable laboratory test values; therefore, specific laboratories should be contacted when evaluating results (Tables 16.1–16.14). Nurses also must be knowledgeable about normal values for the laboratory tests commonly used in the care of newborns and infants.

TABLE 16.1 Common Electrolyte and Chemistry Values	
Parameter	Normal Value
Serum Electrolytes	
Sodium (Na)	135–145 mEq/L
Potassium (K)	4.5–6.8 mEq/L
Chloride (Cl)	95–110 mEq/L
Carbon dioxide (CO_2)	20–25 mmol/L
Serum Chemistries	
Blood urea nitrogen (BUN)	6–30 mg/dL
Calcium (Ca)	7–10 mg/dL
Creatinine (Cr)	0.2–0.9 mg/dL

(continued)

TABLE 16.1 Common Electrolyte and Chemistry Values (*continued*)

Parameter	Normal Value
Glucose (G)	40–97 mg/dL
Magnesium (Mg)	1.5–2.5 mg/dL
Phosphorus (P)	5.4–10.9 mg/dL

TABLE 16.2 Normal Hematologic Values

	Gestational Age (Weeks)						
	28	34	Full-Term Cord Blood	Day 1	Day 3	Day 7	Day 14
Hemoglobin (g/dL)	14.5	15	16.8	18.4	17.8	17	16.8
Hematocrit (%)	45	47	53	58	55	54	52
Red cells (mm³)	4	4.4	5.25	5.8	5.6	5.2	5.1
MCV (mc m³)	120	118	107	108	99	98	96
MCH (pg)	40	38	34	35	33	32.5	31.5
MCHC (%)	31	32	31.7	32.5	33	33	33
Reticulocytes (%)	5–10	3–10	3–7	3–7	1–3	0–1	0–1
Platelets (mc 10³/mm³)			290	192	213	248	252

MCH, mean corpuscular hemoglobin; MCHC, mean corpuscular hemoglobin concentration; MCV, mean corpuscular volume.

Source: Klaus and Fanaroff (2001).

TABLE 16.3 White Cell and Differential Counts in Premature Infants

| | Birth Weight | | | | | |
| | Under 1,500 g | | | 1,500–2,500 g | | |
	1 Week Old	2 Weeks Old	4 Weeks Old	1 Week Old	2 Weeks Old	4 Weeks Old
Total Count (×10³/mm³)						
Mean	16.8	15.4	12.1	13	10	8.4
Range	6.1–32.8	10.4–21.3	8.7–17.2	6.7–14.7	7.0–14.1	5.8–12.4
Percentage of Total Polymorphs						
Segmented	54	45	40	55	43	41
Unsegmented	7	6	5	8	8	6
Eosinophils	2	3	3	2	3	3
Basophils	1	1	1	1	1	1
Monocytes	6	10	10	5	9	11
Lymphocytes	30	35	41	9	36	38

Source: Klaus and Fanaroff (2001).

TABLE 16.4 Summary of Normal Urinary Laboratory Values

	Age of Infant	Normal Value
Ammonia	2–12 months	4–20 mcEq/min/m²
Calcium	1 week	Under 2 mg/dL
Chloride	Infant	1.7–8.5 mEq/24 hr
Creatinine	Newborn	7–10 mg/kg/day
Glucose[a]	Preterm Full-term	60–130 mg/dL 12–32 mg/dL
Glucose (renal threshold)	Preterm Full-term	2.21–2.84 mg/mL 2.20–3.68 mg/mL
Magnesium		180 ± 10 mg/1.73 m²/dL
Osmolality	Infant	50–600 mOsm/kg
Potassium		26–123 mEq/L
Protein		Under 100 mg/m²/dL
Sodium		0.3–3.5 mEq/dL (6–10 mEq/m²)
Specific gravity	Newborn	1.006–1.008

[a]actual blood level.

Source: Ichikawa (1990).

TABLE 16.5 Electrocardiographic Data Pertinent to the Neonate[a]

Parameter	Age				
	Birth to 24 Hours	1–7 Days	8–30 Days	1–3 Months
Heart rate (beats/min)	119 (94–145)	133 (100–175)	163 (115–190)	154 (124–190)
PR interval (sec)	0.1 (0.07–0.12)	0.09 (0.07–0.12)	0.09 (0.07–0.11)	0.1 (0.07–0.13)
P-wave amplitude II	1.5 (0.8–2.3)	1.6 (0.8–2.5)	1.6 (0.08–2.4)	1.6 (0.8–2.4)
QRS duration (sec)	0.065 (0.05–0.08)	0.06 (0.04–0.08)	0.06 (0.04–0.07)	0.06 (0.05–0.08)
QRS axis (degrees)	135 (60–180)	125 (80–160)	110 (60–160)	80 (40–120)
R amplitude V_{4R} (mm)	8.6 (4–14.2)	—	6.3 (3.3–8.5)	5.1 (1.1–10.1)
R amplitude V_1 (mm)	11.9 (4.3–21)	—	11.1 (3.3–18.7)	11.2 (4.5–18)
R amplitude V_5 (mm)	10.2 (4–18)	10.7 (3.4–19)	11.9 (3.5–27)	13.6 (7.3–20.7)
R amplitude V_6 (mm)	3.3 (2.3–7)	5.1 (2.2–13.1)	6.7 (1.7–20.5)	8.4 (3.6–12.9)
S amplitude V_{4R} (mm)	3.8 (0.2–13)	—	1.8 (0.8–4.6)	3.4 (0–9.3)
S amplitude V_1 (mm)	9.7 (1.1–19.1)	—	6.1 (0–15)	7.5 (0.5–17.1)
S amplitude V_5 (mm)	11.9 (0.24)	6.8 (3.6–16.2)	4.8 (2.7–12.3)	4.7 (2–12.7)
S amplitude V_6 (mm)	4.5 (1.6–10.3)	3.3 (0.8–9.9)	2 (0.6–9)	2.4 (0.8–5.8)

[a]Mean (5th–95th percentile).

Source: Fanaroff and Martin (1987); Liebman and Plonsey (1977).

TABLE 16.6 Acid–Base Status

Determination	Sample Source	Birth	1 Hour	3 Hours	24 Hours	2 Days	3 Days
Vigorous Term Infants (Vaginal Delivery)							
pH	Umbilical artery	7.26					
	Umbilical vein	7.29					
PCO_2 (mmHg)	Arterial	54.4	38.8	38.3	33.6	34	35
	Venous	42.8					
O_2 saturation	Arterial	19.8	93.8	94.7	93		
	Venous	47.6					
pH	Left atrial		7.30	7.34	7.41	7.39	7.38
CO_2 content (mEq/L)	—	—	20.6	21.9	21.4	Temporal artery	Temporal artery
Premature Infants							
	Capillary (skin puncture)						
pH	< 1,250 g				7.36	7.35	7.35
PCO_2 (mmHg)					38	44	37
pH	> 1,250 g				7.39	7.39	7.38
PCO_2 (mmHg)					38	39	38

CO_2, carbon dioxide; PCO_2, partial pressure of carbon dioxide; pH, hydrogen ion concentration; O_2, oxygen.

Source: Schaffer (1971).

TABLE 16.7 Selected Chemistry Values in Preterm and Full-Term Infants

Constituent	Preterm Infant	Full-Term Infant
Alkaline phosphatase (U/L) (mean ± SD)[8]	207 ± 60 to 320 ± 142	164 ± 68
Ammonia (mcg/dL)[1]		90–150
Base, excess (mmol/L)[1]		–10 to –2
Bicarbonate, standard (mmol/L)[2]	18–26	20–26
Bilirubin, total (mg/dL)		
Cord[2]	Under 2.8	Under 2.8
24 hours old	1–6	2–6
48 hours old	6–8	6–7
3–5 days old	10–12	4–6
1 month or older	Under 1.5	Under 1.5
Bilirubin, direct (mg/dL)[2]	Under 0.5	Under 0.5
Calcium, total (mg/dL), week 1[3,4]	6–10	8.4–11.6
Ceruloplasmin (mg/dL)[1]		1–3 months: 5–18
Cholesterol (mg/dL)		
Cord[2]		45–98
3 days to 1 year old		65–175
Creatine phosphokinase (U/L)		
Day 1[5]		44–1,150
Day 4		14–97
Creatine (mg/dL)	10 days: 1.3 ± 0.07	1–4 days: 0.3–1

(continued)

TABLE 16.7 Selected Chemistry Values in Preterm and Full-Term Infants (*continued*)		
Constituent	Preterm Infant	Full-Term Infant
	1 month: 0.6 ± 0.05	Over 4 days: 0.2–0.4
Ferritin (mcg/dL)		
Neonate[1]		25–200
1 month old		200–600
2–5 months old		50–200
Over 6 months old		7–142
Gamma-glutamyl transferase (GGT) (U/L)[6]		14–131
Glucose (mg/dL)	20–125	30–125
Under 72 hours old[7,9]	40–125	40–125
Over 72 hours old		357–953
Lactate dehydrogenase (U/L)[6]		1.7–2.4
Magnesium (mg/dL)[4]		275–295 (may be as low as 266)
Osmolality (mOsm/L)[1]		
Phosphorus (mg/dL)		
Birth[4]		4.5–8.7
Day 5		4.2–7.2
1 month old		4.5–6.5
Aspartate aminotransferase (SGOT/AST) (U/L)[7]		24–81
Alanine aminotransferase (SGPT/ALT) (U/L)[7]		10–33

(*continued*)

TABLE 16.7 Selected Chemistry Values in Preterm and Full-Term Infants (*continued*)

Constituent	Preterm Infant	Full-Term Infant
Triglycerides (mg/dL)[2]		10–140
Urea nitrogen (mg/dL)[1]	3–25	4–12
Uric acid (mg/dL)[2]		3–7.5
Vitamin A (mcg/dL) (mean ± SD) (under 10 mcg/dL indicates very low hepatic vitamin A stores)[10]	16 ± 1	23.9 ± 1.8
Vitamin D		
25-hydroxycholecalciferol (ng/mL)[a,11,12]		20–60
1,25-dihydroxycholecalciferol (pg/mL)[a,11,12]		40–90

[a]Serum levels are affected by race, age, season, and diet.

[1]Tietz (1988).

[2]Wallach (1983).

[3]Meites (1975).

[4]Nelson, Finnstrom, and Larsson (1987).

[5]Drummond (1979).

[6]Statland (1979).

[7]Cornblath and Schwartz (1976).

[8]Glass, Hume, Hendry, Strange, and Forfar (1982).

[9]Heck and Erenberg (1987).

[10]Shenai, Chytil, Jhaveri, and Stahlman (1981).

[11]Cooke et al. (1990).

[12]Lichtenstein, Specker, Tsang, Mimouni, and Gormley (1986).

Source: Fanaroff and Martin (2002).

TABLE 16.8 Plasma Albumin and Total Protein in Preterm Infants From Birth to 8 Weeks

Gestation (Weeks)	26	27	28	29	30	31	32	33	34
Albumin (g/dL)									
Reference range (95% confidence limits)	—	1.18–3.06	1.09–2.87	1.20–2.74	1.63–2.75	1.08–3.20	1.38–3.14	1.44–3.34	0.53–3.87
Corrected age									
26–28 weeks gestation		2.13	2.10	2.58	2.29	2.39			
29–31 weeks gestation					2.02	2.14	2.44	2.44	2.54
32–34 weeks gestation								2.35	2.42
Total protein (g/dL)									
Reference range (95% confidence limits)	—	1.28–7.94	3.03–5.03	2.18–5.84	2.64–5.80	3.26–5.66	3.63–5.81	3.57–5.87	3.57–6.59
Corrected age									
26–28 weeks gestation		4.07	4.45	4.84	4.49	4.45			
29–31 weeks gestation					3.93	4.42	4.70	4.82	4.51
32–34 weeks gestation								4.54	4.93

Albumin (g/dL)								
Reference range (95% confidence limits)	1.15–3.87	1.96–3.44	1.50–4.10	1.89–4.15	2.07–4.15	2.07–4.05	2.04–3.90	2.08–3.90
Corrected age								
26–28 weeks gestation	2.73							
29–31 weeks gestation				2.82				
32–34 weeks gestation	2.46	2.38	2.44				3.35	
Total protein (g/dL)								
Reference range (95% confidence limits)	1.52–8.62	3.85–6.91	4.69–6.95	3.32–9.16	4.17–8.25	4.26–8.08	3.73–8.47	3.24–8.76
Corrected age								
26–28 weeks gestation	4.41							
29–31 weeks gestation				4.55				
32–34 weeks gestation	4.78	4.86	4.81				4.96	

Source: Fanaroff and Martin (2002); Reading, Ellis, and Fleetwood (1990).

TABLE 16.9 Plasma-Serum Amino Acid Levels in Premature and Term Newborns (mcmol/L)

Amino Acid	Premature (First Day)	Newborn 16 (Before First Feeding)	16 Days to 4 Months
Taurine	105–255	101–181	
OH-proline	0–80	0	
Aspartic acid	0–20	4–12	17–21
Threonine	155–275	196–238	141–213
Serine	195–345	129–197	104–158
Asp + Glut	655–1,155	623–895	
Proline	155–305	155–305	141–245
Glutamic acid	30–100	27–77	
Glycine	185–735	274–412	178–248
Alanine	325–425	274–384	239–345
Valine	80–180	97–175	123–199
Cystine	55–75	49–75	33–51
Methionine	30–40	21–37	31–47
Isoleucine	20–60	31–47	31–47
Leucine	45–95	55–89	56–98
Tyrosine	20–220	53–85	33–75
Phenylalanine	70–110	64–92	45–65
Ornithine	70–110	66–116	37–61
Lysine	130–250	154–246	117–163

(continued)

TABLE 16.9 Plasma-Serum Amino Acid Levels in Premature and Term Newborns (mcmol/L) (continued)

Amino Acid	Premature (First Day)	Newborn 16 (Before First Feeding)	16 Days to 4 Months
Histidine	30–70	61–93	64–92
Arginine	30–70	37–71	53–71
Tryptophan	15–45	15–45	
Citrulline	8.5–23.7	10.8–21.1	
Ethanolamine	13.4–10.5	32.7–72	
Alpha-amino-n-butyric acid	0–29	8.7–20.4	
Methylhistidine			

Source: Behrman (1977); Dickinson, Rosenblum, and Hamilton (1965, 1970); Klaus and Fanaroff (2001).

TABLE 16.10 Urine Amino Acid Levels in Normal Newborns (mcmol/L)

Amino Acid	mcmol/day
Cysteic acid	Tr–3.32
Phosphoethanolamine	Tr–8.86
Taurine	7.59–7.72
OH-proline	0–9.81
Aspartic acid	Tr
Threonine	0.176–7.99
Serine	Tr–20.7
Glutamic acid	0–1.78

(continued)

TABLE 16.10 Urine Amino Acid Levels in Normal Newborns (mcmol/L) *(continued)*	
Amino Acid	**mcmol/day**
Proline	0–5.17
Glycine	0.176–65.3
Alanine	Tr–8.03
Alpha-aminoadipic acid	
Alpha-amino-*n*-butyric acid	0–0.47
Valine	0–7.76
Cystine	0–7.96
Methionine	Tr–0.892
Isoleucine	0–6.11
Tyrosine	0–1.11
Phenylalanine	0–1.66
Beta-aminoisobutyric acid	0.264–7.34
Ethanolamine	Tr–79.9
Ornithine	Tr–0.554
Lysine	0.33–9.79
1-Methylhistidine	Tr–8.64
3-Methylhistidine	0.11–3.32
Carnosine	0.044–4.01
Beta-aminobutyric acid	
Cystathionine	
Homocitrulline	
Arginine	0.088–0.918
Histidine	Tr–7.04
Sarcosine	
Leucine	Tr–0.918

Source: Fanaroff and Martin (1997); Klaus and Fanaroff (2001); Meites (1997).

TABLE 16.11 Cerebrospinal Fluid Values of Healthy Term Newborns

Component	Age			
	Birth to 24 Hours	1 Day	7 Days	Over 7 Days
Color	Clear or xanthochromic	Clear or xanthochromic	Clear or xanthochromic	
Red blood cells (cells/mm³)	9 (0–1,070)	23 (6–630)	3 (0–48)	
Polymorphonuclear leukocytes (cells/mm³)	3 (0–70)	7 (0–26)	2 (0–5)	
Lymphocytes (cells/mm³)	2 (0–20)	5 (0–16)	1 (0–4)	
Protein (mg/dL)	63 (32–240)	73 (40–148)	47 (27–65)	
Glucose (mg/dL)	51 (32–78)	48 (38–64)	55 (48–62)	
Lactate dehydrogenase (IU/L)	22–73	22–73	22–73	0–40

Source: Klaus and Fanaroff (2002); Naidoo (1968); Neches and Platt (1968).

TABLE 16.12 Cerebrospinal Fluid Values in Very Low-Birth-Weight Infants on Basis of Birth Weight

	≤ 1,000 g		1,001–1,500 g	
	Mean ± SD	Range	Mean ± SD	Range
Birth weight (g)	763 ± 115	550–980	1,278 ± 152	1,020–1,500
Gestational age (weeks)	26 ± 1.3	24–28	29 ± 1.4	27–33
Leukocytes/mm^3	4 ± 3	0–14	6 ± 9	0–44
Erythrocytes/mm^3	1,027 ± 3,270	0–19,050	786 ± 1,879	0–9,750
PMN leukocytes (%)	6 ± 15	0–66	9 ± 17	0–60
MN leukocytes (%)	86 ± 30	34–100	85 ± 28	13–100
Glucose (mg/dL)	61 ± 34	29–217	59 ± 21	31–109
Protein (mg/dL)	150 ± 56	95–370	132 ± 3	45–227

MN, mononuclear; PMN, polymorphonuclear.

Modified from Rodriquez, Kapian, and Mason (1990).

TABLE 16.13 Cerebrospinal Fluid Values in Very-Low-Birth-Weight Infants (1,001–1,500 g) by Chronologic Age

Component	Postnatal Age (Days)					
	0–7		8–28		29–84	
	Mean ± SD	Range	Mean ± SD	Range	Mean ± SD	Range
Birth weight (g)	1,428 ± 107	1,180–1,500	1,245 ± 162	1,020–1,480	1,211 ± 86	1,080–1,300
Gestational age at birth (wk)	31 ± 1.5	28–33	29 ± 1.2	27–31	29 ± 0.7	27–29
Leukocytes/mm³	4 ± 4	1–10	7 ± 11	0–44	8 ± 8	0–23
Erythrocytes/mm³	407 ± 853	0–2,450	1,101 ± 2,643	0–9,750	661 ± 1,198	0–3,800
PMN (%)	4 ± 10	0–28	10 ± 19	0–60	11 ± 19	0–48
Glucose (mg/dL)	74 ± 19	50–96	59 ± 23	39–109	47 ± 13	31–76
Protein (mg/dL)	136 ± 35	85–176	137 ± 46	54–227	122 ± 47	45–187

PMN, polymorphonuclear.

Modified from Rodriquez, Kaplan, and Mason (1990).

TABLE 16.14 Thyroid Function in Full-Term and Preterm Infants

	Serum T$_4$ Concentration in Premature and Term Infants					Serum Free T$_4$ Index in Premature and Term Infants				
	Estimated Gestational Age (Weeks)									
	30–31	32–33	34–35	36–37	Term	30–31	32–33	34–35	36–37	Term
Cord										
Mean	6.5*	7.5***	6.7***	7.5	8.2			5.6	5.6	5.9
SD	1	2.1	1.2	2.8	1.8			1.3	2	1.1
N	3	8	18	17	17			12	10	14
12–72 hours old										
Mean	11.5***	12.3***	12.4***	15.5**	19	13.1†	12.9†	15.5††	17.1	19.7
SD	2.1	3.2	3.1	2.6	2.1	2.4	2.7	3	3.5	3.5
N	12	18	17	15	6	12	14	14	14	6
3–10 days old										

Mean	7.7***	8.5***	10***	12.7**	15.9	8.3†	9†	12††	15.1	16.2
SD	1.8	1.9	2.4	2.5	3	1.9	1.8	2.3	0.7	3.2
N	7	8	9	9	29	6	9	5	4	11
11–20 days old										
Mean	7.5**	8.3***	10.5	11.2	12.2	8‡	9.1†††	11.8	11.3	12.1
SD	1.8	1.6	1.8	2.9	2	1.6	1.9	2.7	1.9	2
N	5	11	9	9	8	5	8	8	5	8
21–45 days old										
Mean	7.8***	8***	9.3***	11.4	12.1	8.4‡	9†††	10.9		11.1
SD	1.5	1.7	1.3	4.2	1.5	1.4	1.6	2.8		1.4
N	11	17	13	5	5	11	17	5		5
46–90 days old			30–73 weeks				34–35 weeks			

(continued)

TABLE 16.14 Thyroid Function in Full-Term and Preterm Infants (*continued*)

	Serum T_4 Concentration in Premature and Term Infants					Serum Free T_4 Index in Premature and Term Infants					
	Estimated Gestational Age (Weeks)										
	30–31	32–33	34–35	36–37	Term	30–31	32–33	34–35	36–37	Term	
Mean		9.6			10.2	9.4				9.7	
SD		1.7			1.9	1.4				1.5	
N		16			17	13				10	

$^*p < 0.05$

$^{**}p < 0.005$

$^{***}p < 0.001$

$^{†}p = 0.001$

$^{††}p = 0.025$

$^{†††}p = 0.01$

$^{‡}p = 0.005$

For comparison of premature and term infants (*t*-test).

Source: Cuestas (1978).

REFERENCES

Behrman, R. E. (1977). *Neonatal–perinatal diseases of the fetus and infant* (2nd ed.). St. Louis, MO: Mosby.

Cooke, R., Hollis, B., Conner, C., Watson, D., Werkman, S., & Chesney, R. (1990). Vitamin D and mineral metabolism in the very low birth weight infant receiving 400 IU of vitamin D. *Journal of Pediatrics, 116,* 423.

Cornblath, M., & Schwartz, R. (Eds.). (1976). *Disorders of carbohydrate metabolism* (2nd ed.). Philadelphia, PA: WB Saunders.

Cuestas, R. A. (1978). Thyroid function in healthy premature infants. *Journal of Pediatrics, 92*(6), 963.

Dickinson, J. C., Rosenblum, H., & Hamilton, P. B. (1965). Ion exchange chromatography of the free amino acids in the plasma of the newborn infant. *Pediatrics, 36,* 2.

Dickinson, J. C., Rosenblum, H., & Hamilton, P. B. (1970). Ion exchange chromatography of the free amino acids in the plasma of infants under 2,500 gm at birth. *Pediatrics, 45,* 606.

Drummond, L. M. (1979). Creatine phosphokinase levels in the newborn and their use in screening for Duchenne muscular dystrophy. *Archives of Disease in Childhood, 54,* 362.

Fanaroff, A. A., & Martin, R. J. (1987). *Neonatal–perinatal medicine: Diseases of the fetus and infant* (4th ed.). St. Louis, MO: Mosby.

Fanaroff, A. A., & Martin, R. J. (Eds.). (1997). *Neonatal–perinatal medicine: Diseases of the fetus and infant* (6th ed.). St. Louis, MO: Mosby.

Fanaroff, A. A., & Martin, R. J. (2002). *Neonatal–perinatal medicine: Diseases of the fetus and infant* (7th ed.). St. Louis, MO: Mosby.

Fanaroff, A. A., & Martin, R. J. (2015). *Fanaroff and Martin's neonatal–perinatal medicine: Diseases of the fetus and infant* (10th ed.). Philadelphia, PA: Elsevier/ Saunders.

Glass, L., Hume, R., Hendry, G. M. A., Strange, R., & Forfar, J. O. (1982). Plasma alkaline phosphatase activity in rickets of prematurity. *Archives of Disease in Childhood, 57,* 373.

Gomella, T. L., Cunningham, M. D., & Eyal, F. G. (2013). *Neonatology: Management, procedures, on-call problems, diseases, and drugs* (7th ed.). New York, NY: McGraw-Hill Professional.

Heck, L. J., & Erenberg, A. (1987). Serum glucose levels in the term neonate during the first 48 hours of life. *Pediatric Research, 110*, 119.

Ichikawa, I. (1990). *Pediatric textbook of fluids and electrolytes*. Baltimore, MD: Lippincott Williams & Wilkins.

Kenner, C., & Lott, J. W. (2014). *Comprehensive neonatal nursing care* (5th ed.). New York, NY: Springer Publishing Company.

Klaus, M. H., & Fanaroff, A. A. (2001). *Care of the high-risk neonate* (5th ed.). Philadelphia, PA: WB Saunders.

Klaus, M. H, & Fanaroff, A. A. (2002). *Neonatal–perinatal medicine: Diseases of the fetus and infant* (6th ed.). St. Louis, MO: Mosby.

Lichtenstein, P., Specker, B. L., Tsang, R. C., Mimouni, F., & Gormley, C. (1986). Calcium-regulating hormones and minerals from birth to 18 months of age: A cross-sectional study. I. Effects of sex, race, age, season, and diet on vitamin D status. *Pediatrics, 77*, 883.

Liebman, J., & Plonsey, R. (1977). Electrocardiography. In A. J. Moss, F. H. Adams, & G. C. Emmanouilides (Eds.), *Heart disease in infants, children and adolescents* (2nd ed.). Baltimore, MD: Lippincott Williams & Wilkins.

Meites, S. (1975). Normal total plasma calcium in the newborn. *Critical Reviews of Clinical Laboratory Science, 6*, 1.

Meites, S. (Ed.). (1997). *Pediatric clinical chemistry: A survey of normals, methods, and instruments*. Washington, DC: American Association for Clinical Chemistry.

Naidoo, B. T. (1968). A history of the Durban Medical School. *South African Medical Journal, 42*, 932.

Neches, W., & Platt, M. (1968). Cerebrospinal fluid LDH in 257 children. *Pediatrics, 41*, 1097.

Nelson, N., Finnstrom, O., & Larsson, L. (1987). Neonatal reference values for ionized calcium, phosphate, and magnesium: Selection of reference population by optimality criteria. *Scandinavian Journal of Clinical Laboratory Investigations, 47*, 111.

Reading, R., Ellis, R., & Fleetwood, A. (1990). Plasma albumin and total protein in preterm babies from birth to eight weeks. *Early Human Development, 22*, 81.

Rodriquez, A. F., Kaplan, S. L., & Mason, E. O. (1990). Cerebrospinal fluid values in the very low birth weight infant. *Journal of Pediatrics, 116*, 971.

Schaffer, A. J. (1971). *Diseases of the newborn* (3rd ed.). Philadelphia, PA: WB Saunders.

Shenai, J. P., Chytil, F., Jhaveri, A., & Stahlman, M. T. (1981). Plasma vitamin A and retinal binding protein in premature and term neonates. *Journal of Pediatrics, 99,* 302.

Statland, B. E. (1979). Fundamental issues in clinical chemistry. *American Journal of Pathology, 95*(1), 243–272.

Tietz, N. W. (Ed.). (1988). *Textbook of clinical chemistry.* Philadelphia, PA: WB Saunders.

Wallach, J. B. (1983). *Interpretation of pediatric tests.* Boston, MA: Little Brown.

ADDITIONAL CHAPTER REFERENCES

Fanaroff, A., & Martin, R. (2015). *Fanaroff and Martin's neonatal–perinatal medicine: Diseases of the fetus and infant* (10th ed.). Philadelphia, PA: Elsevier/ Saunders.

Gomella, T. L., Cunningham, M. D., & Eyal, F. G. (2013). *Neonatology: Management, procedures, on-call problems, diseases, and drugs* (7th ed.). New York, NY: McGraw-Hill Professional.

Kenner, C., & Lott, J. W. (2014). *Comprehensive neonatal nursing care* (5th ed.). New York, NY: Springer Publishing Company.

Common Drugs: Medication Guide

Beth Shields

OVERVIEW

Neonatal patients are not simply "small adults." This unique patient population has a need for specialized care, including the provision of safe and effective medication therapy. With approximately 8% of medications not labeled for use in the neonatal population, weight-based dosing and pharmacokinetic differences must be considered each time a medication is prescribed in this patient population.

MEDICATION GUIDE

Medication guides for neonatal patients are outlined on the following pages.

Neonatal Emergency Parenteral Medications

Medication (Generic Name)	Clinical Indication	Mechanism of Action	Dose/Frequency	Common IV Compatibilities	Administration Instructions/ Comments
Acetaminophen	Analgesia/ antipyretic	Inhibits prostaglandin synthesis in central nervous system	10–15 mg/kg/dose PO/PR q4–6h scheduled or PRN (not to exceed 40 mg/kg/day in preterm infants and 60 mg/kg/day in term infants)	Not applicable	Use with caution in infants with hepatic dysfunction Higher doses required per rectum vs. orally
Acyclovir	Herpes simplex (HSV-1, HSV-2) infections	Inhibits viral DNA polymerase	20 mg/kg/dose IV q8h	Compatible: ampicillin, cefotaxime, dexamethasone, fentanyl, fluconazole, heparin Incompatible: dopamine, dobutamine	IV over 60 min

Ampicillin	Treatment of susceptible bacterial infections including sepsis/meningitis, UTI prophylaxis	50 mg/kg/dose IV/IM < 7 PND q12h < 2 kg & > 7 PND q12h > 2 kg & > 7 PND q6h	Compatible: calcium gluconate, famotidine, heparin Incompatible: dopamine, fentanyl, fluconazole, gentamicin, midazolam sodium bicarbonate	Slow IVP (not more than 100 mg/min) Larger doses for meningitis
Caffeine citrate	Apnea of prematurity	Central nervous system stimulant	Loading dose: 10 mg/kg/dose IV/PO (×1 dose) Maintenance dose: 7–10 mg/kg/dose IV/PO q24h	Compatible: calcium gluconate, gentamicin heparin, potassium chloride, fentanyl, dopamine, dobutamine, morphine Incompatible: furosemide, lorazepam, oxacillin	Maintenance dose 24h after loading dose Loading dose: IV over 30 min Maintenance dose IV: IV over 10–15 min

(continued)

Neonatal Emergency Parenteral Medications (*continued*)

Medication (Generic Name)	Clinical Indication	Mechanism of Action	Dose/Frequency	Common IV Compatibilities	Administration Instructions/ Comments
Cefotaxime	Treatment of susceptible bacterial infections including sepsis/ meningitis	Inhibits bacterial wall synthesis	50 mg/kg/dose IV/IM < 7 PND q12h < 1 kg & > 7 PND q12h > 1 kg & > 7 PND q8h	Compatible: dopamine, fentanyl Incompatible: sodium bicarbonate, fluconazole, vancomycin	Peripheral IV: IV over 30 min Central IV: IV over 3–5 min
Chlorothiazide	Diuresis	Thiazide diuretic, inhibits chloride reabsorption in the distal tubule	PO: 10–20 mg/kg/ dose q12–24h IV: 1–4 mg/kg/dose q12–24h	Compatible: potassium chloride, sodium bicarbonate Incompatible: ampicillin, gentamicin, vancomycin, oxacillin	IV and PO doses are not equivalent

| Dexamethasone | Treatment and prevention of chronic lung disease | Enhance surfactant production, stabilize cell membranes, decrease pulmonary edema | 0.5 mg/kg/day divided IV/PO q12h (× 6 doses); based on clinical indication, a variety of prolonged weaning schedules have been used | Compatible: caffeine, famotidine, fluconazole, furosemide, heparin, morphine, potassium chloride, sodium bicarbonate, vancomycin Incompatible: midazolam | Slow IVP over 1–3 min |
| Dobutamine | Increase myocardial contractility | Direct beta one agonist | 2.5–20 MCG/kg/min continuous infusion; start low and titrate to response | Compatible: calcium gluconate, dopamine, epinephrine, morphine, potassium chloride, vancomycin Incompatible: heparin, piperacillin–tazobactam, sodium bicarbonate | Use large vein for IV administration; short half-life, so must be administered via continuous infusion |

(continued)

Neonatal Emergency Parenteral Medications (*continued*)

Medication (Generic Name)	Clinical Indication	Mechanism of Action	Dose/Frequency	Common IV Compatibilities	Administration Instructions/ Comments
Dopamine	Hypotension secondary to decreased myocardial contractility	Direct beta agonist and release of norepinephrine from storage, alpha-mediated vasoconstriction	2.5–20 MCG/kg/min continuous infusion; start low and titrate to response	Compatible: epinephrine, gentamicin, heparin, midazolam, morphine, potassium chloride Incompatible: ampicillin, furosemide, sodium bicarbonate	Central line preferred; short half-life, so must be administered via continuous infusion
Fentanyl	Analgesia, sedation	Binds to opioid mu receptor	Intermittent dosing: 0.5–1 MCG/kg/dose q2–4h scheduled or PRN (titrate to response) Continuous infusion: 0.5–1 MCG/kg/h (titrate to response)	Compatible: caffeine, dobutamine, epinephrine, furosemide, heparin, midazolam, morphine, potassium chloride	Rapid IVP doses may result in chest wall rigidity Use lower doses in nonventilated and/or opiate naive patients

| Fluconazole | Prophylaxis and treatment of fungal infections | Inhibits cytochrome P450 in susceptible fungi, leading to decreased ergosterol and increased cell membrane permeability | Prophylaxis: 3 mg/kg/dose IV/PO (< 1 kg infants with central lines) twice weekly (until central line out or patient 42 days of age) Systemic treatment: thrush—6 mg/kg/dose (×1) loading dose followed by 3 mg/kg/dose q24h Systemic treatment: 12 mg/kg/dose IV/PO q24h (consider larger loading dose) | Compatible: dexamethasone, dobutamine, gentamicin, heparin, hydrocortisone, midazolam, morphine, potassium chloride, vancomycin Incompatible: ampicillin, cefotaxime, ceftriaxone, furosemide | IV over 60 min |

(continued)

Neonatal Emergency Parenteral Medications (continued)

Medication (Generic Name)	Clinical Indication	Mechanism of Action	Dose/Frequency	Common IV Compatibilities	Administration Instructions/ Comments
Furosemide	Diuresis	Loop diuretic; inhibits resorption of sodium and chloride in the ascending loop of Henle	IV: 1 mg/kg/dose q8–24h PO: 1–2 mg/kg/dose q8–24h	Compatible: calcium gluconate, dexamethasone, dopamine, fentanyl, heparin Incompatible: dobutamine, gentamicin	Slow IVP; maximum rate 0.5 mg/kg/min
Gentamicin	Treatment of susceptible bacterial infections including sepsis, UTI	Inhibits cellular protein synthesis by binding to ribosomal subunits, inhibiting bacterial cell wall membranes	< 700 g: 3 mg/kg/ dose IV q36h 700–2,500 g: 3 mg/kg/dose IV q24h > 2,500 g: 4 mg/kg/dose IV q24h All infants > 34 weeks PCA: 4 mg/kg/dose IV q24h	Compatible: acyclovir, cefotaxime, clindamycin, dopamine, famotidine, fentanyl, fluconazole, midazolam, morphine Incompatible: ampicillin, furosemide	IV over 30 min Prelevel (trough): immediately prior to dose (goal < 1.5 mcg/mL) Post level (peak): 60 min post end of 30-min infusion (6–10 mcg/mL)

Ibuprofen Lysine	Medical closure of patent ductus arteriosus (PDA)	Inhibit prostaglandin synthesis	≤ 32wk GA and birth weight 500–1,500 g 10 mg/kg/dose (×1) initial dose Followed by 5 mg /kg/dose at 24 and 48h after first dose	Compatible: potassium chloride, sodium bicarbonate Incompatible: caffeine, furosemide, midazolam	IV over 15 min, monitor urine output prior to each dose
Indomethacin	Medical closure of PDA	Inhibit prostaglandin synthesis	0.2 mg/kg/dose IV (×1 dose) followed by two additional doses q12h (subsequent doses based on postnatal age) < 48h 0.1 mg/kg/dose 2–7 days: 0.2 mg/kg/dose > 7 days: 0.25 mg/kg/dose	Compatible: furosemide, potassium chloride, sodium bicarbonate Incompatible: calcium gluconate, dobutamine, dopamine, fentanyl gentamicin	IV over 30 min; monitor urine output, serum creatinine, and platelets prior to each dose

(continued)

Neonatal Emergency Parenteral Medications (*continued*)

Medication (Generic Name)	Clinical Indication	Mechanism of Action	Dose/Frequency	Common IV Compatibilities	Administration Instructions/ Comments
Midazolam	Sedation, amnesia	Binds to GABA receptor, inhibitory neurotransmitter	Intermittent dosing IV: 0.05–0.1 mg/kg/dose Continuous infusion: 0.03–0.1 mg/kg/h Intranasal: 0.2 mg/kg/dose preprocedure	Compatible: calcium gluconate, cefotaxime, dobutamine, dopamine, fluconazole, gentamicin Incompatible: ampicillin, dexamethasone, furosemide, sodium bicarbonate	Use lower doses in nonventilated and/ or benzodiazepine naive patients
Morphine	Analgesia, sedation	Binds to opiate receptors in the central nervous system	Intermittent dosing IV: 0.05–0.1 mg/kg/dose q4–8h scheduled or PRN Continuous infusion: 0.01–0.03 mg/kg/h	Compatible: ampicillin, cefotaxime, fluconazole, furosemide, midazolam, vancomycin Incompatible: phenobarbital, sodium bicarbonate	Use lower doses in nonventilated and/ or opiate naive patients Oral doses are typically higher than IV doses

| Vancomycin | Treatment of susceptible bacterial infections including sepsis, pneumonia in skin and soft tissue | Inhibits cell wall synthesis by binding to cell wall precursors | < 29 weeks PCA: 20 mg/kg/dose IV q24h 29–31 weeks PCA: 20 mg/kg/dose IV q18h 31–37 weeks PCA: 20 mg/kg/dose IV q12h > 37 weeks PCA: 15 mg/kg/dose IV q8h | Compatible: calcium gluconate, dopamine, fentanyl, sodium bicarbonate Incompatible: cefotaxime | IV over 60 min Prelevel: immediately prior to dose 10–15 mcg/mL |

(continued)

Neonatal Emergency Parenteral Medications (continued)

Medication (Generic Name)	Dosage Range	Concentration	Comments
Adenosine	0.1 mg/kg/dose	3 mg/mL	Administer rapid bolus over 1–2 seconds; follow each bolus with normal saline flush
Atropine	0.02 mg/kg/dose	0.1 mg/mL	Minimum dose = 0.1 mg = 1 mL
Calcium gluconate	100 mg/kg/dose	100 mg/mL	Dilute with equal volume of dextrose 5% in water injection prior to administration; may be given slow IVP through central line during an arrest; for peripheral line, infuse over 60 minutes
Epinephrine (1:10,000)	0.01 mg/kg/dose	0.1 mg/mL	
Sodium bicarbonate	1–2 meq/kg/dose	0.5 meq/mL	

GA, gestational age; GABA, gamma-aminobutyric acid; PCA, postconceptional days; PND, postnatal days; PO, orally; PR, rectally; PRN, as needed; q, every.

Access the NICU Quick Drip Calculator at
http://www.medcalc.com/drip.html

○ **Dopamine** (2-20 mcg/kg/min)
○ **Dobutamine** (2-20 mcg/kg/min)
○ **Prostaglandin E1** (0.02-0.10 mcg/kg/min)
○ **Fentanyl** (1-5 mcg/kg/hr)
○ **Morphine** (5-15 mcg/kg/hr)
○ **Aminophylline** (0.1-1.0 mg/kg/hr)
○ **Isoproterenol** (0.05-2.0 mcg/kg/min)
○ **Insulin** (0.01-0.20 Units/kg/hr)

Baby's weight (grams): [ ]
Desired rate (cc/hr): [1]
Desired dose: [ ] [ ]

Do not type in this area.

DISCLAIMER: All calculations must be confirmed before use. The authors make no claims of the accuracy of the information contained herein; and these suggested doses are not a substitute for clinical judgement. Neither MedCalc.com nor any other party involved in the preparation or publication of this site shall be liable for any special, consequential, or exemplary damages resulting in whole or part from any user's use of or reliance upon this material.

NEONATAL (0–6 MONTHS) RECOMMENDED IMMUNIZATION SCHEDULE (BASED ON CHRONOLOGIC AGE) UNITED STATES 2014

(Alternative schedule exists for catch-up immunizations)

(Primary series as defined by immunizations given through 6 months of age)

√ = recommended administration age

Vaccine	Birth	1–2 Months	2 Months	4 Months	6 Months	6–18 Months
HBV	√	√				√
DTaP			√	√	√	
Hib			√	√	√[a]	
PCV13			√	√	√	
IPV			√	√	√	√
RV (RV-1 orRV-5)			√	√	√[b]	

Individual vaccine components: HBV, hepatitis B vaccine; Hib, haemophilus influenza type b; DTaP, diptheria, tetanus, and acellular pertussis; PCV 13, pneumococcal conjugate vaccine 13; IPV, inactivated polio vaccine; RV, rotavirus vaccine; RV-1 (Rotarix), RV-5 (Rotateq).

[a] Two- or three-dose primary series depending on vaccine used in primary series.

[b] RV-5 only; RV-1 is a two-dose primary series.

Combination Vaccines (Vaccine Availability Will Vary With Formulary/Contracts)				
(Use of combination vaccines generally preferred over separate injections of its equivalent component vaccines)				
Combination Vaccine by Brand Name	HBV	DTaP	Hib	IPV
Pediatrix	√	√		√
Pentacel		√	√	√
Comvax	√		√	
Kinrix		√		√

REFERENCES

Centers for Disease Control and Prevention (CDC). (2016). Advisory Committee on Immunizations Practices (ACIP). Retrieved from www.cdc.gov/vaccines/acip

Lexi-Comp Online. (2016). *Pediatric and neonatal Lexi-Drugs on line.* Hudson, OH: Lexi-Comp. Retrieved from www.cdc.gov/vaccines/schedules

Appendices

Common Abbreviations

Carole Kenner

AAP	American Academy of Pediatrics
ABE	acute bilirubin encephalopathy
ABG	arterial blood gas
ABR	auditory brainstem response
ACOG	American College of Obstetricians and Gynecologists
AED	automated external defibrillator
aEEG	amplitude-integrated electroencephalogram
AHA	American Heart Association
AIDS	acquired immunodeficiency syndrome
AOP	apnea of prematurity
AP	anteroposterior
ARC	Australian Resuscitation Council
ARF	acute renal failure
ART	antiretroviral therapy
AS	aortic stenosis
ASD	atrial septal defect
ATN	acute tubular necrosis
AV	atrioventricular
BUN	blood urea nitrogen
C3	cervical vertebra at location three
C5	cervical vertebra at location five
C7	cervical vertebra at location seven
CAT	computed axial tomography
CBC	complete blood count
cc	cubic centimeter
CCAM	cystic adenomatous malformation

CCHD	critical congenital heart disease
CCK	cholecystokinin
CDC	Centers for Disease Control and Prevention
CDH	congenital diaphragmatic hernia
CFU	colony-forming units
CHARGE	coloboma, heart defects, atresia of the choanae, retardation of growth and development, genital/urinary abnormalities, ear abnormalities, and/or hearing deficit
CHD	congenital heart disease
CHF	congestive heart failure
CIC	clean intermittent catheterization
CL	chloride
CLABSI	central line associated bloodstream infection
CLAR	Council of Latin America for Resuscitation
CLD	chronic lung disease
cm	centimeter
CMV	cytomegalovirus
CNS	central nervous system
CO$_2$	carbon dioxide
COA	coartation of the aorta
CPAM	congenital pulmonary airway malformation
CPAP	continuous positive airway pressure
CPM	congenital pulmonary malformation
CPR	cardiopulmonary resuscitation
CRIES	crying, requires increased oxygen administration, increased vital signs, expression, sleeplessness
CRP	c-reactive protein
CSF	cerebrospinal fluid
CT	computed tomography
CVC	central venous catheter
CVL	central venous line
CVP	central venous pressure
CXR	chest x-ray
D	daily
DA	ductus arteriosus
DAT	direct antiglobulin test

dB	decibel
DIC	disseminated intravascular coagulation
dL	deciliter
DNA	deoxyribonucleic acid
DTaP	diptheria tetanus and acellular pertussis
EA	esophageal atresia
EBF	erythroblastosis fetalis
EBM	expressed breast milk
ECD	endocardial cushion defect
ECMO	extracorporeal membrane oxygenation
EEG	electroencephalogram
EI	early intervention
EKG	electrocardiogram
ELBW	extremely low birth weight
ENS	enteric nervous system
EOS	early onset sepsis
ERC	European Resuscitation Council
ESPGHAN	European Society for Pediatric Gastroenterology, Hepatology, and Nutrition
ETT	endotracheal tube
ETV	endoscopic third ventriculostomy
EVD	external ventricular device
FCC	family-centered care
FDA	Federal Drug Administration
FFP	fresh frozen plasma
FLACC	face, legs, activity, cry, consolability
FR	French
FRC	function residual capacity
FTC	foot candle
g	gram
G6PD	glucose-6-phosphate dehydrogenase
GA	gestational age
GABA	gamma-aminobutryic acid
GDM	gestational diabetes mellitus
GER	gastroesophageal reflux
GERD	gastroesophageal reflux disease
GFR	glomerular filtration rate

GI	gastrointestinal
G-J	gastro-jejunal
GM	IVH-germinal matrix intraventricular hemorrhage
GU	genitourinary
HBV	hepatitis B vaccine
HC	head circumference
Hg	mercury
Hib	hemophilus influenza type B
HIE	hypoxic-ischemic encephalopathy
HIV	human immunodeficiency virus
HLHS	hypoplastic left heart syndrome
HPA	hypothalamic pituitary adrenal
HSFC	Heart and Stroke Foundation of Canada
HSV	herpes simplex virus
HUS	head ultrasound
IC	intracranial
ICP	increased intracranial pressure
ICU	intensive care unit
IDC	integrative developmental care
IDM	infant of a diabetic mother or idiopathic diabetes mellitus
ILCOR	International Liaison Committee on Resuscitation
IM	intramuscular
iNO	inhaled nitrous oxide
IPAT	Infant Position Assessment Tool
IPV	inactivated polio vaccine
IR	interventional radiologist
IRF	intrinsic renal failure
IUGR	interuterine growth restricted
IV	intravenous
IVC	inferior vena cava
IVH	intraventricular hemorrhage
IVIG	intravenous immunoglobulin
IVP	intravenous push
IWL	insensible water loss
J	jejunostomy
K	potassium

kcal	kilocalorie
kg	kilogram
KMC	kangaroo mother care
L	left
L	liter
L5	lumbar vertebra at location five
LCT	long-chain triglyceride
LES	lower esophageal sphincter
LFT	liver function test
LGA	large for gestational age
LLSB	lower left sternal border
LOS	late onset sepsis
LP	lumbar puncture
MAS	meconium aspiration syndrome
MBS	modified barium swallow
mcg	microgram
mcmol	micromol
MCT	medium-chain triglyceride
MD	medical doctor
mg	milligram
MII	multichannel intraluminal impedance
min	minute
mo	month
M/P	milk-to-plasma ratio
MRI	magnetic resonance imaging
MSAF	meconium stained amniotic fluid
NA	sodium
NALS	neonatal advanced life support
NC	nasal cannula
NG	nasogastric
NGT	nasogastric tube
NIH	National Institutes of Health
NIPPV	noninvasive positive pressure ventilation
NNS	nonnutritive sucking
NP	nurse practitioner
NPO	nothing per os (by mouth)
NREM	nonrapid eye movement

NS	normal saline
NS	nutritive sucking
NSAID	nonsteroidal anti-inflammatory drug
NTD	neural tube defect
NTE	neutral thermal environment
NZRC	New Zealand Resuscitation Council
OFC	occipital frontal circumference
OG	orogastric
OR	operating room
ORL	otolaryngology
oz	ounce
PA	pulmonary artery
$PaCO_2$	partial arterial pressure of carbon dioxide
PaO_2	partial arterial pressure of oxygen
PCA	postconceptional day
PCO_2	partial pressure of carbon dioxide
PCV 13	pneumococcal conjugate vaccine 13
PDA	patent ductus arteriosus
PEEP	positive end expiratory pressure
PEG	percutaneous endoscopic gastrostomy
PFO	patent foramen ovale
PG	phosphatidylglycerol
PGE	prostaglandin E
pH	potential of hydrogen
PICC	peripherally inserted central catheter
PIE	pulmonary interstitial emphysema
PIPP	premature infant pain profile
PND	postnatal day
PO	per os (by mouth)
PO_2	partial pressure of oxygen
POD	postoperative day
PPE	personal protective equipment
PPHN	persistent pulmonary hypertension
PPI	proton pump inhibitor
PR	per rectum (or rectally)
PRBC	packed red blood cells
PRN	pro re nata (as needed)

PS	pulmonary stenosis
PTSD	posttraumatic stress disorder
PVC	polyvinyl chloride
PVL	periventricular leukomalacia
PVR	pulmonary vascular resistance
R	right
RBC	red blood cell
RCSA	Resuscitation Council of Southern Africa
RDS	respiratory distress syndrome
REM	rapid eye movement
RH	relative humidity
RH	right hand
RID	relative infant dose
RN	registered nurse
RNA	ribonucleic acid
ROP	retinopathy of prematurity
RSV	respiratory syncytial virus
RUSP	recommended uniform screening panel
RV	rotovirus vaccine
RV	1-rotarix
RV	5-rotateq
S1	sacral vertebra at location one
SACHDNC	Secretary's Advisory Committee on Heritable Disorders in Newborn and Children
SAH	subarachnoid hemorrhage
SAIE	subacute infective endocarditis
SEM	systolic ejection murmur
SIP	spontaneous intestinal perforation
SiPAP	sign positive airway pressure
SP-A	surfactant protein A
SP-B	surfactant protein B
SpO$_2$	peripheral capillary oxygen saturation
SSB	suck, swallow, breathe
SSC	skin-to-skin contact
SVC	superior vena cava
T1	thoracic vertebra at location one
TcB	transcutaneous bilirubin

TEF	tracheoesophageal fistula
TEWL	transepidermal water loss
TGA	transposition of the great arteries
TOF	tetralogy of fallot
TORCHES CLAP	toxoplasma gondii, rubella, cytomegalovirus, herpes simplex virus, syphilis, chicken pox, lyme disease, acquired immunodeficiency syndrome, parvovirus B9
TPA	tissue plasminogen activator
TPH	transplacental hemorrhage
TSB	total serum bilirubin
TTN	transient tachypnea of the newborn
UAC	umbilical arterial catheter
ULSB	upper left sternal border
US	ultrasound
UTI	urinary tract infection
UVC	umbilical venous catheter
VAP	ventilator associated pneumonia
VCUG	voiding cystourethrogram
VQ	ventilation/perfusion ratio
VS	vital signs
VSD	ventricular septal defect
WBC	white blood cell
WHO	World Health Organization
WMI	white-matter injury
wt	weight
X	times

Expected Increases in Weight, Length/Height, and Head Circumference in the First Year of Life

Parameter	Age (Months)	Expected Increase
Weight	Birth to 3	25–35 g/day
	3–6	12–21 g/day
	6–12	10–13 g/day
Length/height	Birth to 12	25 cm/y
OFC	Birth to 3	2 cm/mo
	4–6	1 cm/mo
	7–12	0.5 cm/mo

Data from Grover (2000) and Ditmyer (2004).

Conversion Table to Standard International (SI) Units

Component	Present Unit	×	Conversion Factor	=	SI Unit
Clinical Hematology					
Erythrocytes	per mm^3		1		10^6/L
Hematocrit	%		0.01		(1)vol RBC/vol whole blood
Hemoglobin	g/dL		10		g/L
Leukocytes	per mm^3		1		10^6/L
Mean corpuscular hemoglobin concentration (MCHC)	g/dL		10		g/L
Mean corpuscular volume (MCV)	mc/m^3		1		fL

(continued)

Component	Present Unit	×	Conversion Factor	=	SI Unit
Platelet count	$10^3/mm^3$		1		$10^9/L$
Reticulocyte count	%		10		10^{-3}
Clinical Chemistry					
Acetone	mg/dL		0.1722		mmol/L
Albumin	g/dL		10		g/L
Aldosterone	ng/dL		27.74		pmol/L
Ammonia (as nitrogen)	mcg/dL		0.7139		mcmol/L
Bicarbonate	mEq/L		1		mmol/L
Bilirubin	mg/dL		17.1		mcmol/L
Calcium	mg/dL		0.2495		mmol/L
Calcium ion	mEq/L		0.50		mmol/L
Carotenes	mcg/dL		0.01836		mcmol/L
Ceruloplasmin	mg/dL		10		mg/L
Chloride	mEq/L		1		mmol/L
Cholesterol	mg/dL		0.02586		mmol/L
Complement, C_3 or C_4	mg/dL		0.01		g/L
Copper	mcg/dL		0.1574		mcmol/L

(*continued*)

Component	Present Unit	×	Conversion Factor	=	SI Unit
Cortisol	mcg/dL		27.59		nmol/L
Creatine	mg/dL		76.25		mcmol/L
Creatinine	mg/dL		88.40		mcmol/L
Digoxin	ng/mL		1.281		nmol/L
Epinephrine	pg/mL		5.458		pmol/L
Fatty acids	mg/dL		10		mg/L
Ferritin	ng/mL		1		mcg/L
α-Fetoprotein	ng/mL		1		mcg/L
Fibrinogen	mg/dL		0.01		g/L
Folate	ng/mL		2.266		nmol/L
Fructose	mg/dL		0.05551		mmol/L
Galactose	mg/dL		0.05551		mmol/L
Gases					
PO_2	mmHg (= torr)		0.1333		kPa
PCO_2	mmHg (= torr)		0.1333		kPa
Glucagon	pg/mL		1		ng/L
Glucose	mg/dL		0.05551		mmol/L

(*continued*)

Component	Present Unit	×	Conversion Factor	=	SI Unit
Glycerol	mg/dL		0.1086		mmol/L
Growth hormone	ng/mL		1		mcg/L
Haptoglobin	mg/dL		0.01		g/L
Hemoglobin	g/dL		10		g/L
Insulin	mcg/L		172.2		pmol/L
	mU/L		7.175		pmol/L
Iron	mcg/dL		0.1791		mcmol/L
Iron-binding capacity	mcg/dL		0.1791		mcmol/L
Lactate	mEq/L		1		mmol/L
Lead	mcg/dL		0.04826		mcmol/L
Lipoproteins	mg/dL		0.02586		mmol/L
Magnesium	mg/dL		0.4114		mmol/L
	mEq/L		0.50		mmol/L
Osmolality	mOsm/ kg H_2O		1		mmol/kg H_2O
Phenobarbital	mg/dL		43.06		mcmol/L
Phenytoin	mg/L		3.964		mcmol/L
Phosphate	mg/dL		0.3229		mmol/L

(*continued*)

Component	Present Unit	×	Conversion Factor	=	SI Unit
Potassium	mEq/L		1		mmol/L
	mg/dL		0.2558		mmol/L
Protein	g/dL		10		g/L
Pyruvate	mg/dL		113.6		mcmol/L
Sodium ion	mEq/L		1		mmol/L
Steroids					
17-hydroxy-corticosteroids	mg/24 hr		2.759		mcmol/day
17-ketoste-roids	mg/24 hr		3.467		mcmol/day
Testosterone	ng/mL		3.467		nmol/L
Theophylline	mg/L		5.550		mcmol/L
Thyroid tests					
Thyroid-stimulating hormone	mcU/mL		1		mU/L
Thyroxine (T_4)	mcg/dL		12.87		nmol/L
Thyroxine free	ng/dL		12.87		pmol/L
Triiodothy-ronine (T_3)	ng/dL		0.01536		nmol/L
Transferrin	mg/dL		0.01		g/L

(*continued*)

Component	Present Unit	×	Conversion Factor	=	SI Unit
Triglycerides	mg/dL		0.01129		mmol/L
Urea nitrogen	mg/dL		0.3570		mmol/L
Uric acid (urate)	mg/dL		59.48		mcmol/L
Vitamin A (retinol)	mcg/dL		0.03491		mcmol/L
Vitamin B_{12}	pg/mL		0.7378		pmol/L
Vitamin C (ascorbic acid)	mg/dL		56.78		mcmol/L
Vitamin D					
Cholecal-ciferol	mcg/mL		2.599		nmol/L
25 OH-cholecal-ciferol	ng/mL		2.496		nmol/L
Vitamin E (alpha-tocopherol)	mg/dL		23.22		mcmol/L
D-xylose	mg/dL		0.06661		mmol/L
Zinc	mcg/dL		0.1530		mcmol/L
Energy	kcal		4.1868		kJ (kilojoule)
Blood pressure	mmHg (= torr)		1.333		mbar

Modified from Young (1987).

International Standards for Newborn Weight, Length, and Head Circumference by Gestational Age and Sex

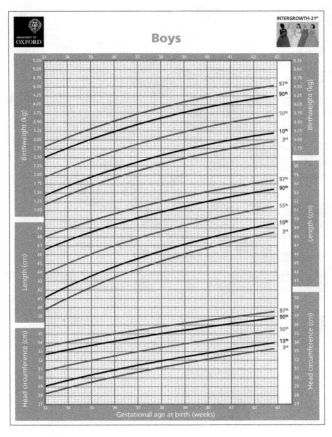

Source: INTERGROWTH-21st newborn size at birth standards. Reprinted by permission from Intergrowth-21st © 2009–2016. https://intergrowth21.tghn.org/articles/category/global-perinatal-package

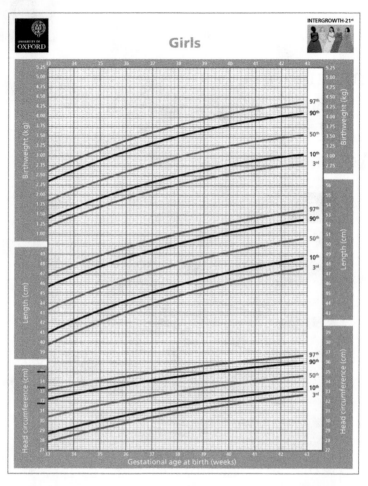

Source: INTERGROWTH-21st newborn size at birth standards. Reprinted by permission from Intergrowth-21st © 2009–2016. https://intergrowth21.tghn.org/articles/category/global-perinatal-package

Web Resources

BILIRUBIN

BiliTool™
http://www.BiliTool.org
Cochrane Library
http://www.cochranelibrary.com
Cochrane Reviews
http://www.cochrane.org/cochrane-reviews
Kernicterus and Newborn Jaundice Online
http://www.kernicterus.org
PICK (Parents of Infants and Children With Kernicterus)
http://pic-k.org

BREASTFEEDING

Desktop reference for drugs during pregnancy and lactation:
  Hale, T. W. (2012). *Medications and mother's milk 2012: A manual of lactational pharmacology* (15th ed.). Plano, TX: Hale Publishing.
Hutchinson, B. (2015). Importance of establishing neonatal BFHI standards in neonatal units. *Newborn and Infant Nursing Reviews*. Retrieved from http://www.sciencedirect.com/science/article/pii/S1527336915001294

IBCLC: International Board of Certified Lactation Consultants: http://iblce.org

LactMed: U.S. National Library of Medicine Drugs and Lactation Database: http://toxnet.nlm.nih.gov/cgi-bin/sis/htmlgen?LACTMED

Neo-BFHI Core Document 2015: http://www.ilca.org/i4a/pages/index.cfm?pagid=4214

Nyqvist, K. H., Maastrup, R., Hansen, M. N., Haggkvist, A. P., Hannula, L., Ezeonodo, A., ... Haiek, L. N. (2015). *Neo-BFHI: The Baby-friendly Hospital Initiative for Neonatal Wards. Core document with recommended standards and criteria.* Nordic and Quebec Working Group.

UNICEF Baby Friendly ten steps: http://www.unicef.org/programme/breastfeeding/baby.htm

UNICEF expanded Baby Friendly ten steps for preterm infants: Nyqvist, K. H., Häggkvist, A.-P., Hansen, M. N., Kylberg, E., Frandsen, A. L., Maastrup, R., ... Baby-Friendly Hospital Initiative Expert Group. Expansion of the Baby-Friendly Hospital Initiative ten steps to successful breastfeeding into neonatal intensive care: Expert group recommendations. *Journal of Human Lactation, 29*(3), 300–309. doi:10.1177/0890334413489775

USA Baby Friendly Hospital Initiative: http://www.babyfriendlyusa .org/about-us/baby-friendly-hospital-initiative/the-ten-steps

CARDIAC SYSTEM

Centers for Disease Control and Prevention. Congenital Heart Defects. Information for Health Care Providers: http://www.cdc.gov/ncbddd/heartdefects/hcp.html

American Academy of Pediatrics Website. Newborn Screening for CCHD. Answers and Resources for Primary Care Pediatricians: http://www.aap.org/en-us/advocacy-and-policy/aap-health-initiatives/PEHDIC/Pages/Newborn-Screening-for-CCHD.aspx

Tennessee Department of Health. Protocol for Critical Congenital Heart Disease (CCHD) Screening:
https://health.state.tn.us/MCH/NBS/PDFs/CCHD_Screening_Protocol_Algorithm.pdf

FAMILY-CENTERED CARE

Institute for Patient and Family Centered Care: http://www.ipfcc.org/advance/topics/better-together-partnering.html

HEARING

Guidelines for Hearing Screening in Childhood From the American Academy of Audiology: www.cdc.gov/ncbddd/hearingloss/documents/AAA_Childhood%20Hearing%20Guidelines_2011.pdf
Guidelines for Pediatric Medical Home Providers for Hearing Screening: http://www.medicalhomeinfo.org/dowloads/pdfs/Algorithm1_2010.pdf

HYDROCELES

Boston Children's Hospital Web:
http://www.childrenshospital.org/conditionsandtreatments/conditions/hydrocele/symptoms-and-causes
Mayo Clinic Web:
http://www.mayoclinic.org/diseases-conditions/hydrocele/basics/definition/con-20024139

INFECTIONS

http://www.sepsisalliance.org/sepsis_and/children
http://www.ncbi.nlm.nih.gov/pubmedhealth/PMH0004557/
www.who.int/maternal_child_adolescent/documents/child_hospital_care/en

INTERNATIONAL GROWTH CURVES

https://intergrowth21.tghn.org/articles/categetory/global-perinatal-
package

KANGAROO MOTHER CARE

Healthy Newborn Network:

http://www.healthynewbornnetwork.org/topic/kangaroo-mother-
care-kmc

Kangaroo Mother Care: Support for Parents & Staff of Premature
Babies:

http://www.kangaroomothercare.com

NEONATAL SURGERY

The Joint Commission: http://www.jointcommission.org/assets/1/6/
2009_clasrelatedstandardshap.pdf

NEONATAL RESUSCITATION AND LIFE SUPPORT
PROGRAMS

American Academy of Pediatrics: https://www.aap.org/en-us/
continuing-medical-education/ life-support/pages/
life-support.aspx

PICC LINE

www.avainfo.org

www.ins1.org

www.nann.org

Videos in Clinical Medicine *PICC Placement in the Neonate*

McCay, A. S., Elliott, E. C., & Walden, M. (2014). Videos in clinical
medicine: PICC placement in the neonate. *New England Journal
of Medicine, 370*, e17. doi:10.1056/NEJMvcm1101914

POSITIONING

Madinger-Lewis, L., Reynolds, L., Zarem, C., Crapnell, T., Inder, T., & Pineda, R. (2014). The effects of alternative positioning on preterm infants in the neonatal intensive care unit: A randomized clinical trial. *Research in Developmental Disabilities, 35*(2), 490–497. Retrieved from http://www.ncbi.nlm.nih.gov/pmc/articles/ PMC3938096

Zarem, C., Crapnell, T., Tiltges, L., Madlinger, L., Reynolds, L., Lukas, K., & Pineda, R. (2013). Neonatal nurses' and therapists' perceptions of positioning for preterm infants in the neonatal intensive care unit. *Neonatal Network, 32*(2), 110–116. Retrieved from http://www.ncbi.nlm.nih.gov/pmc/articles/PMC3953371

RESPIRATORY

www.NICUniversity.org

www.pediatrix.com/PediatrixUniversity

TRACHEOESOPHAGEAL FISTULA/ESOPHAGEAL ATRESIA

The Esophageal Advanced Treatment Program at Boston Children's Hospital offers treatment for all types of disorders of the esophagus. http://www.childrenshospital.org/centers-and-services/programs/ a-_-e/esophageal-atresia-treatment-program

EAT is a European federation of family support groups that focuses on sharing experiences, disseminating information, and raising awareness of LGEA. For additional information, please visit http://www.we.are-eat.org

The Marathon, A True Story by Kerry Sheeran is a written account of one family's experience as they progress through the journey with their child born with LGEA. The author creates a moving parallel with a personal account of running the Boston Marathon. http://www.amazon.com/s/ref=nb_sb_noss?url= search-alias%3Daps&field-keywords=Kerry+Sheerin%2C+The+ marathon

TOFS, a U.K.-based charity providing emotional support to families of children born with tracheo-oesophageal fistula (TOF), esophageal atresia, and associated conditions. The site also links to a range of European TOF groups in other languages.

RESUSCITATION

AAP NRP: http://www.aap.org/nrp

Perinatal Continuing Education Program: http://www.healthsystem.virginia.edu/internet/pcep

The S.T.A.B.L.E.® Program: http://www.thestableprogram.org

REFERENCES

Ditmyer, S. (2004). Hydrocephalus. In P. J. Allen & J. A. Vessey (Eds.), *Primary care of the child with a chronic condition* (4th ed., pp. 543–560). Philadelphia, PA: Mosby.

Grover, G. (2000). Nutritional needs. In C. D. Berkowitz (Ed.), *Pediatrics: A primary care approach* (2nd ed.). Philadelphia, PA: Saunders.

Young, D. S. (1987). Implementation of SI units for clinical laboratory data: Style specifications and conversion tables. *Annals of Internal Medicine, 106*, 114.

Trauma-Informed Age-Appropriate Care

Mary Coughlin

OVERVIEW

- *Traumatic event*: An experience that causes physical, emotional, or psychological distress or harm and is perceived and experienced as a threat to one's safety or to the stability of one's world; a traumatic event overwhelms an individual's ability to cope (Coughlin, 2014).

- *Trauma informed*: The trauma-informed clinician acknowledges that the neonatal intensive care unit (NICU) experience is a traumatic life event associated with deleterious biological and psychological sequelae, and uses this knowledge and understanding of trauma (trauma informed) to mitigate and manage the trauma experience of the hospitalized neonate/infant (Coughlin, 2014).

- *Age-appropriate care*: Recognizes the patient as a person and ensures that the neonatal patient's experience of care aligns with his or her developmental, biological, psychological, and socio-emotional needs (Coughlin, 2014). Proximity to and protection from parents are primal age-appropriate needs of the neonate that are biologically relevant to the infant's developmental continuum.

PHYSIOLOGY

- The brain responds to experiences and environmental stimuli through activation of the stress response system (hypothalamic-pituitary-adrenal [HPA] axis) or allostasis, which means to achieve stability through change (McEwen, 1998a, 1998b).

- Stress mediators promote adaptation to both acute events as well as day-to-day occurrences, such as waking up, moving, and experiences with novel stimuli.

- The developmental trajectory of this mechanism hinges on early life experiences with stress and, in the case of infants and young children, whether or not a caring adult has mediated the stress event.

- Healthy stress responses promote adaptation through activation of the HPA axis, releasing cortisol, which increases cardiovascular tone and serves to enhance the availability and distribution of energy substrates to meet the metabolic demands of the stress situation (Lai & Huang, 2011).

PATHOPHYSIOLOGY

- Healthy development can be derailed by excessive or prolonged activation of stress response systems in the body and the brain (National Scientific Council on the Developing Child [NSCDC], 2014).

- Traumatic events are mediated by the stress response system. When activation of the stress response system in early life is prolonged and there is a paucity of support from a caring adult, the infant is exposed to toxic stress that can lead to long-lasting epigenetic changes in the brain, effecting how the body responds to adversity across the life continuum (Boekelheide et al., 2012; Grasso, Ford, & Briggs-Gowan, 2013).

- Critical illness causes physical, emotional, and psychological distress in the affected individual and overwhelms the individual's ability to cope. Brame and Singer (2010) describe the phenomena of critical illness through the lens of the allostatic model, and describe the deleterious effects of allostatic load (excessive stress) to include:

- Immunosuppression
- Oxidative damage
- Aberrant metabolic modulation
- Stimulation of bacterial growth
- Increased oxygen consumption
- Compromised cardiac function

■ Prematurity has been referred to as a traumatic beginning and requires intensive critical care management (Karr-Morse, 2012).

■ Research has found connections between highly stressful experiences in children and an increased risk for later mental illnesses, including:

- Generalized anxiety disorder
- Major depressive disorders (Blasco-Fontecilla et al., 2013; Nosarti et al., 2012; Rifkin-Graboi, Borelli, & Enlow, 2009; Vanderbilt & Gleason, 2011)

■ Atypical stress responses over a lifetime can also result in increased risk for physical ailments that include:

- Asthma
- Hypertension
- Heart disease
- Diabetes (Finken et al., 2013; Lewandowski et al., 2013; NSCDC, 2004; Thomas, Al Saud, Durighel, Frost, & Bell, 2012)

■ Certain types of stress-induced epigenetic modifications can be reversed and function restored when infants are supported during stressful experiences, facilitating the development of resilience.

ASSESSMENT

■ The preverbal status of the neonate confounded by his or her severity of illness compromises the ability to convey distress consistently and reliably. Behavioral, as well as physiologic, parameters have become the cornerstone of communication between infant and adult caregiver (parent or clinician).

■ Recognizing distress (pain or pain-related stress) in the hospitalized infant requires:

  ■ Attunement to the infant's reality (his or her lived experience of life-threatening illness)

  ■ Astute observational skills grounded in empathy

  ■ An awareness of the infant as a person

■ Whether the infant is experiencing stress or pain, the physiologic sequelae are similar. Context guides the adult caregiver in making a sensitive and accurate assessment that prompts the appropriate prevention and/or management intervention.

CLINICAL MANIFESTATIONS/DIAGNOSIS

Clinical manifestations of stress and pain include:

■ Changes in heart rate, oxygen saturation, and blood pressure, as well as several facial changes, body movements, variance in muscle tone, and vocalizations (Grunau, Johnston, & Craig, 1990; Holsti, Grunau, Oberlander, Whitfield, & Weinberg, 2005; Morison et al., 2003).

■ Again, context must guide the adult caregiver, as there are many instances where the infant is incapable of making facial gestures or vocalizations in response to distress, either because of severity of illness, weakness, or sedation.

■ The absence of clinical manifestations does not exclude the presence of stress or pain and the astute, sensitively attuned adult caregiver must be able to interpret the context of the infant's experience in order to provide age-appropriate support for the infant.

Distress indicators in neonates include:

■ Facial grimace

■ Brow bulge

■ Nasolabial furrow

■ Crying/moaning

■ Clenched toes/fists, finger splay

■ Tense body or limp body

■ Irritability/inconsolability

■ Restlessness

■ Level of arousal (hyper- or hyporesponsive to stimuli)

■ Vital sign variation from baseline related to heart rate, blood pressure, oxygen saturation, tachypnea, or apnea

TREATMENT

■ Parental presence as partners in care of their hospitalized infant is the quintessential best-practice strategy in managing and mitigating the trauma experience. Preserving, protecting, and facilitating parental-role identity impacts both short-term and long-term outcomes for the infant *and* the family.

■ In addition, adoption and implementation of the National Association of Neonatal Nurses (NANN) Practice Guidelines for Age-Appropriate Care of the Premature and Critically Ill Hospitalized Infant (Coughlin, 2011) establish a culture of care committed to managing the neonate's trauma experience.

■ These evidence-based core measures include (Coughlin, Gibbins, & Hoath, 2009, 2014):

■ The healing environment, which encompasses the physical milieu, the human components, and the system dimensions

■ Protected sleep

■ Age-appropriate activities of daily living (posture and movement, feeding, and skin care/hygiene)

■ Prevention and management of pain and stress

■ Family integrated care

PROGNOSIS

■ Integrating family into the care of their infant positively impacts infant outcomes (O'Brien et al., 2013).

■ Caring, supportive relationships with adult caregivers help to regulate stress hormone production (NSCDC, 2014).

■ Standardizing the neonatal patient's experience of care to ensure parental presence and protection along with stable supportive relationships with adult caregivers will reduce the potential damage to developing brain architecture and promote resilience in this vulnerable population (NSCDC, 2014).

REFERENCES

Blasco-Fontecilla, H., Jaussent, I., Olie, E., Garcia, E. B., Beziat, S., Malafosse, A., . . . Courtet, P. (2013). Additive effects between prematurity and postnatal risk factors of suicidal behavior. *Journal of Psychiatric Research, 47*(7), 937–943.

Brame, A. L., & Singer, M. (2010). Stressing the obvious? An allostatic look at critical illness. *Critical Care Medicine, 38*(10), s600–s607.

Boekelheide, K., Blumberg, B., Chapin, R. E., Cote, I., Graziano, J. H., Janesick, A., . . . Rogers, J. M. (2012). Predicting later-life outcomes of early-life exposures. *Environmental Health Perspectives, 120*(10), 1353–1361.

Coughlin, M. (2011). *Age-appropriate care of the premature and critically ill hospitalized infant: Guideline for practice.* Glenview, IL: National Association of Neonatal Nurses.

Coughlin, M. (2014). *Transformative nursing in the NICU: Trauma-informed age-appropriate care.* New York, NY: Springer Publishing Company.

Coughlin, M., Gibbins, S., & Hoath, S. (2009). Core measures for developmentally supportive care in neonatal intensive care: theory, precedence and practice. *Journal of Advanced Nursing, 65*(10), 2239–2248.

Finken, M. J., Meulenbelt, I., Dekker, F. W., Frolich, M., Walther, F. J., Romijn, J. A., . . . Wit, J. M. (2013). Abdominal fat accumulation in adults born preterm exposed antenatally to maternal glucocorticoid treatment is dependent on glucocorticoid receptor gene variation. *Journal of Clinical Endocrinology & Metabolics, 96*, e1650–e1655.

Grasso, D. J., Ford, J. D., & Briggs-Gowan, M. J. (2013). Early life trauma exposure and stress sensitivity in young children. *Journal of Pediatric Psychology, 38*(1), 94–103.

Grunau, R. V., Johnston, C. C., & Craig, K. D. (1990). Neonatal facial and cry responses to invasive and non-invasive procedures. *Pain, 42*(3), 295–305.

Holsti, L., Grunau, R. R., Oberlander, T. F., Whitfield, M. F., & Weinberg, J. (2005). Body movements: An important additional factor in discriminating pain from stress in preterm infants. *Clinical Journal of Pain, 21*(6), 491–498.

Karr-Morse, R. (2012). *Scared sick. The role of childhood trauma in adult disease.* New York, NY: Basic Books.

Lai, M.-C. & Huang, L.-T. (2011). Effects of early life stress on neuroendocrine and neurobehavior: Mechanisms and implications. *Pediatrics & Neonatology, 52*, 122–129.

Lewandowski, A. J., Augustine, D., Lamata, P., Davis, E. F., Lazdam, M., Francis, J., . . . Leeson, P. (2013). Preterm heart in adult life: Cardiovascular magnetic resonance reveals distinct differences in left ventricular mass, geometry, and function. *Circulation, 127*(2), 197–206.

McEwen, B. S. (1998a). Protective and damaging effects of stress mediators. *New England Journal of Medicine, 338*, 171–179.

McEwen, B. S. (1998b). Stress, adaptation, and disease. Allostasis and allostatic load. *Annals of the New York Academy of Sciences, 1*, 33–44.

Morison, S. J., Holsti, L., Grunau, R. E., Whitfield, M. F., Oberlander, T. F., Chan, H. W., & Williams, L. (2003). Are there developmentally distinct motor indicators of pain in preterm infants? *Early Human Development, 72*(2), 131–146.

National Scientific Council on the Developing Child. (2004). *Young children develop in an environment of relationships.* Working Paper No. 1. Retrieved from http://www.developingchild.net

National Scientific Council on the Developing Child. (2005/2014). *Excessive stress disrupts the architecture of the developing brain.* Working Paper 3. Updated Edition. Retrieved from http://www.developingchild.harvard.edu

Nosarti, C., Reichenberg, A., Murray, R. M., Cnattingius, S., Lambe, M. P., Yin, L., . . . Hultman, C. M. (2012). Preterm birth and psychiatric disorders in young adult life. *Archives in General Psychiatry, 69*(6), e1–e8.

O'Brien, K., Bracht, M., Macdonnel, K., McBride, T., Robson, K., O'Leary, L., . . . Lee, S. K. (2013). A pilot cohort analytic study of family integrated care in a Canadian neonatal intensive care unit. *BMC Pregnancy & Childbirth, 13*(Suppl. 1), S12.

Rifkin-Graboi, A., Borelli, J. L., & Enlow, M. B. (2009). Neurobiology of stress in infancy. In C. H. Zeanah, Jr. (Ed.), *Handbook of infant mental health* (3rd ed., pp. 40–58). New York, NY: The Guilford Press.

Thomas, E. L., Al Saud, N. B., Durighel, G., Frost, G., & Bell, J. D. (2012). The effect of preterm birth on adiposity and metabolic pathways and the implications for later life. *Clinical Lipidology, 7*(3), 275–288.

Vanderbilt, D., & Gleason, M. M. (2011). Mental health concerns of the premature infant through the lifespan. *Pediatric Clinics of North America, 58*, 815–832.

Index

Date Due
